IN THE GRIP OF DISEASE

In the Grip of Disease

Studies in the Greek Imagination

G. E. R. LLOYD

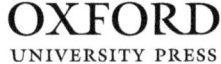

This book has been printed digitally and produced in a standard specification in order to ensure its continuing availability

OXFORD
UNIVERSITY PRESS

Great Clarendon Street, Oxford OX2 6DP

Oxford University Press is a department of the University of Oxford.
It furthers the University's objective of excellence in research, scholarship,
and education by publishing worldwide in

Oxford New York

Auckland Cape Town Dar es Salaam Hong Kong Karachi
Kuala Lumpur Madrid Melbourne Mexico City Nairobi
New Delhi Shanghai Taipei Toronto
With offices in
Argentina Austria Brazil Chile Czech Republic France Greece
Guatemala Hungary Italy Japan South Korea Poland Portugal
Singapore Switzerland Thailand Turkey Ukraine Vietnam

Oxford is a registered trade mark of Oxford University Press
in the UK and in certain other countries

Published in the United States
by Oxford University Press Inc., New York

© G. E. R. Lloyd 2003

The moral rights of the author have been asserted

Database right Oxford University Press (maker)

Reprinted 2008

All rights reserved. No part of this publication may be reproduced,
stored in a retrieval system, or transmitted, in any form or by any means,
without the prior permission in writing of Oxford University Press,
or as expressly permitted by law, or under terms agreed with the appropriate
reprographics rights organization. Enquiries concerning reproduction
outside the scope of the above should be sent to the Rights Department,
Oxford University Press, at the address above

You must not circulate this book in any other binding or cover
And you must impose this same condition on any acquirer

ISBN 978-0-19-925323-4

PREFACE

This study stems in the first instance from a series of lectures that I gave over the three years 1997–2000 in Cambridge to a mixed audience of classicists, historians of medicine, historians of science, and philosophers. But the ideas reflect interests that I have had, and questions that I have puzzled over, going back to my earliest forays into Greek medicine. In general my writings on ancient Greek medicine have, conventionally enough, concentrated on the extant treatises of the medical writers themselves, together with such other direct and indirect sources as we have on medical beliefs and practices at different periods. The present study differs in that I discuss also epic and lyric poetry, tragedy, the historians, and the philosophers, doing so in order to investigate how Greek thought concerning a range of important general issues, including good and evil themselves, was influenced by ideas about disease, about who was in a position to say what that was, to diagnose it in the body or the mind, to identify the causes at work, and to bring about cures or at least to try to alleviate the problems as they were perceived. Issues to do with notions of the self, of authority and control, of claims to knowledge and challenges to those claims, are deeply implicated as also are representations of the best ordering of society and its government. My strategic aim is to throw light on recurrent preoccupations of the Greek imagination.

With such an ambitious project it is clearly not practicable to attempt to be comprehensive. The authors and topics I have chosen for analysis are those that appear most important, most influential on the Greeks themselves, and most interesting from our own perspective. In the Epilogue I discuss briefly some of the modern attitudes to the problems the ancient Greeks faced and some of the more significant repercussions of our Greek inheritance. But I am conscious that the most I can do here is to open up a number of lines of research. It will be for later investigations to pursue them in greater detail.

I have attempted to keep the arguments in my chapters clear and concise. But since I cite a fair number of ancient texts, I have thought it useful to collect the main ones together with my own, or standard, translations at the end of each chapter. The reader can there follow up more of the material that I use than I have cited directly in my text.

It remains to express my thanks to all those who have contributed to this work, to my lecture audiences for many hours of stimulating discussion, and to Hilary O'Shea and her colleagues at Oxford University Press for the exemplary fashion in which they have overseen all the stages in the production this book.

GERL

CONTENTS

List of Texts and Translations		ix
Acknowledgements		xviii
1	Anthropological Perspectives	1
2	Archaic Literature and Masters of Truth	14
3	Secularization and Sacralization	40
4	Tragedy	84
5	The Historians	114
6	Plato	142
7	Aristotle	176
8	After Aristotle: Or Did Anything Change?	202
9	Epilogue	232
Bibliography		247
Index		253

LIST OF TEXTS AND TRANSLATIONS

2.1 Homer, *Iliad* **1. 8–26, and 33–108**, Loeb Classical Library vol. 170, trans. A. T. Murray, rev. William F. Wyatt (Harvard University Press, 1999), modified by G. E. R. Lloyd. Text reproduced from Oxford Classical Texts, *Homer: vol. I, Iliad (Books I–XII)*, ed. D. B. Munro and T. W. Allen, 3rd edn., 1920, Oxford University Press.

2.2 Homer, *Odyssey* **4. 219–32**, trans. Geoffrey E. R. Lloyd. Text reproduced from Oxford Classical Texts, *Homer: vol. III, Odyssey (Books I–XII)*, ed. T. W. Allen, 2nd edn., 1917, Oxford University Press.

2.3 Hesiod, *Works and Days* **70–105**, trans. Geoffrey E. R. Lloyd. Text reproduced from Loeb Classical Library vol. 57 (Harvard University Press, 1914).

2.4 Hesiod, *Works and Days*: **225–47**, trans. Geoffrey E. R. Lloyd. Text reproduced from Loeb Classical Library vol. 57 (Harvard University Press, 1914).

2.5 Sappho, poem 31. 1–16, from *Sappho and Alcaeus: An Introduction to the Study of Ancient Lesbian Poetry*, trans. Denys L. Page (Oxford University Press, 1955).

2.6 Diogenes Laertius: Epimenides, 1. 110 and 112, trans. Geoffrey E. R. Lloyd. Text reproduced from Loeb Classical Library vol. 184 (Harvard University Press, 1925, 1972).

2.7 Empedocles, fragment 111 in *The Presocratic Philosophers: A Critical History with a Selection of Texts* trans. G. S. Kirk, J. E. Raven, and M. Schofield (2nd edn., Cambridge University Press, 1983).

2.8 Empedocles, fragment 112 in *The Presocratic Phil-*

osophers: A Critical History with a Selection of Texts trans. G. S. Kirk, J. E. Raven, and M. Schofield (2nd edn., Cambridge University Press, 1983).

3.1 Hippocrates, *On the Sacred Disease*, **chs. 1–6**, Loeb Classical Library vol. 148, trans. W. H. S. Jones (Harvard University Press, 1923), modified by G. E. R. Lloyd.

3.2 Hippocrates, *On the Sacred Disease*: **ch. 10**, Loeb Classical Library vol. 148, trans. W. H. S. Jones (Harvard University Press, 1923).

3.3 Plato, *The Republic*, **book II, 364b–c5**, Loeb Classical Library vol. 237, trans. Paul Shorey (Harvard University Press, 1930). Text reproduced from Oxford Classical Texts, *Plato: vol. IV*, ed. J. Burnet, 1905, 1978, Oxford University Press.

3.4 Hippocrates, *On the Sacred Disease*: **chs. 21. 1–12** and **22–6**, trans. Geoffrey E. R. Lloyd. Text reproduced from Loeb Classical Library vol. 148 (Harvard University Press, 1923).

3.5 Hippocrates, *On the Diseases of Young Girls*, **ch. 1**, trans. Geoffrey E. R. Lloyd. Text reproduced from *Oeuvres complètes d'Hippocrate*, ed. E. Littré, vol. VIII (J. B. Baillière, Paris, 1853).

3.6 Hippocrates, *De Octimestri Partu* **(*The Eight Month Child*), extracts from chs. 6 and 7**, trans. Geoffrey E. R. Lloyd. Text reproduced from CMG, I 2 1 ed. Hermann Grensemann (Akademie Verlag GmbH, 1968).

3.7 Hippocrates, *On the Diseases of Women I*, **ch. 62**, trans. Geoffrey E. R. Lloyd. Text reproduced from *Oeuvres complètes d'Hippocrate*, ed. E. Littré, vol. VIII (J. B. Baillière, Paris, 1853).

3.8 Hippocrates, *Oath*, Loeb Classical Library vol. 147, trans. W. H. S. Jones (Harvard University Press, 1923).

3.9 Hippocrates, *Law*, **ch. 5**, Loeb Classical Library vol. 148, trans. W. H. S. Jones (Harvard University Press, 1923).

3.10 Pindar, *Pythian* **3. 45–58**, Loeb Classical Library vol. 56, trans. William H. Race (Harvard University Press, 1997).

3.11 Asclepius, *A Collection and Interpretation of the Testimonies*, **vols. 1 and 2**, Epidaurus Inscriptions 22, 23, and 36, pp. 20–1, 25–6, trans. Emma Jeanette Edelstein and Ludwig Edelstein (Johns Hopkins University Press, 1945).

3.12 Hippocrates, *On Regimen*, **IV, ch. 90**, Loeb Classical Library vol. 150, trans. W. H. S. Jones (Harvard University Press, 1923).

3.13 Hippocrates, *Prognosis*: **ch. 1,** Loeb Classical Library vol. 148, trans. W. H. S. Jones (Harvard University Press, 1923).

4.1 Sophocles, *Oedipus Tyrannus* **58–72**, Loeb Classical Library vol. 20, trans. Hugh Lloyd-Jones (Harvard University Press, 1994). Text reproduced from Oxford Classical Texts, *Sophocles: Fabulae*, ed. Hugh Lloyd-Jones and N. G. Wilson, 1990, Oxford University Press.

4.2 Sophocles, *Oedipus Tyrannus* **95–104**, Loeb Classical Library vol. 20, trans. Hugh Lloyd-Jones (Harvard University Press, 1994). Text reproduced from Oxford Classical Texts, *Sophocles: Fabulae*, ed. Hugh Lloyd-Jones and N. G. Wilson, 1990, Oxford University Press.

4.3 Sophocles, *Oedipus Tyrannus* **380–403**, Loeb Classical Library vol. 20, trans. Hugh Lloyd-Jones (Harvard University Press, 1994). Text reproduced from Oxford Classical Texts, *Sophocles: Fabulae*, ed. Hugh Lloyd-Jones and N. G. Wilson, 1990, Oxford University Press.

4.4 Sophocles, *Oedipus at Colonus* **1595–607, and 1620–57**, Loeb Classical Library vol. 21, trans. Hugh Lloyd-Jones (Harvard University Press, 1994). Text reproduced from Oxford Classical Texts, *Sophocles: Fabulae*, ed. Hugh Lloyd-Jones and N. G. Wilson, 1990, Oxford University Press.

4.5 Sophocles, *Philoctetes* **38–47**, Loeb Classical Library vol. 21, trans. Hugh Lloyd-Jones (Harvard University Press, 1994). Text reproduced from Oxford Classical Texts, *Sophocles: Fabulae*, ed. Hugh Lloyd-Jones and N. G. Wilson, 1990, Oxford University Press.

4.6 Aeschylus, *Prometheus Vinctus* 476–500, Loeb Classical Library vol. 145, trans. Herbert Weir-Smyth (Harvard University Press, 1922). Text reproduced from Oxford Classical Texts, *Aeschylus: Tragoediae*, ed. Denys Page, 1972, Oxford University Press.

4.7 Sophocles, *Antigone* 332–64, Loeb Classical Library vol. 21, trans. Hugh Lloyd-Jones (Harvard University Press, 1994), modified by G. E. R. Lloyd. Text reproduced from Oxford Classical Texts, *Sophocles: Fabulae*, ed. Hugh Lloyd-Jones and N. G. Wilson, 1990, Oxford University Press.

4.8 Euripides, *The Bacchae* 135–54, trans. Philip Vellacott from *The Bacchae and Other Plays* (Penguin, 1954). Text reproduced from Oxford Classical Texts, *Euripides: Fabulae, vol. III*, ed. Gilbert Murray, 1st edn., 1913, Oxford University Press.

4.9 Euripides, *The Bacchae* 215–25, and 248–62, trans. Philip Vellacott from *The Bacchae and Other Plays* (Penguin, 1954). Text reproduced from Oxford Classical Texts, *Euripides: Fabulae, vol. III*, ed. Gilbert Murray, 1st edn., 1913, Oxford University Press.

4.10 Euripides, *The Bacchae* 298–305, 309–27, trans. Geoffrey E. R. Lloyd. Text reproduced from Oxford Classical Texts, *Euripides: Fabulae, vol. III*, ed. Gilbert Murray, 1st edn., 1913, Oxford University Press.

4.11 Euripides, *Hippolytus* 176–214, Loeb Classical Library vol. 484, trans. David Kovacs (Harvard University Press, 1995). Text reproduced from Oxford Classical Texts, *Euripides: Fabulae, vol. I*, ed. James Diggle, 1984, Oxford University Press.

5.1 Herodotus, *The Histories*, 4. 202–3. 1 and 205, trans. Aubrey de Sélincourt, (Penguin Classics, 1954). Text reproduced from Oxford Classical Texts, *Herodotus: Historiae vol. I*, ed. K. Hude, 3rd edn., 1927, Oxford University Press.

5.2 Herodotus, *The Histories*, 1. 105. 4, trans. Aubrey de Sélincourt (Penguin Classics, 1954). Text reproduced from

List of Texts and Translations   xiii

Oxford Classical Texts, *Herodotus: Historiae vol. I*, ed. K. Hude, 3rd edn., 1927, Oxford University Press.

5.3 Hippocrates, ***On Airs Waters Places***, ch. 22, Loeb Classical Library vol. 147, trans. W. H. S. Jones (Harvard University Press, 1923).

5.4 Herodotus, ***The Histories***, 3. 28. 2–30. 1, trans. Aubrey de Sélincourt (Penguin Classics 1954). Text reproduced from Oxford Classical Texts, *Herodotus: Historiae Volume I*, ed. K. Hude, 3rd edn., 1927, Oxford University Press.

5.5 Herodotus, ***The Histories***, 6. 75, trans. Aubrey de Sélincourt (Penguin Classics 1954). Text reproduced from Oxford Classical Texts, *Herodotus: Historiae Volume II*, ed. K. Hude, 3rd edn., 1927, Oxford University Press.

5.6 Herodotus, ***The Histories***, 6. 84. 1 and 84. 3, trans. Aubrey de Sélincourt (Penguin Classics 1954). Text reproduced from Oxford Classical Texts, *Herodotus: Historiae Volume II*, ed. K. Hude, 3rd edn., 1927, Oxford University Press.

5.7 Thucydides, ***History*** 1. 22, trans. Geoffrey E. R. Lloyd. Text reproduced from Oxford Classical Texts, *Thucydides: Historiae Volume I*, ed. H. Stuart-Jones and J. E. Powell, 2nd edn., 1942, Oxford University Press.

5.8 Thucydides, ***History*** 2. 47. 1–49.6, 51. 2–4, 51. 6, 53. 1–4, trans. P. J. Rhodes (Aris & Phillips Ltd, 1988), modified by G. E. R. Lloyd. Text reproduced from Oxford Classical Texts, *Thucydides: Historiae Volume I*, ed. H. Stuart-Jones and J. E. Powell, 2nd edn., 1942, Oxford University Press.

5.9 Thucydides, ***History*** 3. 82. 1–2, trans. P. J. Rhodes (Aris & Phillips Ltd, 1994). Text reproduced from Oxford Classical Texts, *Thucydides: Historiae Volume I*, ed. H. Stuart-Jones and J. E. Powell, 2nd edn., 1942, Oxford University Press.

6.1 Plato, ***Gorgias*** 477e7–478c7, Loeb Classical Library vol. 166, trans. W. R. M. Lamb (Harvard University Press,

1925). Text reproduced from Oxford Classical Texts, *Plato: Volume III*, ed. J. Burnet, 1903, Oxford University Press.

6.2 Plato, *Gorgias* 505a6–b12, Loeb Classical Library vol. 166, trans. W. R. M. Lamb (Harvard University Press, 1925). Text reproduced from Oxford Classical Texts, *Plato: Volume III*, ed. J. Burnet, 1903, Oxford University Press.

6.3 Plato, *The Republic*, book II, 372c2–e8, Loeb Classical Library vol. 237, trans. Paul Shorey (Harvard University Press, 1930). Text reproduced from Oxford Classical Texts, *Plato: Volume IV*, ed. J. Burnet, 1905, 1978, Oxford University Press.

6.4 Plato, *The Republic*, book IV, 444c8–e2, Loeb Classical Library vol. 237, trans. Paul Shorey (Harvard University Press, 1930). Text reproduced from Oxford Classical Texts, *Plato: Volume IV*, ed. J. Burnet, 1905, 1978, Oxford University Press.

6.5 Plato, *The Republic*, book V, 459c2–e3, Loeb Classical Library vol. 237, trans. Paul Shorey (Harvard University Press, 1930). Text reproduced from Oxford Classical Texts, *Plato: Volume IV*, ed. J. Burnet, 1905, 1978, Oxford University Press.

6.6 Plato, *The Republic*, book VIII, 563e6–564b2, Loeb Classical Library vol. 276, trans. Paul Shorey (Harvard University Press, 1935). Text reproduced from Oxford Classical Texts, *Plato: Volume IV*, ed. J. Burnet, 1905, 1978, Oxford University Press.

6.7 Plato, *Sophist*, 227c7–228b10, trans. Nicholas P. White (Hackett, 1993). Text reproduced from Oxford Classical Texts, *Plato: Volume I*, ed. J. Burnet, 1905, Oxford University Press.

6.8 Plato, *Laws* Book V 735b1–736a3, Loeb Classical Library vol. 187, trans. R. G. Bury (Harvard University Press, 1926). Text reproduced from Oxford Classical Texts, *Plato: Volume V*, ed. J. Burnet, 1907, Oxford University Press.

6.9 Plato, *Phaedrus* 244a5–b3, 244d5–245a8, trans. R.

List of Texts and Translations xv

Hackforth (Cambridge University Press, 1952 and 1972). Text reproduced from Oxford Classical Texts, *Plato: Volume II*, ed. J. Burnet, 2nd edn. 1915, Oxford University Press.

6.10 Plato, *Phaedrus* 253e5–254e5, trans. R. Hackforth (Cambridge University Press, 1952 and 1972). Text reproduced from Oxford Classical Texts, *Plato: Volume II*, ed. J. Burnet, 2nd edn. 1915, Oxford University Press.

6.11 Plato, *Timaeus* 81e6–82a7, trans. Geoffrey E. R. Lloyd. Text reproduced from Oxford Classical Texts, *Plato: Volume IV*, ed. J. Burnet, 1905, 1978, Oxford University Press.

6.12 Plato, *Timaeus* 82e7–83a5, trans. Geoffrey E. R. Lloyd. Text reproduced from Oxford Classical Texts, *Plato: Volume IV*, ed. J. Burnet, 1905, 1978, Oxford University Press.

6.13 Plato, *Timaeus* 85e2–86a2, trans. Geoffrey E. R. Lloyd. Text reproduced from Oxford Classical Texts, *Plato: Volume IV*, ed. J. Burnet, 1905, 1978, Oxford University Press.

6.14 Plato, *Timaeus* 86b1–7, trans. Geoffrey E. R. Lloyd. Text reproduced from Oxford Classical Texts, *Plato: Volume IV*, ed. J. Burnet, 1905, 1978, Oxford University Press.

6.15 Plato, *Timaeus* 87c4–d3, trans. Geoffrey E. R. Lloyd. Text reproduced from Oxford Classical Texts, *Plato: Volume IV*, ed. J. Burnet, 1905, 1978, Oxford University Press.

7.1 Aristotle, *On the Senses* 436a17–b1, trans. Geoffrey E. R. Lloyd. Text reproduced from Loeb Classical Library vol. 288 (Harvard University Press, 1936).

7.2 Aristotle, *On Respiration* 480b21–30, trans. Geoffrey E. R. Lloyd. Text reproduced from Loeb Classical Library vol. 288 (Harvard University Press, 1936).

7.3 Aristotle, *On the Movement of Animals* 703a28–b2, trans. Geoffrey E. R. Lloyd. Text reproduced from Loeb Classical Library vol. 323 (Harvard University Press, 1937).

7.4 Aristotle, *Politics* 1295a40–b1, trans. Geoffrey E. R. Lloyd. Text reproduced from Loeb Classical Library vol. 264 (Harvard University Press, 1932).

7.5 Aristotle, *Nicomachean Ethics* 1097a11–13, trans. Geoffrey E. R. Lloyd. Text reproduced from Loeb Classical Library vol. 73 (Harvard University Press, 1990).

7.6 Aristotle, *Nicomachean Ethics* 1137a11–17, trans. Geoffrey E. R. Lloyd. Text reproduced from Loeb Classical Library vol. 73 (Harvard University Press, 1990).

7.7 Aristotle, *Nicomachean Ethics* 1104a11–19, trans. Geoffrey E. R. Lloyd. Text reproduced from Loeb Classical Library vol. 73 (Harvard University Press, 1990).

7.8 Aristotle, *Nicomachean Ethics* 1106a29–b7, trans. Geoffrey E. R. Lloyd. Text reproduced from Loeb Classical Library vol. 73 (Harvard University Press, 1990).

7.9 Aristotle, *Nicomachean Ethics* 1114a11–19, trans. Geoffrey E. R. Lloyd. Text reproduced from Loeb Classical Library vol. 73 (Harvard University Press, 1990).

7.10 Aristotle, *Nicomachean Ethics* 1173b22–5, trans. Geoffrey E. R. Lloyd. Text reproduced from Loeb Classical Library vol. 73 (Harvard University Press, 1990).

7.11 Aristotle, *Nicomachean Ethics* 1176a12–16, trans. Geoffrey E. R. Lloyd. Text reproduced from Loeb Classical Library vol. 73 (Harvard University Press, 1990).

7.12 Aristotle, *Politics* 1279a22–31, trans. Geoffrey E. R. Lloyd. Text reproduced from Loeb Classical Library vol. 264 (Harvard University Press, 1932).

7.13 Aristotle, *Politics* 1279b4–10, trans. Geoffrey E. R. Lloyd. Text reproduced from Loeb Classical Library vol. 264 (Harvard University Press, 1932).

7.14 Aristotle, *Poetics* 1449b24–8, trans. Geoffrey E. R. Lloyd. Text reproduced from Loeb Classical Library vol. 199 (Harvard University Press, 1995).

7.15 Aristotle, *Politics* 1341b32–1342a16, trans. Geoffrey E. R. Lloyd. Text reproduced from Loeb Classical Library vol. 264 (Harvard University Press, 1932).

8.1 Celsus, *On Medicine* **1 Prooemium 39**, trans. Geoffrey E. R. Lloyd. Text reproduced from Loeb Classical Library vol. 292 (Harvard University Press, 1935).

8.2 Galen, *On the Opinions of Hippocrates and Plato*, **240. 11–242. 11**, trans. Phillip de Lacy (CMG, V 4 1 2 1980–4).

8.3 Galen, *On the Opinions of Hippocrates and Plato*, **296. 18–27**, trans. Phillip de Lacy (CMG, V 4 1 2 1980–4).

8.4 Galen, 'That the Faculties of the Soul Follow the Mixtures of the Body', ch. 9 in *Selected Works*, trans. with introduction and notes by P. N. Singer (Oxford World Classics, 1997), Oxford University Press. Text is reproduced from Galen, *Scripta Minora*, vol. II, ed. Iwan Mueller (Teubner, Leipzig, 1891).

8.5 Galen, *On the Opinions of Hippocrates and Plato*, **302. 17–30**, trans. Phillip de Lacy (CMG, V 4 1 2 1980–4), Akademie Verlag GmbH.

8.6 Aelius Aristides, *The Sacred Tales*, **47, 62–3 and 65–7**, trans. Charles Allison Behr (Hakkert, Amsterdam 1968). Text reproduced from *Aelii Aristidis Opera Quae Supersunt Omnia*, vol. II ed. Bruno Keil (Weidmann, Berlin, 1898).

8.7 Aelius Aristides, *The Sacred Tales*, **48, 39–43**, trans. Charles Allison Behr (Hakkert, Amsterdam 1968). Text reproduced from *Aelii Aristidis Opera Quae Supersunt Omnia*, vol. II ed. Bruno Keil (Weidmann, Berlin, 1898).

8.8 Lucretius, *On the Nature of Things* **1. 936–50**, Loeb Classical Library vol. 181, trans. W. H. D. Rouse, rev. Martin Ferguson Smith (Harvard University Press, 1975, 1982, 1992).

8.9 Lucretius, *On the Nature of Things*, **6. 1156–81**, Loeb Classical Library vol. 181, trans. W. H. D. Rouse, rev. Martin Ferguson Smith (Harvard University Press, 1975, 1982, 1992).

ACKNOWLEDGEMENTS

The author and publisher are grateful to the following for permission to reproduce copyright material.

Akademie Verlag GmbH for text and translation of extracts [8.2, 8.3, 8.5] from GALEN: *On the Doctrines of Hippocrates and Plato* translated by Phillip de Lacy (CMG, V 4 1 2 1980–1984).

Aris & Phillips Ltd for extract [5.8] from THUCYDIDES: *History* II, translated by P. J. Rhodes (1988), and [5.9] *History* III, translated by P. J. Rhodes (1994).

Cambridge University Press for text and translations of extracts [2.7, 2.8] from DIOGENES LAERTIUS, Book VIII in *The Presocratic Philosophers: A Critical History with a Selection of Texts* translated by G. S. Kirk, J. E. Raven, and M. Schofield (2e Cambridge University Press, 1983); and extracts [6.9, 6.10] from PLATO: *Phaedrus* translated by R. Hackforth (Cambridge University Press, 1952 and 1972).

Hackett Publishing Company, Inc. for extract [6.7] from PLATO: *Sophist* translated by Nicholas P. White (Hackett, 1993), copyright © 1993 by Hackett Publishing Company, Inc. All rights reserved.

Adolf M. Hakkert Publishers for extracts [8.6, 8.7] from AELIUS ARISTIDES: *The Sacred Tales*, XLVII and XLVIII translated by Charles Allison Behr (Hakkert, Amsterdam 1968).

Harvard University Press and the Trustees of the Loeb Classical Library for translations of extract [4.6] from

Acknowledgements

AESCHYLUS: Vol. I: *Prometheus Vinctus*, Loeb Classical Library Vol. 145, translated by Herbert Weir-Smyth (Harvard University Press, 1922); extract [4.11] from EURIPIDES: Vol. II: *Children of Heracles: Hippolytus*, Loeb Classical Library Vol. 484, translated by David Kovacs (Harvard University Press, 1995), copyright © 1995 by the President and Fellows of Harvard College; extracts from HIPPOCRATES: Vol. I: [3.8] *Oath*, and [5.3] *On Airs Waters Places*, Loeb Classical Library Vol. 147, translated by W. H. S. Jones (Harvard University Press, 1923); Vol. II: [3.1, 3.2, 3.4] *On the Sacred Disease*, [3.9] *Law*, and [3.13] *Prognosis*, Loeb Classical Library Vol. 148, translated by W. H. S. Jones (Harvard University Press, 1923); and Vol. IV: [3.12] *On Regimen*: IV, Loeb Classical Library Vol. 150, translated by W. H. S. Jones (Harvard University Press, 1923); extracts [2.1] from HOMER: Vol. 1: *Iliad*, Loeb Classical Library Vol. 170, translated by A. T. Murray, revised by William F. Wyatt (Harvard University Press, 1999), copyright © 1999 by the President and Fellows of Harvard College; extracts from LUCRETIUS: *On the Nature of Things*, Book I: [8.8], and Book VI: [8.9], Classical Library Vol. 181, translated by W. H. D. Rouse, revised by Martin Ferguson Smith (Harvard University Press, 1975, 1982, 1992), copyright © 1975, 1992 by the President and Fellows of Harvard College; extract [3.10] from PINDAR: Vol. I: *Pythian*, Loeb Classical Library Vol. 56, translated by William H. Race (Harvard University Press, 1997), copyright © 1999 by the President and Fellows of Harvard College; extracts from PLATO: Vol. III: [6.1, 6.2] *Gorgias*, Loeb Classical Library Vol. 166, translated by W. R. M. Lamb (Harvard University Press, 1925); Vol. V: [3.3, 6.3, 6.4, 6.5] *The Republic I*, Loeb Classical Library Vol. 237 translated by Paul Shorey (Harvard University Press, 1925); Vol. VI: [6.6] *The Republic II*, Loeb Classical Library Vol. 276, translated by Paul Shorey (Harvard University Press, 1935); and Vol. X: [6.8] *Laws*, Loeb Classical Library Vol. 187, translated by R. G. Bury (Harvard University Press, 1926); and extracts from SOPHOCLES:

Vol. I: [4.1, 4.2, 4.3] *Oedipus Tyrannus*, Loeb Classical Library Vol. 20, translated by Hugh Lloyd-Jones (Harvard University Press, 1994), copyright © 1994 by the President and Fellows of Harvard College; Vol. II [4.4] *Oedipus at Colonus*, [4.5] *Philoctetes*, and [4.7] *Antigone*, Loeb Classical Library Vol. 21, translated by Hugh Lloyd-Jones (Harvard University Press, 1994), copyright © 1994 by the President and Fellows of Harvard College. The Loeb Classical Library ® is a registered trademark of the President and Fellows of Harvard College.

Johns Hopkins University Press for text and translation of extracts [3.11] from ASCLEPIUS: *A Collection and Interpretation of the Testimonies*, Vols. 1 & 2, Epidaurus Inscriptions, translated by Emma Jeanette Edelstein and Ludwig Edelstein (Johns Hopkins University Press, 1945), copyright © 1945, 1998 by Johns Hopkins University Press.

Oxford University Press for text and translation of extract [2.5] from SAPPHO: Poem 31, from *Sappho and Alcaeus: An Introduction to the Study of Ancient Lesbian Poetry* translated by Denys L. Page (OUP, 1955); and translation of extract [8.4] from GALEN: 'That the Faculties of the Soul Follow the Mixtures of the Body', in *Selected Works* translated with an introduction and notes by P. N. Singer (Oxford World Classics, 1997), copyright © P N Singer 1997.

Oxford University Press for texts reproduced from Oxford Classical Texts: [4.6] *Aeschylus: Tragoediae* edited by Denys Page, 1972, © Oxford University Press 1972; [4.11] *Euripides: Fabulae,* Vol. I, edited by James Diggle, 1984, © Oxford University Press 1984, and [4.8, 4.9, 4.10] Vol. III edited by Gilbert Murray, 1e, 1913, © Oxford University Press 1994; [5.1, 5.2, 5.4, 5.5, 5.6] *Herodotus: Historiae* Vol., I edited by K. Hude, 3e, 1927, © Oxford University Press; [2.1] *Homer: Vol. 1, Iliad* (Books I–XII) edited by D. B. Munro and T. W. Allen, 3e, 1920, © Oxford University

Press; and [2.2] *Vol. III, Odyssey* (Books I–XII) edited by T. W. Allen, 2e, 1917, © Oxford University Press; [6.7] *Plato:* Vol. I, edited by J. Burnet, 1e 1905, © Oxford University Press 1995; [6.9, 6.10] Vol. II edited by J. Burnet, 2e 1915, © Oxford University Press; [6.1, 6.2] Vol. III edited by J. Burnet, 1903, © Oxford University Press; [3.3, 6.3, 6.4, 6.5, 6.6, 6.11, 6.12, 6.13, 6.14, 6.15] Vol. IV, edited by J. Burnet, 1905, 1978, © Oxford University Press 1978; and [6.8] Vol. V, edited by J. Burnet, 1907, © Oxford University Press; [4.1, 4.2, 4.3, 4.4, 4.5, 4.7] *Sophocles: Fabulae* edited by Hugh Lloyd-Jones and N. G. Wilson, 1990, © Oxford University Press 1990; and [5.7, 5.8, 5.9] *Thucydides: Historiae* edited by H. Stuart-Jones and J. E. Powell, 2e, 1942, © Oxford University Press 1927, 1942.

Penguin Books Ltd for extracts [4.8, 4.9] from EURIPIDES: *The Bacchae* translated by Philip Vellacott from *The Bacchae and Other Plays* (Penguin, 1954), copyright © Philip Vellacott 1954, 1972; and extracts from HERODOTUS: *The Histories*, Book One [5.2], Book Three [5.4], Book Four [5.1], and Book Six [5.5, 5.6], translated by Aubrey de Sélincourt (Penguin Classics 1954), translation copyright © Aubrey de Sélincourt 1954.

I
Anthropological Perspectives

The ancient Greeks were plagued by plagues real and imaginary. The aim of this study is to explore Greek ideas about disease not just in the narrow sense of what doctors thought was happening to their patients, but also in the broader one of how those and other people's ideas influenced Greek thinking about such questions as causation and responsibility, about the self and the relation between mind and the body, about purification and pollution, about authority and the expert, about reality and appearance, about good and evil. As both social anthropology and the history of medicine have comprehensively shown in recent years, ideas about disease and what it affects are anything but simple cross-cultural universals. Strikingly different ideas on these topics are documented in cultures ancient and modern across the world. My study is intended as a contribution to such work and is driven by the conviction that the investigation of thinking about disease can afford particular insight into the values of the society concerned. While many aspects of the ancient Greek world have been illuminated in studies of individual authors and genres, the full extent of the grip that disease had on the ancient Greek imagination has yet to be revealed. We shall see that it has ramifications far beyond the field of Greek medicine as such, in politics, philosophy, religion, historiography, epic, tragedy, and indeed most genres of literature.

First, however, we should rehearse and take note of some of the methodological and conceptual points that have emerged from medical anthropological studies. We should distinguish between disease and illness. The first is what biomedicine will define as a pathological condition. The second relates to how you feel. The first is, in principle, objective and verifiable by certain tests that are generally agreed. The second is subjective. The distinction remains a useful one, even though it is less rigid than some of its early proponents suggested. There is still plenty of disagreement, among biomedical practitioners, about certain pathological conditions and not just those affecting mental health. Moreover we should not lose sight of the fact that biomedicine as we now know it is a phenomenon of the twentieth and twenty-first centuries. It is a product of the developments of biochemistry and molecular biology (among other sciences) in those centuries, a body of learning that has now been exported to traditional societies across the world. When it first arrives in such societies, it is always a new phenomenon. That is not to deny that there are societies that have their own often sophisticated methods of coping with illness. But over the span of human existence, until very recently there was no understanding, in most cases, of what modern biomedicine categorizes as the diseases in question. That has not prevented plenty of people from claiming—as we do—that some complaints are objective—'disease' in *their* vocabulary—while some are merely subjective.

Medical anthropological findings are crucial to our study of the ancient Greeks in a second respect. That concerns the question of who is represented as being competent to help the sick. In many traditional societies, most people cope with most of what they consider ordinary complaints on their own. Many cultures, but not all, however, have one or more groups of individuals who have or claim a reputation as healers. They may vary from charismatic healers, who cure by the word, by prayer, or the laying on of hands, through those with some experience of drugs or skill in setting fractures or dislocations, to those who can call on all the authority of a learned tradition of medical practice in justification of their own positions. In those societies where there is no such special group, it may simply be up to the individuals concerned to decide first of all that they are ill, and then what to do about it (sometimes of course with the help of friends or relatives); Gilbert Lewis's study of illness in a Sepik society (Lewis 1975) illustrates how this happens among the Gnau. The important point is that both diagnosis and therapy may, or may not, be the responsibility of some experienced or authoritative group or groups. We shall see how contested the question of who can decide who is ill was in ancient Greece.

Two further points follow from those already made. If ideas about sickness vary enormously across different cultures, so too do ideas about what it affects—about our bodies and minds. A further insight from Gilbert Lewis's fieldwork brings out the point. To distract the children who clustered around him as he conducted interviews with native patients and practitioners, he used the tactic of distributing paper and pencils and asking them to do some drawings. At first he ignored and just binned the results, being only too happy that he had secured a little peace and quiet by this device. But he then noticed something strange about the drawings that were made of the human body. While these gave better, or worse, representations, of heads, arms, legs, torsos, every drawing included a visible representation of the 'soul'. Even children knew that this was a vital part of the person, and what distinguished the living from the dead. They varied in their ideas about *where* to put it: some had it more or less in the centre of the body, but others represented it in other parts of the body. But all located it *somewhere*.

The sets of ideas about the human body that are documented across the world exhibit great diversity. In some societies the boundary between the self and what is outside it is strongly marked: in others far less so. Some cultures picture the body itself as constituted by several layers, an inner sanctum (as it were) surrounded by successive coverings, ending at the skin. That often goes with an idea of pathogens as invasive— as hostile forces attacking the body, achieving greatest penetration in the severest complaints. Ruth Padel's excellent study *In and Out of the Mind* (Padel 1992) explores such ideas in ancient Greece, but it is not just there, but also, for example, in ancient China that the notion of disease as invasion plays a prominent role (Kuriyama 1999). In the Chinese case a further leading notion is the association of disease with obstruction and stagnation. Health is then pictured as a matter of the free flow of the vital fluids and *qi* (breath/energy) through the body. If that flow is hindered and there is a blockage, the visible result will be disease (Sivin 1987). Just as Lakoff and Johnson pointed to certain leading images we commonly use to describe argument, emotion, interpersonal exchanges, and so on (Lakoff and Johnson 1980), so the understanding of the topic of health and disease is often a matter of applying concepts drawn from other domains of experience. As the Greeks said, phenomena are the vision of the obscure.

The second and final preliminary point relates to the gap that opens up between popular and more learned traditions. In many cases this will be a difference of degree rather than of kind. Not all learned traditions are mediated through the written rather than the spoken word. Ancient Indian medicine was passed down orally through many generations, so it has been claimed, before it came to be incorporated in the canonical texts of the *Carakasamhita* and *Susrutasamhita*. But literacy can be and often is a powerful weapon in the hands of those who claim special expertise—in medicine as in other fields. Mastery of the writings of earlier authorities can be a necessary condition for entry into the ranks of elite practitioners. The topic of the relations between rival, more or less learned, traditions of medical practice will be a recurrent one in the pages that follow—difficult though some of the ideas of some of the non-literate groups are to reconstruct.

It is important to note, however, that it is not just highly literate groups that exhibit self-consciousness, and that express critical doubts and suspicions about claims to expertise. It was one of Goody's claims in *The Domestication of the Savage Mind* (Goody 1977) that literacy is a crucial determinant in the growth of scepticism, since it is only when speech is written down that what is said can be examined and scrutinized at length and at leisure. However, first it is clear that the writing down of texts can sometimes have the opposite effect, not of encouraging, but of stifling, criticism, since once recognized as a sacred canon a text may be immune to direct challenge.

Second, there are extensive anthropological reports proving that scepticism is frequently expressed concerning those who claim special expertise in many different types of situation and in most societies. Lévi-Strauss highlighted the case of the Kwakiutl called Quesalid (Lévi-Strauss 1968). He doubted that 'shamans' have any special powers or knowledge—though the irony of his experience was that Quesalid's own successful imitation of their practices (to show that they were fraudulent) led him to be acclaimed by his own people as a shaman himself. That is a story from a largely oral culture. Greece in the archaic and classical periods is a culture in the process of transition. What precisely the 'literate revolution' (Havelock 1982) consisted in, and how deep its effects were, are still hotly contested issues. So far as the topics we shall address here are concerned, claims to authority were sometimes backed by appeals to particular bodies of written doctrine, even though this did not happen very frequently until the Hellenistic period. As we shall see, however, it was far from being the case that authority figures always presented themselves as deriving their special status from the mastery of written texts.

The chapters that follow will set out the evidence of the ancient Greek preoccupation with disease from different genres and in different periods. The themes we shall be exploring can be set out under seven interrelated heads.

1. Disease takes us to ideas of the *self*, of the human body and how it works. That includes the views taken on gender difference, which we shall come back to in a variety of different contexts. How the body and mind work normally implies ideas also about their abnormal functioning. Why does disease strike?

2. That takes us to ideas of *causation and responsibility*,

including to theodicy (the justification, or lack of it, for the concept of the divine governance of the cosmos). Who, or what, was responsible for it being the case that you (and your companions) were afflicted with disease, fell ill, went mad, lost their wits? The spectrum of possibilities for an answer ranges from the idea that you must have offended the gods to the conviction that the gods have nothing at all to do with it. Among intermediate positions are that the gods are responsible, but they reward the just and punish the unjust with prosperity and misfortune respectively: so health and disease relate directly to your standing (or that of your ancestors) with the gods who are thought to ensure that good behaviour pays. Again on the profane interpretation of diseases, they may be thought not to be the gods' doing, but to occur by no means simply by chance: they are the outcome of your behaviour and so in that sense you are responsible.

3. Mention of divine interest in disease brings us to the topics of *purification and pollution*. 'Purification' comes in many different varieties (Moulinier 1952, Parker 1996). This may be a matter of ritual cleansing, your making peace with the gods, by prayer and sacrifice, for some guilt or sin. But the purification your body needs may rather consist in clearing it out and purging it, by taking an emetic or a suppository, for instance. The very same vocabulary may be used both of a ritual, and of a physical, purification/purgation.

4. Questions to do with why disease occurred, and what its nature is, lead one to the central topic of who is in a position to answer them, to the issue of *authority and the expert*. Once again there is a spectrum of possibilities, with ritual experts at one end claiming to know what causes the gods to be offended so that they have brought sickness on the individual or the state, and what must be done to placate them and restore well-being. At the other end there are those who claim particular skills in diagnosing the physical origins and natures of diseases and in offering entirely secular advice about how to bring about a cure. The duties of the ritual expert stretch far beyond coping with religious pollution and purification, for

mary, literal, use and other deviant ones. Over and over again the key terms used in relation to health and disease pose severe problems for anyone who seeks an original 'literal' sphere of application. I accordingly prefer to think of all the terms we shall be considering as possessing what I call 'semantic stretch'. Indeed in my view all language exhibits greater or less semantic stretch.

Take, first, the terms already alluded to that deal with purifications of different types. The term *katharsis*, from *katharos* (pure/clean) means 'cleansing'. But what is cleansed can include (*a*) menstrual blood, (*b*) pathogens in the body, (*c*) disturbing emotions in the soul—as in Aristotle's theory of tragedy—and (*d*) ritual pollution.[1] If in each case there is the notion of a return to a clean or pure state, *how* that is construed varies from instance to instance, and so accordingly does the 'purification' in question. As Mary Douglas showed in *Purity and Danger* (Douglas 1966), it would be foolish to think that such an experience as washing your hands is the primary sphere of application from which the religious notion of purity is then derived—but equally foolish to suppose the reverse derivation. Besides what it means to wash your hands

---

[1] *katharsis* and its cognates (*katharmos, kathairein, katharma, katharizo, kathartikos*) are used (1) of the menses (e.g. *On Airs Waters Places*, ch. 4, *CMG* I 1 2, 30. 23, *Aphorisms* V 60, L IV 554. 7); (2) of supposed analogues in other species of animals (Aristotle, *History of Animals* 572^{b}29, *On the Generation of Animals* 775^{b}5); (3) of the after-birth (*On Airs Waters Places* ch. 7, *CMG* I 1 2, 36. 16, *On the Diseases of Women* I ch. 67, L VIII 140. 16, Aristotle, *History of Animals* 574^{b}4); (4) of purgatives generally (*Aphorisms* II 35, L IV 480. 13, *On Regimen in Acute Diseases* ch. 7, Littré, ch. 24 Jones, L II 276. 6 and 7); (5) on getting rid of such feelings as pity and fear—as in Aristotle's account of tragedy, see below Ch. 7 on *Poetics* 1449^{b}24 ff. and cf. *Politics* 1341^{b}38 ff.; (6) of ritual pollution, following murder, for example, and of the rites to remove it (e.g. Aeschylus, *Choephoroi* 968, *Eumenides* 277, 283, Sophocles, *Oedipus Tyrannus* 99, 1228, Euripides, *Bacchae* 77, Herodotus 1. 35, Plato, *Republic* 364e, *Laws* 872e f.); (7) of purifying, in the sense of refining, metals such as gold (Plato, *Politicus* 303d); and (8) of clarifying, in the sense of explaining or resolving, physical problems (Epicurus, *Letter to Pythocles* 86, cf *ekkathairesthai* at 87).

may be, in certain circumstances, no straightforward matter. We are dealing with a term with complex associations and resonances, many of which are directly or indirectly relevant to most occasions of its occurrence. That used to be dealt with under the rubric of the 'interaction' view of metaphor (Black 1962). But that still presupposed a literal/metaphorical dichotomy, and one between primary and transferred uses, whereas it is one of the advantages of the concept of 'semantic stretch' that it does not seek to adjudicate on the limits of the 'strict' sense of terms.

To achieve a *katharsis*, some *katharsis*, Greek healers often had recourse to *pharmaka*—the term from which our own pharmacology is of course derived. But as Derrida (1981), following Artelt (1937), showed, *pharmakon* is used not just of medicinal drugs but also of poisons, and then also of charms or spells. In fact many of the herbal and mineral remedies used by Greek doctors had highly toxic properties and could —and sometimes no doubt did—kill the patients they were supposed to cure. Some of the compounds of arsenic they used, for instance, would qualify as examples of this. The doctors hoped their patients would have confidence in them and their judgement, investing a lot of energy to achieve that effect. But many a patient must have suspected that their doctors did not know what they were doing, even when they accepted that the doctor's motives were benign. Certainly quite a number of other sick people—and not just among the rich and powerful—went further and suspected that their doctors (or others) were actually attempting to poison them.

But a *pharmakon*, we said, need not take the form of something the patient ingested. Spells or charms, recited over a patient, were also called *pharmaka*. In the context of working love magic—the topic of much of the vast collection of extant Greek papyri—the lover used spells not just to persuade the beloved to accept his or her advances, but to force the beloved to do so, compelling them against their will (Betz 1986, Winkler 1990). The negative effects of *pharmaka* are here in evidence as they were in the more purely physical field of drugs. A final example of the ambivalence of this family of terms is provided by the cognate *pharmakos*—used of the scapegoat figure driven from the community to take all its pollution away. The *pharmakos* itself was intensely negatively charged with associations of disease and evil: yet since it brought (supposedly) welfare when it was driven out, it was, in that respect, valued positively, treated generally with awe.

The idea of administering *pharmaka* was often to bring about a cure. They were part of *therapeia* (from which the English 'therapy' comes), one of the regular terms for the 'treatment' that healers of different kinds offered to their various types of 'sick' individual. But here too there are associations in the background that go well beyond the purely medical domain. *Therapeia* and the verb *therapeuo* are commonly used of serving the gods. I do not suggest that Greek doctors consciously or even subconsciously thought of themselves as worshipping their patients, when they offered them therapies or treatments. Yet in the context of temple medicine, the patients (conversely) were supposed to approach the god or the semi-divine hero (such as Asclepius) in a spirit of reverence—and they hoped their piety would be rewarded by a cure.

What the sick hoped to be cured of was sometimes described as a *pathos* (from which our term 'pathology' comes), but that term could include anything that happened to you or that you underwent or suffered (the cognate verb *pascho* has those senses). *Pathe* were not necessarily negative items, ailments that had to be removed. The word is often translated 'affection' or 'feeling' and in Greek psychological theories it is often interpreted by modern scholars as denoting especially what we call the emotions. We shall come eventually, when we discuss Aristotle's views on tragedy and Galen's criticisms of Stoic psychology, to tackle the problem of how Greek philosophers understood what they labelled *pathe*. But one of the tricky questions that involves is just how appropriate it is to match their ideas to those we are used to when we contrast reason and the emotions. How far were those ancient ideas

12   *Anthropological Perspectives*

influenced by the association of *pathe* as affections with *pathe* as illnesses? For now, however, we may simply register that when the doctors dealt with the *pathe* of their patients, they were dealing, potentially, with everything that happened to them, not just what they could identify as specific diseases.

We turn finally to the central terms for disease and health themselves, *nosos* and cognates such as *nosema* on the one hand, *hygieia* on the other. At this point a little elementary lexicography will be enough to illustrate the range of uses and we may leave aside the question of the relationships between them. If we use 'disease' as a conventional rendering of *nosos*, and 'health' as one for *hygieia*, the three questions we need to ask are these: (1) what can be said to suffer disease? (2) what do the diseases they suffer from consist in? And (3) what, conversely, can be said to be healthy?

(1) Among the subjects said to be affected by disease are not just individuals, but also states and constitutions, indeed Greece as a whole. (2) Among the diseases individuals suffer from are 'divine things', 'lack of education', 'love', 'senselessness' (*anoia*), an 'unbridled tongue', 'madness', and 'disorder'. What we find communities suffering from includes faction, injustice, evil, disorder. In Aeschylus there is 'disease' in 'tyranny' and in Demosthenes Greece is 'destroyed and diseased'.[2] (3) Conversely, 'health' and 'healthy' are used not just

---

[2] What is said to suffer from *nosos* or *nosema* may be a city or a state (Sophocles, *Antigone* 1015, 1141, Plato, *Protagoras* 322d, *Republic* 544c, Demosthenes 2. 14), or its affairs (Aristotle, *Constitution of Athens* 6. 4), or a tyranny (Aeschylus, *Prometheus Vinctus,* 224–5), or Greece as a whole (Demosthenes 9. 39), or the worship of the gods (Euripides, *Trojan Women* 27, Poseidon speaks), or a person's eyes, that is their ability to see straight (Euripides, *Helen* 575). What these various subjects may suffer from includes faction (Herodotus 5. 28, cf. Plato, *Sophist* 228a), or folly (Plato, *Laws* 691d), or wickedness (Xenophon, *Memorabilia* 3. 5. 18), or injustice (Plato, *Gorgias* 480b), or an unrestrained tongue (Euripides, *Orestes* 10), or childlessness (Euripides, *Ion* 620), or hatred of enemies (Aeschylus, *Prometheus Vinctus* 978), or love (Euripides, *Hippolytus* 767, Sophocles, *Trachiniae* 491), or madness (Aeschylus, *Persians* 750–1) or any terrible affliction, anguish or distress (Sophocles, *Oedipus Tyrannus* 1293, *Oedipus at Colonus* 544).

Anthropological Perspectives 13

of physical bodies, but of the soul or mind, of wholesome food, of virtuous behaviour. Herodotus speaks of the Greeks being healthy in political and religious matters, Xenophon uses the term of the *kosmos* as a whole, Thucydides uses it of ships that are seaworthy, and Lysias of the statues of the Hermae when they were intact. Opinions and arguments are also regularly said to be healthy (cf. our 'sound'): indeed that antedates philosophical writing since the usage occurs already in Homer.[3]

The interrelated themes we have to consider have repercussions throughout Greek literature, in historiography and philosophy, as well as in medicine itself. The problems have often been addressed in relation to one particular genre at a time. The ambition of this study is to deal with them synoptically. My contention is that, when this is done, we can see that these repercussions are more pervasive and more profound than we generally recognize. Who did the Greeks—different individuals or groups of them—think could pronounce on disease, and cure, and health? What did they truly consist in? These are topics, as we shall see, that are central to their ideas of well-being and good and evil themselves. The divergent answers to those questions take us to the heart of issues to do with authority, with knowledge and understanding, with control, with government, with morality, with values, with the place of humans in the cosmos and the nature of that cosmos itself.

[3] *hygies* and its cognates (*hygieinos, hygieros, hygiaino, hygiazo, hygieia* itself) are used (1) of what is sound in body and mind (Isocrates 12. 7); (2) with respect to the *kosmos* as a whole, of it and its products being kept sound (Xenophon, *Memorabilia* 4. 3. 13); (3) of an (unmutilated) statue of a Herm (Lysias 6. 12); (4) of seaworthy ships (Thucydides 8. 107); (5) of the part of Greece prepared to resist the Persians (Herodotus 7. 157); (6) of sound or sensible opinions (*Iliad* 8. 524, Plato, *Republic* 584e, *Theaetetus* 194b); (7) of statements or orders (one that is not 'healthy' being immoral) (Herodotus 1. 8); (8) of valid proofs (Sextus Empiricus, *Outlines of Pyrrhonism* 1. 116).

2

Archaic Literature and Masters of Truth

Right at the start of Greek literature stands the most famous and most influential text of all, the *Iliad,* a work that every educated Greek of the classical period would know. They would have studied it at school: they would have attended the performances of rhapsodes—professionals who recited the Homeric epics and other poems in public at Athens and elsewhere—and they would in many cases have learnt extensive passages by heart. Homer was reputed to be the educator of the Greeks. What that means exactly is rather unclear. But certainly the *Iliad* was an iconic text, the most highly prized in all Greek literature.

At the beginning of the *Iliad* there is the plague. It is this plague indeed that triggers the entire action of the *Iliad* for with it begins the *wrath* of Achilles. It was Apollo, the poet tells us, *Iliad* 1. 8ff. [T 2.1], who brought about the feud between Achilles and Agamemnon. Apollo's priest Chryses had come to the Achaean camp to ransom his daughter, Chryseis, taken captive in the spoils of war and apportioned to Agamemnon. But while the rest of the Achaeans agreed that she should be returned ('shouting their agreement', 22) Agamemnon refused. Chryses thereupon prays to Apollo to strike the Achaeans. 'If ever I roofed over a pleasing shrine to you, or if ever I burned to you fat thigh pieces of bulls or goats,' Chryses says (37ff.), 'fulfil for me this wish: let the Danaans pay for my tears by your arrows.' The response is swift and deadly. Apollo comes down from Olympus 'like night'. He lets

Archaic Literature and Masters of Truth 15

fly his arrows first on the mules and dogs, then on the men, 'and ever did the pyres of the dead burn thick' (52).

What was to be done? The initiative is taken by Achilles who calls an assembly and addressing Agamemnon he underlines the calamity they face. 'But come,' he says (62 ff.) 'let us ask some seer or priest, or some reader of dreams—for a dream too is from Zeus—who might tell us why Phoebus Apollo has conceived such anger, whether it is because of a vow that he blames us, or a hecatomb; in the hope that perhaps he may accept the savour of lambs and unblemished goats, and be minded to ward off destruction from us.' We may note, straight away, that Achilles himself is represented as in no doubt that it is Apollo who is responsible for the plague. His question is directed solely at what to do to placate him, for which they will need to know why he is angry.

The seer Calchas replies. He is said to be by far the best of diviners, one who 'knew things that are, that will be, and that were before' (70: we shall meet echoes of this expression again). But before he offers his advice, he asks for reassurance, that he will be protected even if he offends a mighty king. To that Achilles replies that he will personally ensure his safety and that no one will lay hands on him 'not even if it is Agamemnon you mean'. Thus reassured Calchas diagnoses the trouble as being Agamemnon's insulting Chryses and refusing to ransom his daughter. For that reason Apollo is afflicting the Achaeans and will not let off doing so until the daughter is returned without ransom and a hecatomb is sacrificed in Apollo's honour.

Agamemnon's opening sally is to call Calchas a 'prophet of evils', who has 'never yet given me a favourable prophecy; always it is dear to your heart to prophesy evil, and no word of good have you ever yet spoken or brought to fulfilment'. Now he speaks his prophecies in public, in front of the Achaeans, blaming Agamemnon for what has happened. He agrees to give back Chryses' daughter ('for I would rather have the army safe than to die', 117) but on condition that he is given Achilles' prize, Briseis, instead. That nearly provokes

Achilles to kill Agamemnon on the spot—but he is restrained by a sudden appearance of Athena. Agamemnon duly restores Chryses' daughter and performs a massive sacrifice, but Achilles has to submit to handing over Briseis. But he swears he will take no further part in the fighting and foresees great devastation for the Achaean army from the Trojans under Hector in his absence. With Chryseis returned to him, Chryses once again prays to Apollo, this time to bring the plague to an end. That duly happens, but the direct and indirect consequences of the quarrel between Achilles and Agamemnon are what the rest of the *Iliad*—on the 'wrath of Achilles' and his eventual setting it aside in reconciliation with the Trojan king Priam—is all about.

Within the framework of the epic it is assumed that the god causes the plague—and can bring about its end—and in both cases he does so at the request of his priest, and for a reason. Disease, on this story, may be sent as a punishment for an offence. There are specialists who know what to do in such predicaments, but their position, their authority, is far from unchallengeable: Calchas is rightly nervous of the response he will get from Agamemnon. Yet it apparently needed no specialist to identify Apollo at work, for Achilles is able to do that on his own. Seers are, however, those who have or claim special gifts of insight—into the past and future as well as into the present. If we could be certain who they were, the real ones that is, we would know better what awaits us. There are levels and levels of understanding, in other words. This whole epic is what the poet has from the Muses, gifted in an analogous way with special knowledge: Hesiod in the *Theogony* (38) uses a very similar expression of them as the one that Homer used of Calchas.

The theme that gods are responsible for diseases and for relief from them is thus strongly developed in the most prominent position in the best known text of Greek literature. Yet we should be careful to note what the first book of the *Iliad* does *not* say as much as what it does. It does not, first, suggest that all diseases everywhere are always sent by the gods. Nor does it develop a universal point of view according to which diseases are a weapon the gods use to ensure justice and punish injustice. This plague is sent by this god on this occasion to punish Agamemnon for slighting his priest.

Other texts in Homer and in Hesiod show that it would be wrong to see any universal implications in the episodes described in *Iliad* 1. This is not particularly surprising, given that Homer is not producing a general statement about disease, nor one that justifies the ways of god to humans. As regards the second of those two points, we shall see in a moment that the first text that attempts a correlation between good behaviour among humans and health and prosperity, and again between injustice and disease and misfortune, is in Hesiod's *Works and Days*. But as regards the first point it is easy to see that elsewhere in the *Iliad* and the *Odyssey* there is no direct link between pain and sickness and the gods. True, Apollo and Artemis are often in action, shooting their arrows: Artemis, who presides over childbirth, is associated especially, though not exclusively, with the diseases of women. But references to disease in the Homeric epics do not necessarily import allusions to gods. In the *Odyssey* (11. 198–201), when Odysseus speaks with his dead mother in the underworld, she contrasts being carried off by Artemis' arrows with dying from hateful consumption, wasting, caused by disease.

More importantly, those who treat disease, called *ieter* or *ietros*, healers/doctors, include several who are in no way represented as ritual specialists. The most famous doctors in the *Iliad*, Machaon and Podalirius, are, it is true, sons of Asclepius, a hero described as a 'blameless healer' (*Il.* 4. 194) who was taught about gentle drugs, *pharmaka*, by the centaur Chiron (*Il.* 4. 218f.). But Asclepius has not yet attained semi-divine status: we shall be looking at how that happened in the next chapter. Machaon and Podalirius themselves know about such matters as the extraction of arrows—shot by mere mortals, this time—and the application of soothing drugs. Their skills as doctors are in addition to their virtues as fighters. Both are engaged, like any other notable warrior, in the battles in the *Iliad*, from which they are called away to perform their feats of medical skill. The clearest recognition of the role of such healers comes in the famous remark that Idomeneus makes at *Iliad* 11. 514f. that 'a healer is worth as much as many others put together when it comes to cutting out arrows and smearing on gentle drugs'.

Just as there are diseases and diseases, ranging from ills sent expressly by the gods, to the complications from the wounds dealt by the blows of mortal warriors, so there are different categories of those called in to cope. We have seen Calchas' diagnosis of the causes of the plague, and Machaon is praised for his skill at treating wounds. But two other groups must also be mentioned (who again will recur in our subsequent studies), namely women and foreigners. A text in the *Odyssey* 4. 219ff. [T 2.2] conveniently alludes to both. Telemachus has arrived at Menelaus' palace to seek news of his father's return. After some opening exchanges where tales of suffering and sadness bring the assembled company to tears, Helen has the idea of spiking the wine with a drug, which, when drunk, takes away all pain and anger. Anyone who drinks this, the poet says, would not weep, even though his mother and his father died or his brother or son was killed before his very eyes. Helen is clearly an expert in such potions, and the source of her expertise is revealed. 'The daughter of Zeus had such cunning drugs, excellent ones, that the Egyptian woman Polydamna, the wife of Thon, gave her, for there the earth, the giver of grain, bears the most drugs, many that are good, when mixed, and many that are baneful. There [in Egypt]—every man is a healer, wise above humankind.'

Three modes of ambivalence are suggested by this text. The potentiality of drugs both for good and for harm, which we noted in Chapter 1, is here explicit. Secondly, when Egypt is said to be the greatest source of drugs—of both kinds—we can detect a sense of awe, wonder, but underlying fear, at the marvels of this foreign place. In other texts, as we shall see, foreigners' ideas about diseases and their cures are strongly disapproved of. But even here in the *Odyssey* the admiration

Archaic Literature and Masters of Truth   19

for the doctors that Egypt produces must be said to be tempered by the realization of the ways in which the drugs their country produces can be used for good or ill.

Thirdly, it is a woman who dispenses this drug in the *Odyssey*, even though Helen is the daughter of Zeus: and she got her knowledge from another foreign woman. That too serves to underline the ambivalence of attitudes towards females in the affair. They are benefactors, no doubt, but also potential dangers.

Our very next text, from Hesiod's *Works and Days*, will confirm the point. At *Works* 42 ff., Hesiod, addressing his brother Perses, tells the story of Prometheus, who stole fire from Zeus and gave it to humans. In revenge (70 ff.) [T 2.3] Zeus causes Hephaestus to make Pandora, the first woman, to whom Athena gives skills and whom Aphrodite makes beautiful. Epimetheus, forgetting his brother's instructions, accepts the gift, with disastrous results. Before Pandora (90 ff.) the tribes of humans lived on earth without ills, without hard work, without terrible diseases. Once Pandora had lifted the lid of the jar in which the gods' gifts were stored, all these evils escaped. 'The earth is full of evils and the sea is full' (101). 'Some diseases come upon men by day and some by night: they roam of their own free will, bringing evils to mortals, silently, since wise Zeus took away speech from them.'

The diseases themselves are personified, wilful, arbitrary. That means there is great unpredictability in their coming. Yet humans would have lived without diseases, so the myth would have it, but for the action of Pandora. As things are now, it is not as if males can do without females, of course. Pandora is full of grace and her skills, in weaving especially, are invaluable. Yet she is a bane *(pema,* 82) to males that eat bread—because females consume what the males produce. Evidently in the judgement of this male poet—addressing no doubt a largely male audience—the ambivalence towards women is heavily tilted towards the negative, a view echoed in lyric poetry by Semonides in his account of the various tribes of women, bitch, sow, vixen, all females marked by destructive characters. Even the female bee, praised at least for her industry, and said to be the best for males, even she is no exception to the generalization that comes immediately after her description, namely that Zeus made women as an evil.[1]

The second respect in which Hesiod goes well beyond Homer—over and above his fantastic myth of woman as the source of all evil—relates to a further passage in the *Works* which maintains that justice is rewarded by health and prosperity, injustice by the opposite. Hesiod's own great banes are the 'bribe-devouring kings' (e.g. 264) against whom he warns his brother Perses (with whom he is locked in a family dispute that would very probably have to be settled by those very kings). In the end, Hesiod claims (217ff.) [T 2.4], Justice wins. 'But they who give straight judgements to strangers and to the men of the land,' he says (225 ff.), '. . . their city flourishes and the people prosper in it. Peace, the nurse of children, is abroad in their land, and all-seeing Zeus never decrees cruel war against them. Neither famine nor disaster (*ate*, ruin, and especially the delusion that leads to it) ever haunt men who do true justice . . . The earth bears an abundant livelihood . . . their women bear children like their parents.' So much for the just city, but for those who practise *hubris,* violence, and wicked deeds, Zeus decrees a penalty (*dike*, here in the sense of punishment, rather than of justice itself). Often a whole city suffers on account of a bad man who sins and does evil deeds. 'On them the son of Cronos brings great bane (*pema*, 242 cf. Pandora), both famine and plague (*loimos*). And the people waste away and their women do not bear children.' The moral is immediately spelt out: 'You kings, pay attention, you too, to *dike.*' For Zeus has 30,000 spirits on watch for the wrong-doing that is done on earth (248–55).

Piecing together these ideas in Hesiod, we can see him first blaming women for the hard life that males have to live, but then also claiming that it is injustice that brings disaster, and in both cases a prominent place is assigned to diseases among the misfortunes that he is trying to account for. Diseases roam

[1] Semonides 7, on which see Loraux 1993.

freely among humans: but they are not natural. It took certain important and polemical developments that we shall be studying in the next chapter for the idea to be established that diseases all have natural causes and indeed for the idea of nature itself to be, as I shall argue, *invented*. If Homer describes a sphere of competence for human doctors, the picture Hesiod paints in the myths of Pandora and of the Just and Unjust Cities is one of diseases as the instruments of divine retribution. 'There is no way to escape the will [or mind] of Zeus' (*Works* 105). If Zeus is the just god that Hesiod wants Perses and us to believe, all well and good. But what kind of justice does he dispense? That question can hardly be avoided, insofar as a whole city may suffer from the wrongdoing of just one person. The diseases that fly out of Pandora's jar roam at random among humans. That too seems to problematize the idea of cosmic justice.[2]

Besides, on whose authority are we to accept these stories? On Hesiod's, of course, and he got them from the Muses. But the way that Calchas' divine inspiration was challenged in the *Iliad* already suggests that there is no unassailable authority to which anyone, priests, prophets, the poets themselves, can appeal to secure acceptance of their ideas. We may well wonder just how far Hesiod himself imagined that either his brother Perses or those bribe-devouring kings would take his advice and reform.

We have already seen the variety of ideas expressed in Homer and Hesiod concerning diseases, their origins, what should be done to cure or to avoid them, and who can pronounce on such questions, ideas which in Hesiod's case (at least) are endorsed by the poet speaking on his own account. But three other early figures can now be used to extend even further the range of beliefs entertained on these and related topics. These are the seventh-century lyric poet Sappho, the 'sage' Epimenides, and the philosopher Empedocles, who will serve as a bridge to our discussion of fifth-century ideas in the next chapter.

Sappho offers a rare and precious opportunity to listen to

[2] Contrast Lloyd-Jones 1983.

a Greek woman speaking for herself, and it is a very different voice we hear from those of Hesiod and Semonides. 'Fortunate as the gods he seems to me', her poem 31 [T 2.5] begins, 'the man who sits opposite you and listens to your sweet voice and your lovely laughter; that, I vow, has set my heart within my breast a-flutter. For when I look at you a moment, then I have no longer power to speak. But my tongue keeps silence: straightway a subtle flame has stolen beneath my flesh, with my eyes I see nothing, my ears are humming, a cold sweat covers me, and a trembling seizes me all over, I am paler than grass, I seem to be not far short of death.'

The power of the poem lies in the detail with which Sappho describes her feelings. Of course this is high poetry: but that detail reflects, one is tempted to say, an almost clinical observation of her own condition, the cold sweat, the trembling, the aphonia (as the Greek doctors were to say), the fire or flame (where *pur* is a regular term in Greek medicine for fever) that creeps beneath the skin, even the palpitating heart. There is not a single item in that list that does not have Greek medical parallels. But does Sappho believe she is ill? That is the kind of question to which we shall learn to resist giving a simple answer. *Eros* is, as we have already seen in Chapter 1, often described as a *nosos*, but then *nosos*, as we are discovering, does not just cover disease but is used of many other misfortunes. What is certain, however, is that the vocabulary Sappho uses for her passion is continuous with that of common later descriptions of diseases.

Did she believe Aphrodite was responsible? Certainly her relationship with the goddess is an intimate love–hate one. Certainly Aphrodite is often thought to be at work when mere mortals fall in love. But again at the level of this text, as we have it, we may note there is no mention of Aphrodite. The immediate cause of Sappho's speechlessness is the girl. But having said that, we must add a note of caution. This relates to the common archaic and classical Greek notion of what has been called double determination.[3] An act may be at once the

[3] See Dodds 1951, ch. 1

Archaic Literature and Masters of Truth 23

responsibility of a human agent, *and* ascribed to a divinity. A famous case that makes the point is Agamemnon's eventual acceptance of responsibility, in the *Iliad*, for having taken Briseis from Achilles, in the sense that he agrees to offer compensation, even though, as he puts it, Zeus and *ate* (delusion) took away his senses (*Il*.19.137ff. cf. 86ff., where he begins by saying he was *not* himself *aitios*, responsible, precisely because he was deluded). So the fact that Sappho clearly describes the girl as the cause as well as the object of her passion does not mean that we can infer that the goddess has nothing to do with it.

Epimenides is a legendary figure whose very date is disputed. Some put him in the seventh century, though Plato places him a century later.[4] Among the stories that circulated about him is one reminiscent of Rip Van Winkle, namely that he became famous in part because he fell asleep for fifty-seven years. But another story introduces him as the man who purified Athens when it was afflicted by a plague. Diogenes Laertius (1.110) [T 2.6] reports two versions of this, both of them starting with the Athenians summoning Epimenides from Crete when the Pythian priestess commanded them to purify (*katherai*) the city. In the first version he let sheep, some black, some white, loose on the Areopagus and told men to follow them and wherever each of them lay down, there to sacrifice to a local god. The story has an aetiological ring to it, as Diogenes continues by remarking that even in his day (third century CE) there are anonymous altars in various parts of Attica set up as memorials of the atonement. But in the second version of the story Epimenides declares the cause of the plague to be the pollution caused at the time when Cylon seized the Acropolis and certain suppliants who had taken refuge in a temple were nevertheless killed. In that version Diogenes has the plague ending only after the sacrifice of two young men.

---

[4] Plato, *Laws* 642d puts his purification of Athens ten years before the Persian Wars.

The discrepancies in the stories are what we should expect when we are dealing with legend. But whatever the truth of either version, Epimenides occupies a familiar, ambivalent, role that we shall see recurs in other contexts (Teiresias, Philoctetes). This is of the person who has special insight and special powers, often including the ability to cure diseases. Epimenides is able to say what should be done to remove the pollution. In other evidence about him we are told he collected herbs (Diogenes Laertius 1. 112). So he was not just a purifier, but also a healer, though the tale of his commanding human sacrifice underlines that his was an authority to be feared. Anyone who had the reputation of having slept for fifty-seven years had indeed to be thought, as Diogenes puts it, 'most dear to the gods'.

My third and final figure bears important resemblances to Epimenides, though now we are dealing with a definite historical individual. Empedocles is often given pride of place in histories of so-called Presocratic philosophy, for, among other things, the first clear statement that other physical bodies consist of different combinations of earth, water, air, and fire. He does not use the word later adopted for 'elements' (*stoicheion*) but calls these four the 'roots' (*rizomata*) of things. However, to treat them just as elements already oversimplifies matters, for these four roots are divine and are brought together and separated by two further divine cosmic forces he names Love and Strife.

But whatever his other interests were, Empedocles presents himself as a wonder-worker and a purifier (cf. Kingsley 1995): indeed one of his poems, or, according to some his whole output, went by the title of the *Purifications*. In one of the quotations from his work (Fr. 111) [T 2.7] he says that his listener will be able to control the winds and rain and drought, and even will bring the dead back to life. He promises also to teach *pharmaka*, drugs/remedies that are a defence for ills and old age. In another text (Fr. 112) [T 2.8] he addresses his fellow-citizens, the inhabitants of Acragas. 'An immortal god, mortal no more, I go about honoured by all, as is fitting, crowned with ribbons and fresh garlands: and by all whom I come upon as I enter their prospering towns, by men and women, I am revered. They follow me in their thousands, asking where lies the road to profit, some desiring prophecies, while others ask to hear the word of healing for every kind of illness, long transfixed by harsh pains.'

Now Galen's view of Empedocles, often repeated by modern scholars, was that he was a leading figure in what he calls the Sicilian or Italian school of doctors,[5] a group he thinks of as analogous to the Coans and Cnidians represented in our extant Hippocratic treatises and reported in the medical history known as *Anonymus Londinensis*. We shall be reviewing the doubts that may be expressed about Coans and Cnidians being organized in established schools in due course. As for the Italians, we certainly hear of fifth- and fourth-century medical writers based in Magna Graecia who put forward medical theories based on physical principles of one type or another, elements, humours, or whatever. Two of the most famous of these are the Pythagorean Philolaus of Croton and Philistion of Locri.

But what kind of doctor was Empedocles? He dispensed *pharmaka*, but we have seen that that could include charms and spells as well as drugs. On his own account he was accepted by his contemporaries as no mere ordinary mortal. They thought of him (or so he says) as a god. Certainly the advice he offers in the *Purifications* mainly relates to keeping yourself ritually clean. He warns against the consequences of behaviour he considers polluting, and that includes such ordinary practices as meat eating. He believes that all creatures have an immortal soul, even though this is normally condemned to the misery of reincarnation in cycles of rebirth from which only the purest will escape. We should certainly not underestimate the radical nature of Empedocles' rejection of one of the principal institutions of the city religion—blood sacrifice—as well as a deeply ingrained dietary custom.

---

[5] Galen, *On the Method of Healing* I ch. 1, K X 6.

Those who went to him for advice—to return to the text of Fr. 112—received oracles and the 'word of healing' for every kind of disease. Empedocles here uses the term *baxis* for 'word', and that was particularly associated with oracular pronouncements. There is no reason to think that Empedocles just offered charms and incantations. But there is every reason to believe that he operated as a wonder-worker. His healing was under the aegis not of the Olympian gods, but rather of the deities he introduces in his poem under their names— Aphrodite, Hephaestus, and so on. But Hephaestus was elemental fire, and Aphrodite, as the principle of Love that acts on the roots, was hardly the goddess with whom Sappho seemed so intimate.

Empedocles thus stands as a prototype of a very Greek holy man or sage. He claimed divine inspiration and divine powers. At the same time he was a consummate self-publicist.

CHAPTER 2 TEXTS

2.1 Homer, *Iliad* 1. 8–26, 33–108

Τίς τ' ἄρ σφωε θεῶν ἔριδι ξυνέηκε μάχεσθαι;
Λητοῦς καὶ Διὸς υἱός· ὁ γὰρ βασιλῆι χολωθεὶς
νοῦσον ἀνὰ στρατὸν ὦρσε κακήν, ὀλέκοντο δὲ λαοί,   10
οὕνεκα τὸν Χρύσην ἠτίμασεν ἀρητῆρα
Ἀτρεΐδης· ὁ γὰρ ἦλθε θοὰς ἐπὶ νῆας Ἀχαιῶν
λυσόμενός τε θύγατρα φέρων τ' ἀπερείσι' ἄποινα,
στέμματ' ἔχων ἐν χερσὶν ἑκηβόλου Ἀπόλλωνος
χρυσέῳ ἀνὰ σκήπτρῳ, καὶ λίσσετο πάντας Ἀχαιούς,   15
Ἀτρεΐδα δὲ μάλιστα δύω, κοσμήτορε λαῶν·
"Ἀτρεΐδαι τε καὶ ἄλλοι ἐυκνήμιδες Ἀχαιοί,
ὑμῖν μὲν θεοὶ δοῖεν Ὀλύμπια δώματ' ἔχοντες
ἐκπέρσαι Πριάμοιο πόλιν, εὖ δ' οἴκαδ' ἱκέσθαι·
παῖδα δ' ἐμοὶ λύσαιτε φίλην, τὰ δ' ἄποινα δέχεσθαι,   20
ἁζόμενοι Διὸς υἱὸν ἑκηβόλον Ἀπόλλωνα."
   Ἔνθ' ἄλλοι μὲν πάντες ἐπευφήμησαν Ἀχαιοὶ
αἰδεῖσθαί θ' ἱερῆα καὶ ἀγλαὰ δέχθαι ἄποινα·
ἀλλ' οὐκ Ἀτρεΐδῃ Ἀγαμέμνονι ἥνδανε θυμῷ,
ἀλλὰ κακῶς ἀφίει, κρατερὸν δ' ἐπὶ μῦθον ἔτελλε·   25

Detienne (1967/1996) introduced the term Masters of Truth for those archaic leaders who made special claims to Wisdom, and certainly Empedocles presents himself in a way that fits that label. These were charismatic leaders, but ones whose reputation was not just for special holiness, special purity, but also for superior knowledge of the truth. As we shall see, however, that claim, so often made, was just as often contested. The trouble about Masters of Truth was: could you believe them? There were rather a lot of them and they came in different guises. While the claims they made for themselves—or that were made for them—were that they had special powers, their being special immediately posed problems: what was the origin of these powers? Was it entirely benign? How could they be understood? Could they indeed be believed?

We shall see these themes return in our next study.

CHAPTER 2 TEXTS

2.1 Homer, *Iliad* 1. 8–26, 33–108

Who then of the gods was it that brought these two together to contend? The son of Leto and Zeus; for he, angered at the king, roused throughout the army an evil pestilence, and the men were perishing, because to Chryses his priest the son of Atreus had done dishonor. For he had come to the swift ships of the Achaeans to free his daughter and he brought with him ransom past counting; and in his hands he held the ribbons of Apollo, who strikes from afar, on a staff of gold, and he implored all the Achaeans, but most of all the two sons of Atreus, the marshalers of armies: 'Sons of Atreus, and you other well-greaved Achaeans, to you may the gods who have dwellings on Olympus grant that you sack the city of Priam, and return home safely; but set my dear child free for me, and accept the ransom in reverence for the son of Zeus, Apollo, who strikes from afar.'

Then all the rest of the Achaeans shouted their agreement, to respect the priest and accept the glorious ransom; yet this did not please the heart of Agamemnon, son of Atreus, but he sent him

"μή σε, γέρον, κοίλῃσιν ἐγὼ παρὰ νηυσὶ κιχείω."

Ὣς ἔφατ', ἔδεισεν δ' ὁ γέρων καὶ ἐπείθετο μύθῳ·
βῆ δ' ἀκέων παρὰ θῖνα πολυφλοίσβοιο θαλάσσης·
πολλὰ δ' ἔπειτ' ἀπάνευθε κιὼν ἠρᾶθ' ὁ γεραιὸς   35
Ἀπόλλωνι ἄνακτι, τὸν ἠΰκομος τέκε Λητώ·
"κλῦθί μευ, ἀργυρότοξ', ὃς Χρύσην ἀμφιβέβηκας
Κίλλαν τε ζαθέην Τενέδοιό τε ἶφι ἀνάσσεις,
Σμινθεῦ, εἴ ποτέ τοι χαρίεντ' ἐπὶ νηὸν ἔρεψα,
ἢ εἰ δή ποτέ τοι κατὰ πίονα μηρί' ἔκηα   40
ταύρων ἠδ' αἰγῶν, τόδε μοι κρήηνον ἐέλδωρ·
τίσειαν Δαναοὶ ἐμὰ δάκρυα σοῖσι βέλεσσιν."

Ὣς ἔφατ' εὐχόμενος, τοῦ δ' ἔκλυε Φοῖβος Ἀπόλλων,
βῆ δὲ κατ' Οὐλύμποιο καρήνων χωόμενος κῆρ,
τόξ' ὤμοισιν ἔχων ἀμφηρεφέα τε φαρέτρην.   45
ἔκλαγξαν δ' ἄρ' ὀϊστοὶ ἐπ' ὤμων χωομένοιο,
αὐτοῦ κινηθέντος. ὁ δ' ἤϊε νυκτὶ ἐοικώς.
ἕζετ' ἔπειτ' ἀπάνευθε νεῶν, μετὰ δ' ἰὸν ἕηκε·
δεινὴ δὲ κλαγγὴ γένετ' ἀργυρέοιο βιοῖο.
οὐρῆας μὲν πρῶτον ἐπῴχετο καὶ κύνας ἀργούς,   50
αὐτὰρ ἔπειτ' αὐτοῖσι βέλος ἐχεπευκὲς ἐφιεὶς
βάλλ'· αἰεὶ δὲ πυραὶ νεκύων καίοντο θαμειαί.

Ἐννῆμαρ μὲν ἀνὰ στρατὸν ᾤχετο κῆλα θεοῖο,
τῇ δεκάτῃ δ' ἀγορήνδε καλέσσατο λαὸν Ἀχιλλεύς·
τῷ γὰρ ἐπὶ φρεσὶ θῆκε θεὰ λευκώλενος Ἥρη·   55
κήδετο γὰρ Δαναῶν, ὅτι ῥα θνήσκοντας ὁρᾶτο.
οἱ δ' ἐπεὶ οὖν ἤγερθεν ὁμηγερέες τ' ἐγένοντο,
τοῖσι δ' ἀνιστάμενος μετέφη πόδας ὠκὺς Ἀχιλλεύς·
"Ἀτρεΐδη, νῦν ἄμμε παλιμπλαγχθέντας ὀΐω
ἂψ ἀπονοστήσειν, εἴ κεν θάνατόν γε φύγοιμεν,   60
εἰ δὴ ὁμοῦ πόλεμός τε δαμᾷ καὶ λοιμὸς Ἀχαιούς.
ἀλλ' ἄγε δή τινα μάντιν ἐρείομεν ἢ ἱερῆα,
ἢ καὶ ὀνειροπόλον, καὶ γάρ τ' ὄναρ ἐκ Διός ἐστιν,
ὅς κ' εἴποι ὅ τι τόσσον ἐχώσατο Φοῖβος Ἀπόλλων,
εἴτ' ἄρ' ὅ γ' εὐχωλῆς ἐπιμέμφεται εἴθ' ἑκατόμβης,   65
αἴ κέν πως ἀρνῶν κνίσης αἰγῶν τε τελείων
βούλεται ἀντιάσας ἡμῖν ἀπὸ λοιγὸν ἀμῦναι."

Ἤτοι ὅ γ' ὣς εἰπὼν κατ' ἄρ' ἕζετο· τοῖσι δ' ἀνέστη
Κάλχας Θεστορίδης, οἰωνοπόλων ὄχ' ἄριστος,
ὃς ᾔδη τά τ' ἐόντα τά τ' ἐσσόμενα πρό τ' ἐόντα,   70

away harshly, and laid on him a stern command: 'Let me not find you, old man, by the hollow ships.'

So he spoke, and the old man was seized with fear and obeyed his words. He went in silence along the shore of the loud-resounding sea; and then, when he had gone apart, the old man prayed earnestly to the lord Apollo, whom fair-haired Leto bore: 'Hear me, you of the silver bow, who have under your protection Chryse and sacred Cilla, and who rule mightily over Tenedos, Smintheus, if ever I roofed over a pleasing shrine for you, or if ever I burned to you fat thigh pieces of bulls or goats, fulfil for me this wish: let the Danaans pay for my tears by your arrows.'

So he spoke in prayer, and Phoebus Apollo heard him. Down from the peaks of Olympus he strode, angry at heart, with his bow and covered quiver on his shoulders. The arrows rattled on the shoulders of the angry god as he moved; and his coming was like the night. Then he sat down apart from the ships and let fly an arrow; terrible was the twang of the silver bow. The mules he attacked first and the swift dogs, but then on the men themselves he let fly his stinging arrows, and struck; and ever did the pyres of the dead burn thick.

For nine days the missiles of the god ranged through the army, but on the tenth Achilles called the army to the place of assembly, for the goddess, white-armed Hera, had put it in his heart; for she pitied the Danaans because she saw them dying. So, when they were assembled and met together, among them rose and spoke Achilles, swift of foot: 'Son of Atreus, now I think we shall be driven back and return home, our plans thwarted—if we should escape death, that is—if indeed war and pestilence alike are to subdue the Achaeans. But come, let us ask some seer or priest, or some reader of dreams— for a dream too is from Zeus—who might tell us why Phoebus Apollo has conceived such anger, whether it is because of a vow that he blames us, or a hecatomb; in the hope that perhaps he may accept the savour of lambs and unblemished goats, and be minded to ward off destruction from us.'

When he had thus spoken he sat down, and among them rose up Calchas, son of Thestor, far the best of diviners, who had knowledge of all things that are, and that will be, and that were before, and who

καὶ νήεσσ' ἡγήσατ' Ἀχαιῶν Ἴλιον εἴσω
ἣν διὰ μαντοσύνην, τήν οἱ πόρε Φοῖβος Ἀπόλλων.
ὅ σφιν ἐϋφρονέων ἀγορήσατο καὶ μετέειπεν·
"ὦ Ἀχιλεῦ, κέλεαί με, διίφιλε, μυθήσασθαι
μῆνιν Ἀπόλλωνος ἑκατηβελέταο ἄνακτος· 75
τοιγὰρ ἐγὼν ἐρέω· σὺ δὲ σύνθεο καί μοι ὄμοσσον
ἦ μέν μοι πρόφρων ἔπεσιν καὶ χερσὶν ἀρήξειν·
ἦ γὰρ ὀΐομαι ἄνδρα χολωσέμεν, ὃς μέγα πάντων
Ἀργείων κρατέει καί οἱ πείθονται Ἀχαιοί·
κρείσσων γὰρ βασιλεύς, ὅτε χώσεται ἀνδρὶ χέρηϊ. 80
εἴ περ γάρ τε χόλον γε καὶ αὐτῆμαρ καταπέψῃ,
ἀλλά τε καὶ μετόπισθεν ἔχει κότον, ὄφρα τελέσσῃ
ἐν στήθεσσιν ἑοῖσι. σὺ δὲ φράσαι εἴ με σαώσεις."
  Τὸν δ' ἀπαμειβόμενος προσέφη πόδας ὠκὺς Ἀχιλλεύς·
"θαρσήσας μάλα εἰπὲ θεοπρόπιον ὅ τι οἶσθα· 85
οὐ μὰ γὰρ Ἀπόλλωνα Διΐ φίλον, ᾧ τε σύ, Κάλχαν,
εὐχόμενος Δαναοῖσι θεοπροπίας ἀναφαίνεις,
οὔ τις ἐμεῦ ζῶντος καὶ ἐπὶ χθονὶ δερκομένοιο
σοὶ κοίλῃς παρὰ νηυσὶ βαρείας χεῖρας ἐποίσει
συμπάντων Δαναῶν, οὐδ' ἢν Ἀγαμέμνονα εἴπῃς, 90
ὃς νῦν πολλὸν ἄριστος Ἀχαιῶν εὔχεται εἶναι."
  Καὶ τότε δὴ θάρσησε καὶ ηὔδα μάντις ἀμύμων·
"οὔτ' ἄρ' ὅ γ' εὐχωλῆς ἐπιμέμφεται οὔθ' ἑκατόμβης,
ἀλλ' ἕνεκ' ἀρητῆρος, ὃν ἠτίμησ' Ἀγαμέμνων
οὐδ' ἀπέλυσε θύγατρα καὶ οὐκ ἀπεδέξατ' ἄποινα, 95
τοὔνεκ' ἄρ' ἄλγε' ἔδωκεν ἑκηβόλος ἠδ' ἔτι δώσει·
οὐδ' ὅ γε πρὶν Δαναοῖσιν ἀεικέα λοιγὸν ἀπώσει,
πρίν γ' ἀπὸ πατρὶ φίλῳ δόμεναι ἑλικώπιδα κούρην
ἀπριάτην ἀνάποινον, ἄγειν θ' ἱερὴν ἑκατόμβην
ἐς Χρύσην· τότε κέν μιν ἱλασσάμενοι πεπίθοιμεν." 100
  Ἤτοι ὅ γ' ὣς εἰπὼν κατ' ἄρ' ἕζετο· τοῖσι δ' ἀνέστη
ἥρως Ἀτρεΐδης εὐρὺ κρείων Ἀγαμέμνων
ἀχνύμενος· μένεος δὲ μέγα φρένες ἀμφὶ μέλαιναι
πίμπλαντ', ὄσσε δέ οἱ πυρὶ λαμπετόωντι ἐΐκτην.
Κάλχαντα πρώτιστα κάκ' ὀσσόμενος προσέειπε· 105
"μάντι κακῶν, οὐ πώ ποτέ μοι τὸ κρήγυον εἶπας·
αἰεί τοι τὰ κάκ' ἐστὶ φίλα φρεσὶ μαντεύεσθαι,
ἐσθλὸν δ' οὔτε τί πω εἶπας ἔπος οὔτ' ἐτέλεσσας."

2.2 Homer, *Odyssey* 4. 219–32

Then Helen, daughter of Zeus, had another plan. Straightway she put into the wine which they were drinking a drug to quiet all pain and anger and bring forgetfulness of every evil. Whoever should drink this down, when mixed in the bowl, would not in the course of that day let fall a tear on his cheeks, not even if his mother and father died, or his brother or dear son were killed by the sword and his own eyes saw it. The daughter of Zeus had such cunning drugs, excellent ones, that the Egyptian woman Polydamna, the wife of Thon, gave her, for there the earth, the giver of grain, bears the most drugs, many that are good, when mixed, and many that are baneful. There every man is a healer, wise above humankind: for they are of the race of Paieon.

2.3 Hesiod, *Works and Days* 70–105

Straightway the famous Lame God moulded from the earth a likeness of a modest girl, on the plans of the son of Cronos. And grey-eyed Athene clothed and adorned her, and the divine Graces and lady Persuasion put golden necklaces on her, and the fair-tressed Seasons crowned her with spring flowers. And Pallas Athene adorned her in every way. And the Slayer of Argus, the guide, put lies and crafty words and a deceitful character in her breast according to the plans of Zeus the thunderer: and the herald of the gods put speech in her. And he named this woman Pandora, because all those who lived on Olympus gave her a gift, a bane for men who eat bread.

And when he had completed the sheer, hopeless, snare, the father sent the famous Argus-Slayer, the swift messenger of the gods, to take it to Epimetheus as a gift. And Epimetheus did not think of what Prometheus had told him, namely not to receive a gift from Olympian Zeus, but to send it back, lest it prove an evil for mortals. But he took the gift, and only then realized that it was evil.

For before this the tribes of men lived on earth free from evils and hard toil and grievous diseases, which bring the Fates on men: for

νούσων τ' ἀργαλέων, αἵ τ' ἀνδράσι Κῆρας ἔδωκαν.
αἶψα γὰρ ἐν κακότητι βροτοὶ καταγηράσκουσιν.
ἀλλὰ γυνὴ χείρεσσι πίθου μέγα πῶμ' ἀφελοῦσα
ἐσκέδασ'· ἀνθρώποισι δ' ἐμήσατο κήδεα λυγρά.   95
μούνη δ' αὐτόθι Ἐλπὶς ἐν ἀρρήκτοισι δόμοισιν
ἔνδον ἔμιμνε πίθου ὑπὸ χείλεσιν, οὐδὲ θύραζε
ἐξέπτη· πρόσθεν γὰρ ἐπέλλαβε πῶμα πίθοιο
αἰγιόχου βουλῇσι Διὸς νεφεληγερέταο.
ἄλλα δὲ μυρία λυγρὰ κατ' ἀνθρώπους ἀλάληται·   100
πλείη μὲν γὰρ γαῖα κακῶν, πλείη δὲ θάλασσα·
νοῦσοι δ' ἀνθρώποισιν ἐφ' ἡμέρῃ, αἳ δ' ἐπὶ νυκτὶ
αὐτόματοι φοιτῶσι κακὰ θνητοῖσι φέρουσαι
σιγῇ, ἐπεὶ φωνὴν ἐξείλετο μητίετα Ζεύς.
οὕτως οὔτι πῃ ἔστι Διὸς νόον ἐξαλέασθαι.   105

2.4 Hesiod, *Works and Days* 225–47

Οἳ δὲ δίκας ξείνοισι καὶ ἐνδήμοισι διδοῦσιν   225
ἰθείας καὶ μή τι παρεκβαίνουσι δικαίου,
τοῖσι τέθηλε πόλις, λαοὶ δ' ἀνθεῦσιν ἐν αὐτῇ·
εἰρήνη δ' ἀνὰ γῆν κουροτρόφος, οὐδέ ποτ' αὐτοῖς
ἀργαλέον πόλεμον τεκμαίρεται εὐρύοπα Ζεύς·
οὐδὲ ποτ' ἰθυδίκῃσι μετ' ἀνδράσι λιμὸς ὀπηδεῖ   230
οὐδ' ἄτη, θαλίῃς δὲ μεμηλότα ἔργα νέμονται.
τοῖσι φέρει μὲν γαῖα πολὺν βίον, οὔρεσι δὲ δρῦς
ἄκρη μέν τε φέρει βαλάνους, μέσση δὲ μελίσσας·
εἰροπόκοι δ' ὄιες μαλλοῖς καταβεβρίθασιν·
τίκτουσιν δὲ γυναῖκες ἐοικότα τέκνα γονεῦσιν·   235
θάλλουσιν δ' ἀγαθοῖσι διαμπερές· οὐδ' ἐπὶ νηῶν
νίσσονται, καρπὸν δὲ φέρει ζείδωρος ἄρουρα.
   Οἷς δ' ὕβρις τε μέμηλε κακὴ καὶ σχέτλια ἔργα,
τοῖς δὲ δίκην Κρονίδης τεκμαίρεται εὐρύοπα Ζεύς.
πολλάκι καὶ ξύμπασα πόλις κακοῦ ἀνδρὸς ἀπηύρα,   240
ὅς κεν ἀλιτραίνῃ καὶ ἀτάσθαλα μηχανάαται.
τοῖσιν δ' οὐρανόθεν μέγ' ἐπήγαγε πῆμα Κρονίων
λιμὸν ὁμοῦ καὶ λοιμόν· ἀποφθινύθουσι δὲ λαοί.
οὐδὲ γυναῖκες τίκτουσιν, μινύθουσι δὲ οἶκοι
Ζηνὸς φραδμοσύνῃσιν Ὀλυμπίου· ἄλλοτε δ' αὖτε   245
ἢ τῶν γε στρατὸν εὐρὺν ἀπώλεσεν ἢ ὅ γε τεῖχος
ἢ νέας ἐν πόντῳ Κρονίδης ἀποαίνυται αὐτῶν.

mortals grow old swiftly in misery. But the woman took off the great lid of the jar with her hands and scattered dire sorrows for men. Only Hope remained there within in an unbreakable home under the rim of the jar and did not fly out of the door. For before that the lid of the jar stopped her, by the designs of Zeus the cloud-gatherer who wields the aegis. But the other countless miseries wander among men. The earth is full of evils and the sea is full. Some diseases come upon men by day and some by night: they roam of their own free will, bringing evils to mortals, silently, for wise Zeus took away speech from them. Thus there is no way to escape the will of Zeus.

2.4 Hesiod, *Works and Days* 225–47

But they who give straight judgements to strangers and to the men of the land, and who do not go astray from what is just, their city flourishes and the people prosper in it. Peace, the nurse of children, is abroad in their land, and all-seeing Zeus never decrees cruel war against them. Neither famine nor disaster ever haunt men who do true justice, but in good cheer they tend the fields they care for. The earth bears them an abundant livelihood, and on the mountains the oaks bear acorns on their tops and bees in their midst. Their woolly sheep are laden with fleeces: their women bear children like their parents. They flourish continually with good things and do not travel on ships, for the grain-giving earth bears them fruit.

But for those who practise evil violence and wicked deeds, for them the far-seeing son of Cronos decrees a penalty. Often a whole city suffers on account of a bad man who sins and contrives evil deeds. On them the son of Cronos brings great bane, both famine and plague down from heaven. And the people waste away and their women do not bear children, and the houses decline, through the plans of Olympian Zeus. Again at another time the son of Cronos either destroys their broad army, or their walls, or demolishes their ships on the sea.

Chapter 2 Texts

2.5 Sappho, Fr. 31. 1–16

φαίνεταί μοι κῆνος ἴcoc θέοιcιν
ἔμμεν' ὤνηρ, ὄττις ἐνάντιός τοι
ἰcδάνει καὶ πλάcιον ἆδυ φωνεί-
cαc ὑπακούει   4

καὶ γελαίcαc ἰμέροεν, τό μ' ἦ μὰν
καρδίαν ἐν cτήθεcιν ἐπτόαιcεν·
ὡς γὰρ ἔc c' ἴδω βρόχε', ὤc με φώναι-
c' οὐδ' ἒν ἔτ' εἴκει,   8

ἀλλ' ἄκαν μὲν γλῶccα †ἔαγε†, λέπτον
δ' αὔτικα χρῶι πῦρ ὑπαδεδρόμηκεν,
ὀππάτεccι δ' οὐδ' ἒν ὄρημμ', ἐπιρρόμ-
βειcι δ' ἄκουαι,   12

κὰδ' δέ μ' ἴδρωc ψῦχρος ἔχει, τρόμος δὲ
παῖcαν ἄγρει, χλωροτέρα δὲ ποίας
ἔμμι, τεθνάκην δ' ὀλίγω 'πιδεύης
φαίνομαι   16

2.6 Epimenides (Diogenes Laertius 1. 110, 112)

110   Τότε καὶ Ἀθηναίοις [τότε] λοιμῷ κατεχομένοις ἔχρησεν ἡ Πυθία καθῆραι τὴν πόλιν· οἱ δὲ πέμπουσι ναῦν τε καὶ Νικίαν τὸν Νικηράτου εἰς Κρήτην, καλοῦντες τὸν Ἐπιμενίδην. καὶ ὃς ἐλθὼν Ὀλυμπιάδι τεσσαρακοστῇ ἕκτῃ ἐκάθηρεν αὐτῶν τὴν πόλιν καὶ ἔπαυσε τὸν λοιμὸν τοῦτον τὸν τρόπον. λαβὼν πρόβατα μέλανά τε καὶ λευκὰ ἤγαγε πρὸς τὸν Ἄρειον πάγον· κἀκεῖθεν εἴασεν ἰέναι οἷ βούλοιντο, προστάξας τοῖς ἀκολούθοις ἔνθα ἂν κατακλίνοι αὐτῶν ἕκαστον, θύειν τῷ προσήκοντι θεῷ· καὶ οὕτω λῆξαι τὸ κακόν. ὅθεν ἔτι καὶ νῦν ἔστιν εὑρεῖν κατὰ τοὺς δήμους τῶν Ἀθηναίων βωμοὺς ἀνωνύμους, ὑπόμνημα τῆς τότε γενομένης ἐξιλάσεως. οἱ δὲ τὴν αἰτίαν εἰπεῖν τοῦ λοιμοῦ τὸ Κυλώνειον ἄγος σημαίνειν τε τὴν ἀπαλλαγήν· καὶ διὰ τοῦτο ἀποθανεῖν δύο νεανίας, Κρατῖνον καὶ Κτησίβιον, καὶ λυθῆναι τὴν συμφοράν.

112   λέγεται δὲ καὶ πρῶτος οἰκίας καὶ ἀγροὺς καθῆραι καὶ ἱερὰ ἱδρύσασθαι. εἰσὶ δ' οἳ μὴ κοιμηθῆναι αὐτὸν λέγουσιν, ἀλλὰ χρόνον τινὰ ἐκπατῆσαι ἀσχολούμενον περὶ ῥιζοτομίαν.

2.5 Sappho, Fr. 31. 1–16

Fortunate as the gods he seems to me, that man who sits opposite you, and listens nearby to your sweet voice

And your lovely laughter; that, I vow, has set my heart within my breast a-flutter. For when I look at you a moment, then I have no longer power to speak,

But my tongue keeps silence, straightway a subtle flame has stolen beneath my flesh, with my eyes I see nothing, my ears are humming,

A cold sweat covers me, and a trembling seizes me all over, I am paler than grass, I seem to be not far short of death . . .

2.6 Epimenides (Diogenes Laertius 1. 110, 112)

Then when the Athenians were attacked by plague, the Pythian priestess commanded them to purify the city. They sent a ship commanded by Nicias the son of Niceratus to Crete, to summon Epimenides. And he came in the forty-sixth Olympiad and purified the city and stopped the plague in the following way. He took sheep, some black, some white, and brought them to the Areopagus. There he let them loose to go wherever they liked, and he told men to follow them, and wherever each one lay down, to sacrifice to the local god. And thus the evil was stopped. And so even today one may find anonymous altars in different Athenian demes, which are memorials of the atonement. But some say that he declared the cause of the plague to be the pollution that Cylon brought and showed how to remove it: and in consequence two young men, Cratinus and Ctesibis, were put to death and the city was delivered from disaster. 110

He is said to have been the first to purify houses and fields and to establish temples. Some say that he did not go to sleep but withdrew himself for a period engaged in collecting roots. 112

2.7 Empedocles, Fr. 111 (Diogenes Laertius 8. 59)

φάρμακα δ' ὅσσα γεγᾶσι κακῶν καὶ γήραος ἄλκαρ
πεύσῃ, ἐπεὶ μούνῳ σοὶ ἐγὼ κρανέω τάδε πάντα.
παύσεις δ' ἀκαμάτων ἀνέμων μένος οἵ τ' ἐπὶ γαῖαν
ὀρνύμενοι πνοιαῖσι καταφθινύθουσιν ἀρούρας·
καὶ πάλιν, ἢν ἐθέλῃσθα, παλίντιτα πνεύματ⟨α⟩ ἐπάξεις·
θήσεις δ' ἐξ ὄμβροιο κελαινοῦ καίριον αὐχμόν
ἀνθρώποις, θήσεις δὲ καὶ ἐξ αὐχμοῖο θερείου
ῥεύματα δενδρεόθρεπτα, τά τ' αἰθέρι ναιετάουσιν,
ἄξεις δ' ἐξ Ἀίδαο καταφθιμένου μένος ἀνδρός.

2.8 Empedocles, Fr. 112 (Diogenes Laertius 8. 62 (lines 1–10) and Clement, *Strom*. 6. 30 (lines 9–11))

ὦ φίλοι, οἳ μέγα ἄστυ κάτα ξανθοῦ Ἀκράγαντος
ναίετ' ἀν' ἄκρα πόλεος, ἀγαθῶν μελεδήμονες ἔργων,
χαίρετ'· ἐγὼ δ' ὑμῖν θεὸς ἄμβροτος, οὐκέτι θνητὸς
πωλεῦμαι μετὰ πᾶσι τετιμένος, ὥσπερ ἔοικα,
ταινίαις τε περίστεπτος στέφεσίν τε θαλείοις· 5
⟨πᾶσι δὲ⟩ τοῖς ἂν ἵκωμαι ἐς ἄστεα τηλεθάοντα,
ἀνδράσιν ἠδὲ γυναιξί, σεβίζομαι· οἱ δ' ἅμ' ἕπονται
μυρίοι ἐξερέοντες, ὅπῃ πρὸς κέρδος ἀταρπός,
οἱ μὲν μαντοσυνέων κεχρημένοι, οἱ δ' ἐπὶ νούσων
παντοίων ἐπύθοντο κλύειν εὐηκέα βάξιν, 10
δηρὸν δὴ χαλεπῇσι πεπαρμένοι ⟨ἀμφ' ὀδύνῃσιν⟩.

2.7 Empedocles, Fr. 111 (Diogenes Laertius 8. 59)

You shall learn all the remedies that there are for ills and defence against old age, since for you alone will I accomplish all this. And you shall stay the force of the unwearied winds which sweep over the earth and lay waste the fields with their blasts; and then, if you wish, you shall bring back breezes in requital. After black rain you shall cause drought for men in due season, and then after summer drought cause air-inhabiting tree-nourishing streams. And you shall bring from Hades the strength of a dead man.

2.8 Empedocles, Fr. 112 (Diogenes Laertius 8. 62 (lines 1–10) and Clement, *Strom.* 6. 30 (lines 9–11))

Friends, who live in the great city of the yellow Acragas, up on the heights of the citadel, caring for good deeds, I give you greetings. An immortal god, mortal no more, I go about honoured by all, as is fitting, crowned with ribbons and fresh garlands; and by all whom I come upon as I enter their prospering towns, by men and women, I am revered. They follow me in their thousands, asking where lies the road to profit, some desiring prophecies, while others ask to hear the word of healing for every kind of illness, long transfixed by harsh pains.

3
Secularization and Sacralization

One of the biggest challenges to understanding Greek medicine in the fifth century BCE is that of accounting for two remarkable concurrent developments. On the one hand there is the move made by some Hippocratic authors to insist that all diseases have natural causes, on the other there is the growth of the cults of Asclepius and other healing gods and heroes. Earlier positivist historians of medicine liked to represent the former as superseding the latter. First there was religious medicine, the type represented in the shrines of Asclepius at Epidaurus, Athens, Cos, and elsewhere. Then came naturalistic accounts of diseases and their cures. Science, in a word, on this view, overtook religion as the basis of medical practice.

That view is well wide of the mark. In fact the rise of temple medicine dates to the same period as that of those Hippocratic accounts that advocate naturalistic explanations of diseases. The great shrines we now see at Epidaurus and Pergamum are Hellenistic foundations. Yet in the case of Epidaurus at least the cult of Asclepius there goes back certainly into the classical period. But it was in the fifth century that that cult 'took off', just the period when many of the Hippocratic authors were active.

Even more importantly, it was not as if the rise of secular medicine spelt the demise of that practised in the shrines and temples. Any such idea is refuted by the continued popularity of the latter throughout Graeco-Roman antiquity, down to the second century CE, for instance, and beyond. Moreover temple medicine was popular not just with ordinary people or

Secularization and Sacralization

among the uneducated. It numbered among its enthusiastic supporters prominent members of the literate elite. We shall be discussing Sophocles' role in the acceptance of the cult at Athens in the fifth century BCE in the next chapter. We shall be coming back, in Chapter 8, to the evidence provided by Aelius Aristides. He was a famous orator of the second century CE, and as ardent and articulate an advocate of Asclepius' powers of healing as any in the ancient world. So one of our major questions is the *concurrent* rise of two sharply contrasting attitudes and approaches to disease and cure.

I shall deal first with the evidence from the Hippocratic writers and then turn in the second part of this chapter to the data we have for the practices of temple medicine. But the pluralism of Greek medicine stretches, as we shall see, well beyond those two traditions to include several others as well, from the practices of itinerant sellers of charms and incantations, to those of the root-cutters, drug-sellers, the midwives, and a variety of other women healers.

Before we turn to the principal Hippocratic text we need to consider, namely *On the Sacred Disease*, it is worth underlining the heterogeneity to be found within what we call the Hippocratic Corpus. This consists of some seventy treatises ranging in date from the late sixth to the third century BCE, with most falling in the period 450–350. None can reliably be attributed to Hippocrates himself, the famous doctor mentioned by both Plato and Aristotle,[1] whose name came to be attached to this collection when its main components came to be put together for the first time probably in Alexandria at the end of the fourth century BCE. Many treatises are, in any case, compilations, the work of several different writers. We know that to be the case with one that is no longer extant, the *Cnidian Sentences*, where our chief source (*On Regimen in Acute Diseases*) speaks not just of its authors, in the plural, but

[1] Plato, *Phaedrus* 270c and *Protagoras* 311bc, show that already in the 5th cent. Hippocrates was a famous doctor, as also does Aristotle, *Politics* 1326^{a}14ff. But none of these texts gives us any determinate information on his theory of diseases or on the treatments he favoured.

also of its revisers. Only one work, or the main part of it at least, can be ascribed to a known author, and this is the treatise *On the Nature of Man*, sections of which are assigned to Polybus, the son-in-law of Hippocrates, by both Aristotle and the author of *Anonymus Londinensis*.[2]

What is more important than the name of any author is the content of the works. The variety is very great. We have individual case histories, the clinical notes contained in the *Epidemics*, discussions of surgical interventions (mostly the treatment of fractures and dislocations), accounts of women's diseases and reproductive problems, general theories of disease or of medical method (evidently a highly disputed topic), and discussions of medical ethics and etiquette (some of those works are among the latest in the Corpus: we shall have something to say about the famous *Oath* and the *Law* in due course). Some works show little concern for literary style or polish, but others are general lectures, exhibition speeches or *epideixeis*, on such topics as the status of medicine and its claims to be an art (*On the Art*) or the constitution of the human body (*On the Nature of Man*).

The material found in one or other treatise covers problems we would think of as falling under the heads of pathology, physiology, surgery, embryology, gynaecology, pharmacology, but we have to recognize that such terms are inappropriate in two respects. First, no such disciplinary boundaries were drawn by the ancients and, second, in every case what we mean by those subject areas is something very different from ancient theories and practices. Above all we should not think of the Corpus as a homogeneous whole. Different authors represented in these works disagreed not just about the causes

---

[2] The question of the authentic works of Hippocrates continues to exercise scholars (see Lloyd 1991, ch. 9) even though conclusions on that subject have, more often than not, merely reflected their authors' preconceptions about what is best in 'Hippocratic' medicine. That is not true of the recent attempt by Smith (1979) to associate the treatise *On Regimen* with Hippocrates, though his arguments have not commanded any more general agreement among scholars than previous identifications (see Lloyd 1991, 194–7).

of diseases, but also about how to go about diagnosing and treating them—as well as on how the doctor should behave towards his patients. Thus some of the rules laid down in the *Oath*—such as not to procure abortion—are ignored elsewhere in the Corpus.

These points are relevant to our understanding of the attack on the idea that the gods intervene to cause diseases or bring about their cures in the treatise *On the Sacred Disease*. While this treatise and others such as *On Airs Waters Places* adopt a severely naturalistic approach to medicine, the tone of some works is, as we shall see, rather different.

The author of *On the Sacred Disease* states his thesis at the outset in no uncertain terms (ch. 1) [T 3.1]. 'I am about to discuss the disease called "sacred". It is not, in my opinion, any more divine or more sacred than other diseases, but has a nature and a cause. But humans have considered it a divine thing through their inexperience and their wonder at its peculiar character.' The description that we are later given of the disease in question makes it clear that the writer principally has in mind what we should call epileptic fits. Whatever we may think about the author's own theories and treatments, he certainly shows keen skills of observation in his account of the onset of the disease. He refers to what we call the 'aura' that may precede an attack, and his description of the behaviour and symptoms of those affected includes loss of voice, choking, foaming at the mouth, clenching of the teeth, convulsive movements of the hands, eyes fixed, loss of consciousness, occasional defecation (ch. 7, Littré vi. 372. 4 ff., ch. 10, Jones) [T 3.2].

Those who first called this a sacred disease are, he says, like the mages, purifiers, charlatans, and quacks who claim to be very pious and to have superior knowledge. 'Being at a loss, and having no treatment that would help, they concealed and sheltered themselves behind the divine and called this disease sacred in order that their utter ignorance might not be manifest' (ch. 1, Littré vi. 354. 15 ff., ch. 2, Jones) [T 3.1]. They prescribed purifications and incantations along with abstinence from baths and certain dietary and other rules. The patients were not to wear goat-skin or sleep on goat-skin blankets, for instance. They deployed a battery of arguments and pretexts, so that if the patient got better, their own reputation for cleverness was enhanced, while if the patient died, they could excuse themselves by explaining that the gods were to blame.

Some of the prescriptions the writer ascribes to the 'purifiers' correspond to rules of behaviour that other sources associate with the Pythagoreans. Yet there is this difference, that the Pythagoreans were laying down general norms, while the purifiers were dealing, or trying to deal, with the problems posed by particular diseases. The connection with Empedocles (often described as a Pythagorean and indeed one who shared their belief in the transmigration of souls) is, however, closer—not that we should think of him as the direct target of the Hippocratic work. Empedocles composed, as we saw, a work called *Purifications*; he said that people came to him seeking the 'word of healing' for every kind of disease, and in Fr. 111 he claimed that his knowledge would enable people to control the wind and rain and drought. *On the Sacred Disease* specifies those who assert that they understand how to 'bring down the moon, to eclipse the sun, to make storm and sunshine, rain and drought, the sea impassable and the earth barren'—claims that the author duly dismisses as nonsense (ch. 1, Littré vi. 358. 19ff., ch. 4, Jones). But if the purifiers in *On the Sacred Disease* certainly seem to make claims that tally with those Empedocles puts into his poem, it is still not the case that Empedocles himself should be seen as the target. At least there is this difference between him and the purifiers, that he expressed a supreme self-confidence that goes far beyond even the most extravagant pretensions the purifiers laid claim to. Rather the practitioners attacked in the Hippocratic treatise resemble those whom we hear of from Plato who went from door to door selling charms and incantations to whoever they could persuade to buy them (*Republic* 364bc [T 3.3], cf. *Laws* 909a–d).

Secularization and Sacralization 45

The criticisms the author makes are extraordinarily comprehensive. First he attacks his opponents' inexperience and their motives. They have no idea about the real causes of the disease. They invent excuses to conceal their ignorance and try to cover themselves whatever the outcome of their treatment. As to their basic motivation, these are 'men in need of a livelihood' (ch. 1, Littré vi. 360. 10, ch. 4, Jones) [T 3.1]: they are in it for the money that they can extract from their gullible clientele.

Secondly he shows that their treatments cannot be effective by the repeated use of arguments that take the form of a reductio ad absurdum (if A, then B: but not B: so not A). If wearing goatskins and eating goat is unhealthy, then it would follow that none of those who live in Libya could enjoy good health since they do just that. But, he implies, they are healthy enough: so the goat connection must be wrong. Actually, with a good deal of exaggeration he says that the Libyans have no clothing, no footwear, no blankets that are not made from goatskin.

Thirdly he attacks the consistency of his opponents' views. They cannot have it that their account of the origins of the disease and how to cure it is correct and still maintain that the gods are at work. 'But if to eat or use these things engenders and increases the disease, while to refrain works a cure, then neither is the god to blame nor are the purifications beneficial: it is the foods that cure and hurt, and the power of the god vanishes' (ch. 1, Littré vi. 358. 1ff., ch. 2, Jones). Again, if the stuff they 'purify' away is holy, they ought to preserve it and not abandon it on the mountains (ch. 1, Littré vi. 362. 13ff., ch. 4, Jones).

Fourthly he goes into the attack on the religious front itself. Those who attempt to cure these diseases cannot consider them sacred or divine (ch. 1, Littré vi. 358. 5ff., ch. 3, Jones). If their purifications and treatment can remove the disease, then presumably the disease could equally well be brought about by such means. In which case, the divine is not responsible, but rather something all too human. Instead of being particularly holy, they are, in reality, quite impious, for they claim to be able to *control* the gods and they are committed to the idea that a man's body is actually defiled by the god (ch. 1, Littré vi. 362. 16ff., ch. 4, Jones), that is when the god causes the disease. In the author's view the human body is itself corruptible, but god perfectly holy. What is divine is able to purify us (the author uses the term *kathairein* here too) when we enter the gods' temples: so it is quite irreligious to accuse the gods of causing defilement.

The cunning of his own position is that he does not argue that the notion of the divine is totally irrelevant. His view is not that no disease has anything to do with the divine, but rather that all are *equally* divine—evidently because nature itself is divine. At one stroke he is able to neutralize his opponents' view that there is something special about the 'sacred disease'—and their attempts to assign different varieties of the disease to different individual deities (ch. 1, Littré vi. 360. 13ff., ch. 4, Jones)—and at the same time to claim the high spiritual ground for himself. They are wrong because they introduce the notion of the intervention of personal gods in individual complaints. He has a far superior notion of the divine, manifest throughout nature, and itself the source of purity. He accuses them of claiming to be particularly pious: implicitly he does the same himself.

This battery of arguments is impressive, even though the rhetorical elements are easy to see. We have noted the exaggeration in the idea that all Libyan clothes are made of goatskin. But if he is merciless in his demolition of the purifiers' practices, we must now ask how well he himself got on, in his diagnoses, explanations, and treatments. I have already remarked on the exactness of his description of the onset of epilepsy. But as to its cause, he identifies that as the blocking of the veins in the head, claiming that this happens because of phlegm and particularly affects those of a phlegmatic disposition. This incidentally provides him with a further argument against invoking gods. His differential view that the sacred disease attacks the phlegmatic rather than the bilious allows him to argue that if its origin were divine, all types would be affected without distinction: 'if it were more divine than others, this disease ought to have attacked all equally, without making any difference between bilious and phlegmatic' (ch. 2, Littré vi. 366. 2ff., ch. 5, Jones).[3]

Yet first his own idea of the veins or blood-vessels in the body is quite schematic. It is certainly not based on anatomical dissection, even though at one point (ch. 11, Littré vi. 382. 6ff., ch. 14, Jones) he suggests one might open the head of a goat supposedly suffering from the disease and inspect its brain to verify that the cause is not a god, but the fluid with which the brain is swamped. Like almost all the other Hippocratic writers his ideas about the insides of the human body were derived from external observation and what could be inferred from such practices as venesection.[4]

Secondly his claim that the sacred disease—like every other kind—can be cured by adjustments to 'regimen' (diet and exercise) at the end of the treatise (ch. 18, Littré vi. 394. 9ff., 396. 5ff., ch. 21, Jones) [T 3.4] is just wishful thinking. The purifiers, if they had had the chance (which they now do not), might well have accused the Hippocratic writer of being in practice just as much at a loss as he said they were, both in terms of understanding the causes of epilepsy and in bringing about any alleviation, let alone cure. And they might have followed that up by pointing out that he was in medical practice for the money—in search of a livelihood—just as much as they were.

From several points of view we might say that there was little to choose between the Hippocratic author and the

[3] *On the Sacred Disease* ch. 15, Littré vi. 388. 12ff., ch. 18, Jones, further uses phlegm/bile analysis as a way of differentiating between different types of madness.

[4] The one exception is the treatise *On the Heart* but as Lonie (1973) showed, this is a product of the Hellenistic period. Aristotle was the first systematically to dissect animals, but human dissection was not undertaken until the work of Herophilus and Erasistratus (von Staden 1989). On the early history of dissection and other sources of knowledge of the insides of the body, see Lloyd 1991, ch. 8, 164ff.

purifiers he lambasts. Yet there is one chief exception to this, which takes us to the heart of the matter and is the key to the confidence of his attack. The purifiers must be wrong, he thinks, because all diseases have a nature and natural causes. If that is the case, then it is superfluous to invoke the individual interventions of gods or divinities of any kind in the account of disease. All diseases may be divine, in the sense explained, but that means none is especially so. There can be no question of invoking Apollo or Artemis or Zeus to explain why this person suffered from this or that disease, let alone why a group of people did.

A short digression is in order to underline the significance of this concept of nature. Nature, *phusis*, had been used only once in Homer of the way the magical plant *molu* grows—which Athena points out to Odysseus and he then uses as an antidote to the charms of Circe (*Od.* 10. 302 ff.). Not everything happens because of the gods in Homer, for sure: there is a clear sense of certain regularities in the phenomena, expressed especially in the similes that refer to animal behaviour or changes in the weather. However, Homer has no concept that picks out the domain of nature as such. It was that notion that constitutes the chief innovation in the kinds of accounts of phenomena such as earthquakes, or thunder and lightning, or eclipses, or the rainbow, that we find in the Presocratic philosophers—however much they disagreed about the actual—natural—causes at work.[5] The thinkers, both philosophers and medical writers, whom Aristotle came to label the 'naturalists', *phusikoi*, used that concept to mark out the domain in which they had particular expertise. Their types of account were superior, in their view, to traditional beliefs that had invoked Zeus as responsible for lightning, Poseidon for earthquakes, and so on, precisely because what

---

[5] Presocratic philosophers further differed in their views on the gods and the divine. While in Plato, *Laws* 10, those who advocated naturalistic explanations of the phenomena and in cosmology were accused of atheism, more often the naturalists took the view that nature itself is divine.

often asked by other states to supply doctors to serve as 'public physicians' (Cohn-Haft 1956, Sherwin-White 1978). It evidently helped young practitioners to have been associated with one or other teacher on Cos—not that we should think of any Coan school of medicine as an official establishment teaching a set medical curriculum. Those doctors we know to have come from Cos or to have been trained there certainly adopted widely contrasting views both on pathology and on therapeutics. They may have been the chief reason for the fame of Cos in some quarters: but in the fourth century at least no lay institution that we can identify was as firmly established as the shrine.

The origins of temple medicine go back to practices that can be traced to local shrines of healing gods and heroes for which we have evidence from many parts of Greece. They were common in Attica, for example (Kutsch 1913), and we know of an important shrine dedicated to Amphiaraus at Oropus and others to Machaon and Podalirius. But during the fifth century, as Edelstein and Edelstein especially 1945 showed (cf. Graf 1992), the cult of Asclepius acquired far more than just local significance, for it came to vie with, even in some quarters surpass, the importance of Apollo, the chief Olympian associated with healing, who was, in any case, represented as Asclepius' father. Asclepius had figured, as we saw, as a healer in the *Iliad*, where his sons are both warriors and doctors. But he was not deified until much later. Pindar tells the story of Asclepius' overstepping the mark by bringing a dead person back to life (*Pythian* 3) [T 3.10]—for which he was punished by Zeus with death. Yet that did not prevent him from being invoked as the supreme healer. The transformation may be compared with that of Heracles, incinerated on a pyre, but cast thereafter in the role of protector. Indeed Heracles was another hero to whom shrines were dedicated to which the faithful came to be healed.

Apart from the literary references that enable us to trace how the legend of Asclepius grew, we have direct evidence of the cult from the inscriptions that come from one or other of his shrines, especially but by no means solely the one at Epidaurus. We must repeat that these inscriptions mostly date from the fourth century onwards. Moreover their purpose is clear: they were set up in prominent locations in the sanctuaries to record the successes achieved, as an advertisement, in other words, for the powers of Asclepius. In these circumstances we can understand better why the success rate claimed is 100 per cent in very marked contrast to the performance that some of the Hippocratic authors recorded. Of the individual case histories contained in the first and third books of the *Epidemics*, indeed, some 60 per cent of the patients died. We shall be returning to this later.

But in the shrines it is not just diseases that are cured. People are described as being guided by the god to find lost treasure, even a lost child. The only occasions when immediate success was not forthcoming are when the patient expressed doubts about the god's power, or—worse still—refused the payment due. Hermon of Thasos is one such case (22 on Stele B) [T 3.11]. His blindness was cured by Asclepius. But since afterwards he did not bring the thank-offerings, the god made him blind again. But when he came back and slept again in the temple, the god made him well. Cephisias' story contains another warning (36) [T 3.11]. He laughed at the cures of Asclepius, saying that if he says he could cure lame people that is a lie, for if he could do so he would surely have healed Hephaestus. The god punishes him by bringing it about that he was struck by his horse and became a cripple himself. But 'later on, after he had entreated him earnestly, the god made him well'.

We can gather a little from the inscriptions themselves, and more from the later accounts in Aelius Aristides (cf. Ch. 8), about what went on in these shrines. The sick came and were encouraged to sleep in the sanctuary (this is the theme of a hilarious comic scene in Aristophanes' *Plutus*, 659–747, which focuses on stealing the food offerings placed on the altar). The patient then had a dream which contained the god's instructions for treatment: or, better still, the

Secularization and Sacralization

patient woke already cured. As for the instructions, they no doubt often needed the interpretations of the staff at the shrine.

The inscriptions contain some frankly miraculous cures. One such is the case of Aristagora of Troezen (23) [T 3.11]. She had a tapeworm in her belly and when she came and had a dream in the temple at Troezen, the god happened to be away at Epidaurus. His sons cut off her head but were unable to put it back again. So they summoned Asclepius to come. 'Meanwhile day breaks and the priest (*hiareus*) clearly sees her head cut off from the body.' But that did not stop Aristagora from going to sleep again the following night, when this time she had a vision. The god arrived back from Epidaurus and fastened the head back on to her neck. Then he cut open her belly, took the tapeworm out, and stitched her up again.

This episode shows the god exercising truly supernatural powers. The operation he undertakes on Aristagora's belly has no parallel in our Hippocratic surgical treatises, even though we know that attempts were made to excise kidney and bladder stones, for otherwise there would have been no need for the *Oath* to prohibit them. But elsewhere in the activities described in the inscriptions, the god's treatments are more mundane and indeed follow the patterns found in the Hippocratic Corpus, for example the use of herbal remedies. The god makes considerable use of emetics, for instance, just as ordinary doctors did.

Two points are striking about this shrine-based treatment. First, the god often acts very much in the way that many of the Hippocratic doctors would—only with this difference, that the god is infallible. But secondly we can detect a certain tension between the recommendations in the inscriptions and what some of the Hippocratics would have prescribed. We have seen how some of the Hippocratic writers attack the whole idea of gods being involved in diseases and their cures. But it may not be too fanciful to see the temple healers offering oblique criticisms of standard Hippocratic treatments. In one case, for instance, the inscription says that cauterization is to be avoided (48, Herzog 1931, p. 28, and cf. many cases of human prescriptions being contradicted by the god which we shall come to in Chapter 8 when dealing with Aelius Aristides).

There is more of an overlap between these divergent medical traditions than the rivalry between them might lead us to expect. This relates both to the image of the doctor's role and how the doctor behaves, and to the vocabulary used to describe medical procedures. Three examples are particularly noteworthy.

First we have seen that dreams were a key part of the practice of temple medicine: they were the way the god conveyed his advice about cure. Yet dreams were also accepted as diagnostic tools in many Hippocratic texts. Indeed the fourth book of *On Regimen* is devoted to the interpretation of the dreams of patients—only these are now understood in purely physical terms. To dream of 'springs and cisterns', for instance (ch. 90, *CMG* I 2 4, 226. 17ff.) [T 3.12] indicates 'some trouble of the bladder; it should be thoroughly purged by diuretics. A troubled sea indicates disease of the belly; it should be thoroughly purged by light, soft aperients'.

Secondly, there is common ground in the terminology used to describe what the doctor should aim to achieve. We saw that in *On the Sacred Disease* the purifiers who are attacked there claimed to bring about their kind of *katharsis*, in their case a ritual cleansing. But the Hippocratic naturalists also worked to bring about *katharsis*, though in their instance this was a matter of physical purgation, getting rid of pathogens in the body through the excreta. A woman's monthly periods were a natural *katharsis*, but if they were interrupted or irregular, they had to be stimulated by medical intervention. If the *katharsis* did not happen as it should, drugs needed to be used to bring it about.

My third example is that of prognosis. Much Greek medicine, of all types, was preoccupied with forecasting the likely outcome of a complaint. More attention was paid to prognosis than to diagnosis as such. It is possible that the detailed case

Secularization and Sacralization

histories in the *Epidemics* were recorded in part to enable doctors to anticipate the courses of the diseases they were likely to encounter. Certainly studying those cases would provide them with useful information about the correlations between signs and outcomes, especially about the all-important issue of whether the patient was going to survive or die. The Hippocratic treatise *Prognosis* reveals the author's awareness of the psychological, as well as the purely medical, functions of prognosis. 'I hold that it is an excellent thing for a physician to practise forecasting', the work begins (ch. 1, L II 110. 1 ff.) [T 3.13]. 'For if he discover and declare unaided by the side of his patients the present, the past and the future, and fill in the gaps in the account given by the sick, he will be the more believed to understand the cases, so that men will confidently entrust themselves to him for treatment.' That sets out the authority-enhancing role of prognosis. But there is also a defensive one. 'For the longer time you plan to meet each emergency the greater your power to save those who have a chance of recovery, while you will be blameless if you learn and declare beforehand those who will die and those who will get better' (112. 6 ff.).

We can see that this writer is very realistic about the need to handle the doctor–patient relationship with tact. But the extra factor that we should not miss is how, when the doctor is encouraged to pronounce on past, present, and future, his role immediately conjures up analogies with that of the prophet Calchas in the *Iliad* or that of the Muses in Hesiod's *Theogony*. Foreknowledge is a key element in the claim of a Master of Truth: but now the naturalistic doctors hope to get this, not by divine inspiration, but by staring at the patient's face (*Prognosis* ch. 2) or investigating what can be learned from his or her urine.

We began this chapter by pointing to the apparent puzzle of the concomitant development both of naturalistic medicine and of the cult of Asclepius—both of secularization and of sacralization. Our study has revealed just how complex the interrelations between the several traditions of Greek medicine were. First some of the procedures used span both Hippocratic naturalism and temple medicine. Dreams are diagnostic tools in both, prognosis is practised in both: the god prescribes foods and drugs and practises surgical interventions (in dreams) just as ordinary doctors did. But secondly there are covert or overt criticisms from within one tradition of other rival ones. The god warns against cautery. *On the Sacred Disease* attacks any idea of personal divine intervention in the causes or cures of diseases. Yet thirdly the vocabulary used to describe medical practice shows many common features. In particular *katharsis* does double service in Hippocratic naturalism and healing that invoked the divine. It is as if both those traditions expected patients to respond positively to the idea that what they needed was a 'cleansing'. Yet the kind of cleansing they received proved to be very different in the two cases, for the Hippocratics used laxatives and emetics, not charms, spells, and incantations. If the common vocabulary suggests certain assumptions widely shared by healers and patients, the divergent meanings and uses of the terms in question point to the struggle to appropriate the concepts in question and give them the interpretation favoured by one tradition against its rivals.

None of these healers, we should emphasize again in conclusion, could do much to cure complaints such as epilepsy or many other of the acute diseases for which we have graphic descriptions in the Hippocratic case histories and elsewhere. Indeed several Hippocratic writers record their failures, register their own helplessness, and even say that their own treatments were at fault.[7] Part of the reassurance that naturalistic

---

[7] In a remarkable sequence of chapters (63–7) *On Joints* especially repeatedly warns that the attempt to reduce intractable lesions does more harm than good (L IV 268. 12 ff., 274. 8 ff., 20 ff., 276. 12 ff., 278. 5 ff.). *Epidemics* 3 case 9 of the first series (L III 58. 7 ff.) and case 5 of the second (118. 8) record that treatment was ineffectual. *On Joints* ch. 47 (L IV 210. 9 ff.) goes into the author's failure to reduce humpback in some detail, so that others can learn from his mistakes, and perhaps most strikingly in *Epidemics* 5 we have a series of instances where the doctor in charge iden-

Secularization and Sacralization 59

doctors offered their patients—if indeed it can be considered reassuring—was the image they presented of themselves as entirely honest. They were not in business, as the temple healers were, to make extravagant claims for their own successes.

Religious healing, for its part, offered solace of a different kind. If you pray to the god, he will help. What you dream indicates that you are in touch with the god and you should put your trust in him—and his mortal representatives. Naturalistic medicine, for those who believed in it, insisted that you look elsewhere. At least those who accepted the arguments of *On the Sacred Disease* were relieved of the anxiety that went with the idea that diseases are a punishment for sin—your own or that of your ancestors. Maybe naturalistic medicine was ineffective in many cases. But it had some success in such areas as the setting of fractures and dislocations, and the advice to let nature effect a cure was often sensible. In other more difficult cases, even if the actual treatments used did not get results, believers could reassure themselves that the attempted explanations of diseases and the kinds of remedies applied were along the right lines.

As for religious healing, who could tell whether or not prayers were answered? If cures occurred, did that suggest they were? If not, could it not be claimed that other factors were in play, that meant that the gods were still displeased? We know from the evidence not just of the Hippocratic authors, but also of Thucydides (whom we shall be considering in Chapter 5), that faced with the plague that struck Athens at the start of the Peloponnesian War in 429 BCE, patients and their relatives and friends despaired. Ordinary doctors were quite unable to help: those who went to the temples were no better off.

The equal and concomitant development of two quite dis-

---

tifies errors in the treatments administered, including those for which he was personally responsible himself (chs. 27–30, L V 226. 10ff., 20ff., 228. 5ff., 10ff.). These texts are discussed in detail in Lloyd 1987, 124–35.

tinct, but overlapping, medical traditions, is thus, in one respect at least, more readily understandable. In the bid to secure the support of their patients, who would have good cause to be doubtful, if not suspicious, of both, the proponents of each tradition relied on the plausibility of their approach to the whole question of the nature of health and

CHAPTER 3 TEXTS

3.1 *On the Sacred Disease* chs. 1–6 (Jones), 1–3 (Littré)

I Περὶ τῆς ἱερῆς νούσου καλεομένης ὧδ' ἔχει. οὐδέν τί μοι δοκεῖ τῶν ἄλλων θειοτέρη εἶναι νούσων οὐδὲ ἱερωτέρη, ἀλλὰ φύσιν μὲν ἔχει καὶ πρόφασιν, οἱ δ' ἄνθρωποι ἐνόμισαν θεῖόν τι πρῆγμα εἶναι ὑπὸ ἀπειρίης καὶ θαυμασιότητος, ὅτι οὐδὲν ἔοικεν ἑτέροισι· καὶ κατὰ μὲν τὴν ἀπορίην αὐτοῖσι τοῦ μὴ γινώσκειν τὸ θεῖον διασῴζεται, κατὰ δὲ τὴν εὐπορίην τοῦ τρόπου τῆς ἰήσιος ᾧ ἰῶνται, ἀπόλλυται, ὅτι καθαρμοῖσί τε ἰῶνται καὶ ἐπαοιδῇσιν. εἰ δὲ διὰ τὸ θαυμάσιον θεῖον νομιεῖται, πολλὰ τὰ ἱερὰ νοσήματα ἔσται καὶ οὐχὶ ἕν, ὡς ἐγὼ ἀποδείξω ἕτερα οὐδὲν ἧσσον ἐόντα θαυμάσια οὐδὲ τερατώδεα, ἃ οὐδεὶς νομίζει ἱερὰ εἶναι. τοῦτο μὲν οἱ πυρετοὶ οἱ ἀμφημερινοὶ καὶ οἱ τριταῖοι καὶ οἱ τεταρταῖοι οὐδὲν ἧσσόν μοι δοκέουσιν ἱεροὶ εἶναι καὶ ὑπὸ θεοῦ γίνεσθαι ταύτης τῆς νούσου, ὧν οὐ θαυμασίως ἔχουσιν· τοῦτο δὲ ὁρῶ μαινομένους ἀνθρώπους καὶ παραφρονέοντας ἀπὸ οὐδεμιῆς προφάσιος ἐμφανέος, καὶ πολλά τε καὶ ἄκαιρα ποιέοντας, ἔν τε τῷ ὕπνῳ οἶδα πολλοὺς οἰμώζοντας καὶ βοῶντας, τοὺς δὲ πνιγομένους, τοὺς δὲ καὶ ἀναΐσσοντάς τε καὶ φεύγοντας ἔξω καὶ παραφρονέοντας μέχρι ἐπέγρωνται, ἔπειτα δὲ ὑγιέας ἐόντας καὶ φρονέοντας ὥσπερ καὶ πρότερον, ἐόντας τ' αὐτοὺς ὠχρούς τε καὶ ἀσθενέας, καὶ ταῦτα οὐχ ἅπαξ, ἀλλὰ πολλάκις. ἄλλα τε πολλά ἐστι καὶ παντοδαπὰ ὧν περὶ ἑκάστου λέγειν πολὺς ἂν εἴη λόγος.

II Ἐμοὶ δὲ δοκέουσιν οἱ πρῶτοι τοῦτο τὸ νόσημα ἱερώσαντες τοιοῦτοι εἶναι ἄνθρωποι οἷοι καὶ νῦν εἰσι μάγοι τε καὶ καθάρται καὶ ἀγύρται καὶ ἀλαζόνες, οὗτοι δὲ καὶ προσποιέονται σφόδρα θεοσεβέες εἶναι καὶ πλέον τι εἰδέναι. οὗτοι τοίνυν παραμπεχόμενοι καὶ προβαλλόμενοι τὸ θεῖον τῆς ἀμηχανίης τοῦ μὴ ἔχειν ὅ τι προσενέγκαντες ὠφελήσουσι, καὶ ὡς μὴ κατάδηλοι ἔωσιν οὐδὲν ἐπιστάμενοι, ἱερὸν ἐνόμισαν τοῦτο τὸ πάθος εἶναι· καὶ λόγους ἐπιλέξαντες ἐπιτηδείους τὴν ἴησιν κατεστήσαντο ἐς τὸ ἀσφαλὲς σφίσιν αὐτοῖσι, καθαρμοὺς προσφέροντες καὶ ἐπαοιδάς, λουτρῶν

disease, rather than on any obviously verifiable record of success in producing cures. But when the issue was about such approaches, the attractiveness or the lack of it of those rival traditions, to different constituents of the general public they served, were more evenly balanced than we moderns might initially suspect.

CHAPTER 3 TEXTS

3.1 *On the Sacred Disease* chs. 1–6 (Jones), 1–3 (Littré)

I I am about to discuss the disease called 'sacred'. It is not, in my opinion, any more divine than other diseases, but has a nature and a cause. But humans have considered it a divine thing through their inexperience and their wonder at its peculiar character. Now while men continue to believe in its divine origin because they are at a loss to understand it, they really disprove its divinity by the facile method of healing which they adopt, consisting as it does of purifications and incantations. But if it is to be considered divine just because it is wonderful, there will be not one sacred disease but many, for I will show that other diseases are no less wonderful and portentous, and yet nobody considers them sacred. For instance, quotidian fevers, tertians and quartans seem to me to be no less sacred and god-sent than this disease, but nobody wonders at them. Then again one can see men who are mad and delirious from no obvious cause, and committing many strange acts; while in their sleep, to my knowledge, many groan and shriek, others choke, others dart up and rush out of doors, being delirious until they wake, when they become as healthy and rational as they were before, though pale and weak; and this happens not once but many times. Many other instances, of various kinds, could be given, but time does not permit us to speak of each separately.

II My own view is that those who first attributed a sacred character to this malady were like the mages, purifiers, charlatans and quacks of our own day, men who claim great piety and superior knowledge. Being at a loss, and having no treatment which would help, they concealed and sheltered themselves behind the divine, and called this illness sacred, in order that their utter ignorance might not be manifest. They added a plausible story, and established a method of treatment that secured their own position. They

τε ἀπέχεσθαι κελεύοντες καὶ ἐδεσμάτων πολλῶν καὶ ἀνεπιτηδείων ἀνθρώποισι νοσέουσιν ἐσθίειν· θαλασσίων μὲν τρίγλης, μελανούρου, κεστρέος, ἐγχέλυος (οὗτοι γὰρ ἐπικηρότατοί εἰσιν), κρεῶν δὲ αἰγείων καὶ ἐλάφων καὶ χοιρίων καὶ κυνὸς (ταῦτα γὰρ κρεῶν ταρακτικώτατά ἐστι τῆς κοιλίης), ὀρνίθων δὲ ἀλεκτρυόνος καὶ τρυγόνος καὶ ὀτίδος, ἔτι δὲ ὅσα νομίζεται ἰσχυρότατα εἶναι, λαχάνων δὲ μίνθης, σκορόδου καὶ κρομμύων (δριμὺ γὰρ ἀσθενέοντι οὐδὲν συμφέρει), ἱμάτιον δὲ μέλαν μὴ ἔχειν (θανατῶδες γὰρ τὸ μέλαν), μηδὲ ἐν αἰγείῳ κατακεῖσθαι δέρματι μηδὲ φορεῖν, μηδὲ πόδα ἐπὶ ποδὶ ἔχειν, μηδὲ χεῖρα ἐπὶ χειρὶ (πάντα γὰρ ταῦτα κωλύματα εἶναι). ταῦτα δὲ τοῦ θείου εἵνεκα προστιθέασιν, ὡς πλέον τι εἰδότες, καὶ ἄλλας προφάσιας λέγοντες, ὅπως, εἰ μὲν ὑγιὴς γένοιτο, αὐτῶν ἡ δόξα εἴη καὶ ἡ δεξιότης, εἰ δὲ ἀποθάνοι, ἐν ἀσφαλεῖ καθισταῖντο αὐτῶν αἱ ἀπολογίαι καὶ ἔχοιεν πρόφασιν ὡς οὐδὲν αἴτιοί εἰσιν, ἀλλ' οἱ θεοί· οὔτε γὰρ φαγεῖν οὔτε πιεῖν ἔδοσαν φάρμακον οὐδέν, οὔτε λουτροῖσι καθήψησαν, ὥστε δοκεῖν αἴτιοι εἶναι. ἐγὼ δὲ δοκῶ Λιβύων ἂν τῶν τὴν μεσόγειον οἰκεόντων οὐδέν' ἂν ὑγιαίνειν, ὅτι ἐπ' αἰγείοισι δέρμασι κατακέονται καὶ κρέασιν αἰγείοισι χρέονται, ἐπεὶ οὐκ ἔχουσιν οὔτε στρῶμα οὔτε ἱμάτιον οὔτε ὑπόδημα ὅ τι μὴ αἴγειόν ἐστιν· οὐ γάρ ἐστιν αὐτοῖς ἄλλο προβάτιον οὐδὲν ἢ αἶγες καὶ βόες. εἰ δὲ ταῦτα ἐσθιόμενα καὶ προσφερόμενα τὴν νοῦσον τίκτει τε καὶ αὔξει καὶ μὴ ἐσθιόμενα ἰῆται, οὐκέτι ὁ θεὸς αἴτιος ἐστιν, οὐδὲ οἱ καθαρμοὶ ὠφελέουσιν, ἀλλὰ τὰ ἐδέσματα τὰ ἰώμενά ἐστι καὶ τὰ βλάπτοντα, τοῦ δὲ θεοῦ ἀφανίζεται ἡ δύναμις.

III Οὕτως οὖν ἔμοιγε δοκέουσιν οἵτινες τῷ τρόπῳ τούτῳ ἐγχειρέουσιν ἰῆσθαι ταῦτα τὰ νοσήματα οὔτε ἱερὰ νομίζειν εἶναι οὔτε θεῖα· ὅπου γὰρ ὑπὸ καθαρμῶν τοιούτων μετάστατα γίνεται καὶ ὑπὸ θεραπείης τοιῆσδε, τί κωλύει καὶ ὑφ' ἑτέρων τεχνημάτων ὁμοίων τούτοισιν ἐπιγίνεσθαί τε τοῖσιν ἀνθρώποισι καὶ προσπίπτειν; ὥστε τὸ θεῖον μηκέτι αἴτιον εἶναι, ἀλλά τι ἀνθρώπινον. ὅστις γὰρ οἷός τε περικαθαίρων ἐστὶ καὶ μαγεύων ἀπάγειν τοιοῦτον πάθος, οὗτος κἂν ἐπάγοι ἕτερα τεχνησάμενος, καὶ ἐν τούτῳ τῷ λόγῳ τὸ θεῖον ἀπόλλυται. τοιαῦτα λέγοντες καὶ μηχανώμενοι προσποιέονται πλέον τι εἰδέναι, καὶ ἀνθρώπους ἐξαπατῶσι προστιθέμενοι αὐτοῖς ἁγνείας τε καὶ καθάρσιας, ὅ τε πολὺς αὐτοῖς τοῦ λόγου ἐς τὸ θεῖον ἀφήκει καὶ τὸ δαιμόνιον. καίτοι ἔμοιγε οὐ περὶ εὐσεβείης τοὺς λόγους δοκέουσι ποιεῖσθαι, ὡς οἴονται, ἀλλὰ περὶ ἀσεβείης μᾶλλον, καὶ ὡς οἱ θεοὶ οὐκ εἰσί, τὸ δὲ εὐσεβὲς αὐτῶν καὶ τὸ θεῖον ἀσεβές ἐστι καὶ ἀνόσιον, ὡς ἐγὼ διδάξω.

IV Εἰ γὰρ σελήνην καθαιρεῖν καὶ ἥλιον ἀφανίζειν καὶ χειμῶνά τε καὶ

Chapter 3 Texts 63

used purifications and incantations; they forbade the use of baths, and of many foods that are unsuitable for sick folk—of sea fishes: red mullet, blacktail, hammer and the eel (these are the most harmful sorts); the flesh of goats, deer, pigs and dogs (meats that disturb most the digestive organs); the cock, pigeon and bustard, with all birds that are considered substantial foods; mint, leek and onion among the vegetables, as their pungent character is not at all suited to sick folk; the wearing of black (black is the sign of death); not to lie on or wear goat-skin, not to put foot on foot or hand on hand (all which conduct is inhibitive). These observances they impose because of the divine origin of the disease, claiming superior knowledge and alleging other causes, so that, should the patient recover, the reputation for cleverness may be theirs; but should he die, they may have a sure fund of excuses, with the defence that they are not at all to blame, but the gods. Having given nothing to eat or drink, and not having steeped their patients in baths, no blame can be laid, they say, upon them. So I suppose that no Libyan dwelling in the interior can enjoy good health, since they lie on goat-skins and eat goats' flesh, possessing neither coverlet nor cloak nor footgear that is not from the goat; in fact they possess no cattle save goats and oxen. But if to eat or use these things engenders and increases the disease, while to refrain works a cure, then neither is the god to blame nor are the purifications beneficial; it is the foods that cure or hurt, and the power of the god disappears.

III Accordingly I hold that those who attempt in this manner to cure these diseases cannot consider them either sacred or divine; for when they are removed by such purifications and by such treatment as this, there is nothing to prevent the production of attacks in men by devices that are similar. If so, something human is to blame, and not the divine. He who by purifications and magic can take away such an affection can also by similar means bring it on, so that by this argument the action of the divine is disproved. But these sayings and devices they claim superior knowledge, and deceive men by prescribing for them cleansings and purifications, most of their talk turning on the intervention of gods and spirits. Yet in my opinion their discussions show not piety, as they think, but impiety rather, implying that the gods do not exist, and what they call piety and the divine is, as I shall prove, impious and unholy.

IV For if they profess to know how to bring down the moon, to eclipse the sun, to make storm and sunshine, rain and drought, the

εὐδίην ποιεῖν καὶ ὄμβρους καὶ αὐχμοὺς καὶ θάλασσαν ἄπορον καὶ γῆν ἄφορον καὶ τἄλλα τὰ τοιουτότροπα πάντα ὑποδέχονται ἐπίστασθαι, εἴτε καὶ ἐκ τελετέων εἴτε καὶ ἐξ ἄλλης τινὸς γνώμης καὶ μελέτης φασὶ ταῦτα οἷόν τ᾽ εἶναι γενέσθαι οἱ ταῦτ᾽ ἐπιτηδεύοντες, δυσσεβεῖν ἔμοιγε δοκέουσι καὶ θεοὺς οὔτε εἶναι νομίζειν οὔτε ἰσχύειν οὐδὲν οὔτε εἴργεσθαι ἂν οὐδενὸς τῶν ἐσχάτων. ἃ ποιέοντες πῶς οὐ δεινοὶ αὐτοῖς εἰσίν; εἰ γὰρ ἄνθρωπος μαγεύων καὶ θύων σελήνην καθαιρήσει καὶ ἥλιον ἀφανιεῖ καὶ χειμῶνα καὶ εὐδίην ποιήσει, οὐκ ἂν ἔγωγέ τι θεῖον νομίσαιμι τούτων εἶναι οὐδέν, ἀλλ᾽ ἀνθρώπινον, εἰ δὴ τοῦ θείου ἡ δύναμις ὑπὸ ἀνθρώπου γνώμης κρατεῖται καὶ δεδούλωται. ἴσως δὲ οὐχ οὕτως ἔχει ταῦτα, ἀλλ᾽ ἄνθρωποι βίου δεόμενοι πολλὰ καὶ παντοῖα τεχνῶνται καὶ ποικίλλουσιν ἔς τε τἄλλα πάντα καὶ ἐς τὴν νοῦσον ταύτην, ἑκάστῳ εἴδει τοῦ πάθεος θεῷ τὴν αἰτίην προστιθέντες. καὶ ἢν μὲν γὰρ αἶγα μιμῶνται, καὶ ἢν βρύχωνται, ἢ τὰ δεξιὰ σπῶνται, μητέρα θεῶν φασὶν αἰτίην εἶναι. ἢν δὲ ὀξύτερον καὶ εὐτονώτερον φθέγγηται, ἵππῳ εἰκάζουσι, καὶ φασὶ Ποσειδῶνα αἴτιον εἶναι. ἢν δὲ καὶ τῆς κόπρου τι παρῇ, ὅσα πολλάκις γίνεται ὑπὸ τῆς νούσου βιαζομένοισιν, Ἐνοδίῃ πρόσκειται ἡ ἐπωνυμίη· ἢν δὲ πυκνότερον καὶ λεπτότερον, οἷον ὄρνιθες, Ἀπόλλων νόμιος. ἢν δὲ ἀφρὸν ἐκ τοῦ στόματος ἀφίῃ καὶ τοῖσι ποσὶ λακτίζῃ, Ἄρης τὴν αἰτίην ἔχει. οἷσι δὲ νυκτὸς δείματα παρίσταται καὶ φόβοι καὶ παράνοιαι καὶ ἀναπηδήσιες ἐκ τῆς κλίνης καὶ φεύξιες ἔξω, Ἑκάτης φασὶν εἶναι ἐπιβολὰς καὶ ἡρώων ἐφόδους. καθαρμοῖσί τε χρέονται καὶ ἐπαοιδῇσι, καὶ ἀνοσιώτατόν τε καὶ ἀθεώτατον πρῆγμα ποιέουσιν, ὡς ἔμοιγε δοκεῖ· καθαίρουσι γὰρ τοὺς ἐχομένους τῇ νούσῳ αἵματί τε καὶ ἄλλοισι τοιούτοις ὥσπερ μίασμά τι ἔχοντας, ἢ ἀλάστορας, ἢ πεφαρμακευμένους ὑπὸ ἀνθρώπων, ἤ τι ἔργον ἀνόσιον εἰργασμένους, οὓς ἐχρῆν τἀναντία τούτων ποιεῖν, θύειν τε καὶ εὔχεσθαι καὶ ἐς τὰ ἱερὰ φέροντας ἱκετεύειν τοὺς θεούς· νῦν δὲ τούτων μὲν ποιέουσιν οὐδέν, καθαίρουσι δέ. καὶ τὰ μὲν τῶν καθαρμῶν γῇ κρύπτουσι, τὰ δὲ ἐς θάλασσαν ἐμβάλλουσι, τὰ δὲ ἐς τὰ ὄρεα ἀποφέρουσιν, ὅπῃ μηδεὶς ἅψεται μηδὲ ἐμβήσεται· τὰ δ᾽ ἐχρῆν ἐς τὰ ἱερὰ φέροντας τῷ θεῷ ἀποδοῦναι, εἰ δὴ ὁ θεός ἐστιν αἴτιος· οὐ μέντοι ἔγωγε ἀξιῶ ὑπὸ θεοῦ ἀνθρώπου σῶμα μιαίνεσθαι, τὸ ἐπικηρότατον ὑπὸ τοῦ ἁγνοτάτου· ἀλλὰ καὶ ἢν τυγχάνῃ ὑπὸ ἑτέρου μεμιασμένον ἤ τι πεπονθός, ὑπὸ τοῦ θεοῦ καθαίρεσθαι ἂν αὐτὸ καὶ ἁγνίζεσθαι μᾶλλον ἢ μιαίνεσθαι. τὰ γοῦν μέγιστα τῶν ἁμαρτημάτων καὶ ἀνοσιώτατα τὸ θεῖόν ἐστι τὸ καθαῖρον καὶ ἁγνίζον καὶ ῥύμμα γινόμενον ἡμῖν, αὐτοί τε ὅρους τοῖσι θεοῖσι τῶν ἱερῶν καὶ τῶν τεμενέων ἀποδείκνυμεν, ὡς ἂν μηδεὶς ὑπερβαίνῃ ἢν μὴ ἁγνεύῃ, ἐσιόντες τε ἡμεῖς

sea impassable and the earth barren, and all such wonders, whether it be by rites or by some cunning or practice that they can, according to the adepts, be effected, in any case I am sure that they are impious, and cannot believe that the gods exist or have any strength, and that they would not refrain from the most extreme actions. Wherein surely they are terrible in the eyes of the gods. For if a man by magic and sacrifice will bring the moon down, eclipse the sun, and cause storm and sunshine, I shall not believe that any of these things is divine, but human, seeing that the power of the divine is overcome and enslaved by the cunning of man. But perhaps what they profess is not true, the fact being that men, in need of a livelihood, contrive and devise many fictions of all sorts, about this disease among other things, putting the blame, for each form of the affection, upon a particular god. If the patient imitate a goat, if he roar, or suffer convulsions in the right side, they say that the Mother of the Gods is to blame. If he utter a piercing and loud cry, they liken him to a horse and blame Poseidon. Should he pass excrement, as often happens under the stress of the disease, the surname Enodia is applied. If it be more frequent or thinner, like that of birds, it is Apollo Nomius. If he foam at the mouth and kick, Ares has the blame. When at night occur fears and terrors, delirium, jumpings from the bed and rushings out of doors, they say that Hecate is attacking or that heroes are assaulting. In making use, too, of purifications and incantations they do what I think is a very unholy and irreligious thing. For the sufferers from the disease they purify with blood and such like, as though they were polluted, blood-guilty, bewitched by men, or had committed some unholy act. All such they ought to have treated in the opposite way; they should have brought them to the sanctuaries, with sacrifices and prayers, in supplication to the gods. As it is, however, they do nothing of the kind, but merely purify them. Of the purifying objects some they hide in the earth, others they throw into the sea, others they carry away to the mountains, where nobody can touch them or tread on them. Yet, if a god is indeed the cause, they ought to have taken them to the sanctuaries and offered them to him. However, I hold that a man's body is not defiled by a god, the one being utterly corruptible, the other perfectly holy. No, even should it have been defiled or in any way injured through some different agency, a god is more likely to purify and sanctify it than he is to cause defilement. At least it is the divine that purifies, sanctifies and cleanses us from the greatest and

περιρραινόμεθα οὐχ ὡς μιαινόμενοι, ἀλλ' εἴ τι καὶ πρότερον ἔχομεν μύσος, τοῦτο ἀφαγνιούμενοι. καὶ περὶ μὲν τῶν καθαρμῶν οὕτω μοι δοκεῖ ἔχειν.

v Τὸ δὲ νόσημα τοῦτο οὐδέν τί μοι δοκεῖ θειότερον εἶναι τῶν λοιπῶν, ἀλλὰ φύσιν ἔχει ἣν καὶ τὰ ἄλλα νοσήματα, καὶ πρόφασιν ὅθεν ἕκαστα γίνεται· καὶ ἰητὸν εἶναι, καὶ οὐδὲν ἧσσον ἑτέρων, ὅ τι ἂν μὴ ἤδη ὑπὸ χρόνου πολλοῦ καταβεβιασμένον ᾖ, ὥστε ἤδη ἰσχυρότερον εἶναι τῶν φαρμάκων τῶν προσφερομένων. ἄρχεται δὲ ὥσπερ καὶ τἄλλα νοσήματα κατὰ γένος· εἰ γὰρ ἐκ φλεγματώδεος φλεγματώδης, καὶ ἐκ χολώδεος χολώδης γίνεται, καὶ ἐκ φθινώδεος φθινώδης, καὶ ἐκ σπληνώδεος σπληνώδης, τί κωλύει ὅτῳ πατὴρ ἢ μήτηρ εἴχετο νοσήματι, τούτῳ καὶ τῶν ἐκγόνων ἔχεσθαί τινα; ὡς ὁ γόνος ἔρχεται πάντοθεν τοῦ σώματος, ἀπό τε τῶν ὑγιηρῶν ὑγιηρός, καὶ ἀπὸ τῶν νοσερῶν νοσερός. ἕτερον δὲ μέγα τεκμήριον ὅτι οὐδὲν θειότερόν ἐστι τῶν λοιπῶν νοσημάτων· τοῖσι γὰρ φλεγματώδεσι φύσει γίνεται· τοῖσι δὲ χολώδεσιν οὐ προσπίπτει· καίτοι εἰ θειότερόν ἐστι τῶν ἄλλων, τοῖσιν ἅπασιν ὁμοίως ἔδει γίνεσθαι τὴν νοῦσον ταύτην, καὶ μὴ διακρίνειν μήτε χολώδεα μήτε φλεγματώδεα.

vi Ἀλλὰ γὰρ αἴτιος ὁ ἐγκέφαλος τούτου τοῦ πάθεος, ὥσπερ καὶ τῶν ἄλλων νοσημάτων τῶν μεγίστων·

3.2 *On the Sacred Disease* ch. 10 (Jones), ch. 7 (Littré)

x Ἢν δὲ τούτων μὲν τῶν ὁδῶν ἀποκλεισθῇ, ἐς δὲ τὰς φλέβας, ἃς προείρηκα, τὸν κατάρροον ποιήσηται, ἄφωνος γίνεται καὶ πνίγεται, καὶ ἀφρὸς ἐκ τοῦ στόματος ἐκρεῖ, καὶ οἱ ὀδόντες συνηρείκασι, καὶ αἱ χεῖρες συσπῶνται, καὶ τὰ ὄμματα διαστρέφονται, καὶ οὐδὲν φρονέουσιν, ἐνίοισι δὲ καὶ ὑποχωρεῖ ἡ κόπρος κάτω. ὅπως δὲ τούτων ἕκαστον πάσχει ἐγὼ φράσω· ἄφωνος μέν ἐστιν ὅταν ἐξαίφνης τὸ φλέγμα ἐπικατελθὸν ἐς τὰς φλέβας ἀποκλείσῃ τὸν ἠέρα καὶ μὴ παραδέχηται μήτε ἐς τὸν ἐγκέφαλον μήτε ἐς τὰς φλέβας τὰς κοίλας μήτε ἐς τὰς κοιλίας, ἀλλ' ἐπιλάβῃ τὴν ἀναπνοήν· ὅταν γὰρ λάβῃ ἄνθρωπος κατὰ τὸ στόμα καὶ τοὺς μυκτῆρας τὸ πνεῦμα, πρῶτον μὲν ἐς τὸν ἐγκέφαλον ἔρχεται, ἔπειτα δὲ ἐς τὴν κοιλίην τὸ πλεῖστον μέρος, τὸ δὲ ἐπὶ τὸν πλεύμονα, τὸ δὲ ἐπὶ τὰς φλέβας. ἐκ τούτων δὲ σκίδναται ἐς τὰ λοιπὰ μέρεα κατὰ τὰς φλέβας· καὶ ὅσον μὲν ἐς τὴν κοιλίην ἔρχεται, τοῦτο μὲν τὴν κοιλίην διαψύχει, καὶ ἄλλο οὐδὲν συμ-

most impious of our sins; and we ourselves fix boundaries to the sanctuaries and precincts of the gods, so that nobody may cross them unless he be pure; and when we enter we sprinkle ourselves, not as defiling ourselves thereby, but to wash away any pollution we may already have contracted. Such is my opinion about purifications.

v But this disease is in my opinion no more divine than any other; it has the same nature as other diseases, and the cause that gives rise to individual diseases. It is also curable, no less than other illnesses, unless by long lapse of time it be so ingrained as to be more powerful than the remedies that are applied. Its origin, like that of other diseases, lies in heredity. For if a phlegmatic parent has a phlegmatic child, a bilious parent a bilious child, a consumptive parent a consumptive child, and a splenetic parent a splenetic child, there is nothing to prevent some of the children suffering from this disease when one or the other of the parents suffered from it; for the seed comes from every part of the body, healthy seed from the healthy parts, diseased seed from the diseased parts. Another strong proof that this disease is no more divine than any other is that it affects the naturally phlegmatic, but does not attack the bilious. Yet, if it were more divine than others, this disease ought to have attacked all equally, without making any difference between bilious and phlegmatic.

vi The fact is that the cause of this affection, as of the more serious diseases generally, is the brain.

3.2 *On the Sacred Disease* ch. 10 (Jones), ch. 7 (Littré)

x If the phlegm be cut off from these passages but makes its descent into the veins I have mentioned above, the patient becomes speechless and chokes; froth flows from the mouth; he gnashes his teeth and twists his hands; the eyes roll and intelligence fails, and in some cases excrement is discharged. I will now explain how each symptom occurs. The sufferer is speechless when suddenly the phlegm descends into the veins and intercepts the air, not admitting it either into the brain, or into the hollow veins, or into the cavities, thus checking respiration. For when a man takes in breath by the mouth or nostrils, it first goes to the brain, then most of it goes to the belly, though some goes to the lungs and some to the veins. From these parts it disperses, by way of the veins, into the others. The portion that goes into the belly cools it, but has no further use; but the air that goes into the lungs and the veins is of use when it enters

βάλλεται· ὁ δ' ἐς τὸν πλεύμονά τε καὶ τὰς φλέβας ἀὴρ συμβάλλεται ἐς τὰς κοιλίας ἐσιὼν καὶ ἐς τὸν ἐγκέφαλον, καὶ οὕτω τὴν φρόνησιν καὶ τὴν κίνησιν τοῖσι μέλεσι παρέχει, ὥστε, ἐπειδὰν ἀποκλεισθῶσιν αἱ φλέβες τοῦ ἠέρος ὑπὸ τοῦ φλέγματος καὶ μὴ παραδέχωνται, ἄφωνον καθιστᾶσι καὶ ἄφρονα τὸν ἄνθρωπον. αἱ δὲ χεῖρες ἀκρατεῖς γίνονται καὶ σπῶνται, τοῦ αἵματος ἀτρεμίσαντος καὶ οὐ διαχεομένου ὥσπερ εἰώθει. καὶ οἱ ὀφθαλμοὶ διαστρέφονται, τῶν φλεβίων ἀποκλειομένων τοῦ ἠέρος καὶ σφυζόντων. ἀφρὸς δὲ ἐκ τοῦ στόματος προέρχεται ἐκ τοῦ πλεύμονος· ὅταν γὰρ τὸ πνεῦμα μὴ ἐσίῃ ἐς αὐτόν, ἀφρεῖ καὶ ἀναβλύει ὥσπερ ἀποθνῄσκων. ἡ δὲ κόπρος ὑπέρχεται ὑπὸ βίης πνιγομένου· πνίγεται δὲ τοῦ ἥπατος καὶ τῆς ἄνω κοιλίης πρὸς τὰς φρένας προσπεπτωκότων καὶ τοῦ στομάχου τῆς γαστρὸς ἀπειλημμένου· προσπίπτει δ' ὅταν τὸ πνεῦμα μὴ ἐσίῃ ἐς τὸ στόμα ὅσον εἰώθει. λακτίζει δὲ τοῖσι ποσὶν ὅταν ὁ ἀὴρ ἀποκλεισθῇ ἐν τοῖσι μέλεσι καὶ μὴ οἷός τε ᾖ διεκδῦναι ἔξω ὑπὸ τοῦ φλέγματος· ἀΐσσων δὲ διὰ τοῦ αἵματος ἄνω καὶ κάτω σπασμὸν ἐμποιεῖ καὶ ὀδύνην, διὸ λακτίζει. ταῦτα δὲ πάσχει πάντα, ὁπόταν τὸ φλέγμα παραρρυῇ ψυχρὸν ἐς τὸ αἷμα θερμὸν ἐόν· ἀποψύχει γὰρ καὶ ἵστησι τὸ αἷμα· καὶ ἢν μὲν πολὺ ᾖ τὸ ῥεῦμα καὶ παχύ, αὐτίκα ἀποκτείνει· κρατεῖ γὰρ τοῦ αἵματος τῷ ψύχει καὶ πήγνυσιν· ἢν δὲ ἔλασσον ᾖ, τὸ μὲν παραυτίκα κρατεῖ ἀποφράξαν τὴν ἀναπνοήν· ἔπειτα τῷ χρόνῳ ὁπόταν σκεδασθῇ κατὰ τὰς φλέβας καὶ μιγῇ τῷ αἵματι πολλῷ ἐόντι καὶ θερμῷ, ἢν κρατηθῇ οὕτως, ἐδέξαντο τὸν ἠέρα αἱ φλέβες, καὶ ἐφρόνησαν.

3.3 Plato, *The Republic*, Book 2, 364b2–c5

364b τούτων δὲ πάντων οἱ περὶ θεῶν τε λόγοι καὶ ἀρετῆς θαυμασιώτατοι λέγονται, ὡς ἄρα καὶ θεοὶ πολλοῖς μὲν ἀγαθοῖς δυστυχίας τε καὶ βίον κακὸν ἔνειμαν, τοῖς δ' ἐναντίοις ἐναντίαν μοῖραν. ἀγύρται δὲ καὶ μάντεις ἐπὶ πλουσίων θύρας ἰόντες πείθουσιν ὡς ἔστι παρὰ σφίσι δύναμις ἐκ θεῶν
c ποριζομένη θυσίαις τε καὶ ἐπῳδαῖς, εἴτε τι ἀδίκημά του γέγονεν αὐτοῦ ἢ προγόνων, ἀκεῖσθαι μεθ' ἡδονῶν τε καὶ ἑορτῶν, ἐάν τέ τινα ἐχθρὸν πημῆναι ἐθέλῃ, μετὰ σμικρῶν δαπανῶν ὁμοίως δίκαιον ἀδίκῳ βλάψει ἐπαγωγαῖς τισιν καὶ καταδέσμοις, τοὺς θεούς, ὥς φασιν, πείθοντές σφισιν ὑπηρετεῖν.

the cavities and the brain, thus causing intelligence and movement of the limbs, so that when the veins are cut off from the air by the phlegm and admit none of it, the patient is rendered speechless and senseless. The hands are paralysed and twisted when the blood is still, and is not distributed as usual. The eyes roll when the minor veins are shut off from the air and pulsate. The foaming at the mouth comes from the lungs; for when the breath fails to enter them they foam and boil as though death were near. Excrement is discharged when the patient is violently compressed, as happens when the liver and the upper bowel are forced against the diaphragm and the mouth of the stomach is intercepted; this takes place when the normal amount of breath does not enter the mouth. The patient kicks when the air is shut off in the limbs, and cannot pass through to the outside because of the phlegm; rushing upwards and downwards through the blood it causes convulsions and pain; hence the kicking. The patient suffers all these things when the phlegm flows cold into the blood which is warm; for the blood is chilled and arrested. If the flow be copious and thick, death is immediate, for it masters the blood by its coldness and congeals it. If the flow be less, at the first it is master, having cut off respiration; but in course of time, when it is dispersed throughout the veins and mixed with the copious, warm blood, if in this way it be mastered, the veins admit the air and intelligence returns.

3.3 Plato, *The Republic*, Book 2, 364b2–c5

But the strangest of all these speeches are the things they say about the gods and virtue, how so it is that the gods themselves assign to many good men misfortunes and an evil life, but to their opposites a contrary lot; and begging priests and soothsayers go to rich men's doors and make them believe that they by means of sacrifices and incantations have accumulated a treasure of power from the gods that can expiate and cure with pleasurable festivals any misdeed of a man or his ancestors, and that if a man wishes to harm an enemy, at slight cost he will be enabled to injure just and unjust alike, since they are masters of spells and enchantments that constrain the gods to serve their end.

3.4 On the Sacred Disease ch. 21 (Jones), ch. 18 (Littré)

XXI Αὕτη δὲ ἡ νοῦσος ἡ ἱερὴ καλεομένη ἀπὸ τῶν αὐτῶν προφασίων γίνεται ἀφ' ὧν καὶ αἱ λοιπαὶ ἀπὸ τῶν προσιόντων καὶ ἀπιόντων, καὶ ψύχεος καὶ ἡλίου καὶ πνευμάτων μεταβαλλομένων τε καὶ οὐδέποτε ἀτρεμιζόντων. ταῦτα δ' ἐστὶ θεῖα, ὥστε μηδὲν δεῖ ἀποκρίνοντα τὸ νόσημα θειότερον τῶν λοιπῶν νομίσαι, ἀλλὰ πάντα θεῖα καὶ πάντα ἀνθρώπινα· φύσιν δὲ ἕκαστον ἔχει καὶ δύναμιν ἐφ' ἑωυτοῦ, καὶ οὐδὲν ἄπορόν ἐστιν οὐδὲ ἀμήχανον· ἀκεστά τε τὰ πλεῖστά ἐστι τοῖς αὐτοῖσι τούτοισιν ἀφ' ὧν καὶ γίνεται.

ὅστις δὲ ἐπίσταται ἐν ἀνθρώποισι ξηρὸν καὶ ὑγρὸν ποιεῖν, καὶ ψυχρὸν καὶ θερμὸν, ὑπὸ διαίτης, οὗτος καὶ ταύτην τὴν νοῦσον ἰῷτο ἄν, εἰ τοὺς καιροὺς διαγινώσκοι τῶν συμφερόντων, ἄνευ καθαρμῶν καὶ μαγείης.

3.5 On the Diseases of Young Girls ch. 1

Πρῶτον περὶ τῆς ἱερῆς νούσου καλεομένης, καὶ περὶ τῶν ἀποπλήκτων, καὶ περὶ τῶν δειμάτων, ὁκόσα φοβεῦνται οἱ ἄνθρωποι ἰσχυρῶς, ὥστε παραφρονέειν καὶ ὁρῆν δοκέειν δαίμονάς τινας ἐφ' ἑωυτῶν δυσμενέας, ὁκότε μὲν νυκτός, ὁκότε δὲ ἡμέρης, ὁκότε δὲ ἀμφοτέρῃσι τῇσιν ὥρῃσιν· ἔπειτα ἀπὸ τῆς τοιαύτης ὄψιος πολλοὶ ἤδη ἀπηγχονίσθησαν, πλέονες δὲ γυναῖκες ἢ ἄνδρες· ἀθυμοτέρη γὰρ καὶ ὀλιγωτέρη ἡ φύσις ἡ γυναικείη. Αἱ δὲ παρθένοι, ὁκόσῃσιν ὥρη γάμου, παρανδρούμεναι, τοῦτο μᾶλλον πάσχουσιν ἅμα τῇ καθόδῳ τῶν ἐπιμηνίων, πρότερον οὐ μάλα ταῦτα κακοπαθέουσαι· ὕστερον γὰρ τὸ αἷμα ξυλλείβεται ἐς τὰς μήτρας, ὡς ἀπορρευσόμενον· ὁκόταν οὖν τὸ στόμα τῆς ἐξόδου μὴ ᾖ ἀνεστομωμένον, τὸ δὲ αἷμα πλέον ἐπιρρέῃ διά τε τὰ σιτία καὶ τὴν αὔξησιν τοῦ σώματος, τηνικαῦτα οὐκ ἔχον τὸ αἷμα ἔκρουν ἀναΐσσει ὑπὸ πλήθεος ἐς τὴν καρδίην καὶ ἐς τὴν διάφραξιν· ὁκόταν οὖν ταῦτα πληρωθέωσιν, ἐμωρώθη ἡ καρδίη· εἶτα ἐκ τῆς μωρώσιος νάρκη· εἶτ' ἐκ τῆς νάρκης παράνοια ἔλαβεν.

Ἐχόντων δὲ τουτέων ὧδε, ὑπὸ μὲν τῆς ὀξυφλεγμασίης μαίνεται, ὑπὸ δὲ τῆς σηπεδόνος φονᾷ, ὑπὸ δὲ τοῦ ζοφεροῦ φοβέεται καὶ δέδοικεν, ὑπὸ δὲ τῆς περὶ τὴν καρδίην πιέξιος ἀγχόνας κραίνουσιν, ὑπὸ δὲ τῆς κακίης τοῦ αἵματος ἀλύων καὶ ἀδημονέων ὁ θυμὸς κακὸν ἐφέλκεται· ἕτερον δὲ καὶ

3.4 On the Sacred Disease ch. 21 (Jones), ch. 18 (Littré)

This so-called 'sacred' disease is due to the same causes as all other diseases, to the things we see come and go [i.e. to and from the body], the cold and the sun too, the changing and inconstant winds. These things are divine. So that there is no need to separate this disease from the others and consider it more divine than them. Rather they are all divine and all human. Each has its own nature and power, and there is nothing in any disease that is unintelligible or insusceptible to treatment. Most are cured by the same things that caused them.

A man with the knowledge of how to produce by regimen dryness and moisture, cold and heat in the human body, could cure this disease too provided he could distinguish the right moment for the application of what is beneficial, without recourse to purifications and magic.

3.5 On the Diseases of Young Girls ch. 1

First I shall deal with the so-called 'sacred' disease, with apoplectic fits and with terrors, that humans are afraid of so much that they go mad and think they see spirits that are hostile to them, some by night, some by day, some at both times. Then as a result of visions of such a kind, many have already hanged themselves, though more women than men, because the female nature is less courageous and weaker. Young girls especially are affected by this at the onset of menstruation, when they are of an age to marry but do not go with a man, even though before they did not suffer from this severely. Yet later, the blood collects in the womb, to flow out: but when the mouth of the exit is not opened, and when the blood flows in all the more because of the nourishment and the growth of the body, when the blood has no way to flow out, it rises up from this abundance to the heart and the diaphragm. When these are filled, the heart becomes sluggish, and numbness results from this sluggishness, and then madness comes from the numbness.

In this state [the woman] becomes mad from the violent inflammation, she is murderous from the putrefaction, she fears and is terrified from the darkness, she plots hanging from the pressure around her heart; her spirit is distraught and dismayed from the bad quality of the blood, and it attracts evil to itself. On other occasions

φοβερὰ ὀνομάζει· καὶ κελεύουσιν ἅλλεσθαι καὶ καταπίπτειν ἐς τὰ φρέατα καὶ ἄγχεσθαι, ἅτε ἀμείνονά τε ἐόντα καὶ χρείην ἔχοντα παντοίην· ὁκότε δὲ ἄνευ φαντασμάτων, ἡδονή τις, ἀφ' ἧς ἐρᾷ τοῦ θανάτου ὥσπέρ τινος ἀγαθοῦ. Φρονησάσης δὲ τῆς ἀνθρώπου, τῇ Ἀρτέμιδι αἱ γυναῖκες ἄλλα τε πολλά, ἀλλὰ δὴ καὶ τὰ πουλυτελέστατα τῶν ἱματίων καθιεροῦσι τῶν γυναικείων, κελευόντων τῶν μάντεων, ἐξαπατεώμεναι. Ἡ δὲ τῆσδε ἀπαλλαγή, ὁκόταν τι μὴ ἐμποδίζῃ τοῦ αἵματος τὴν ἀπόρρυσιν. Κελεύω δ' ἔγωγε τὰς παρθένους, ὁκόταν τὸ τοιοῦτον πάσχωσιν, ὡς τάχιστα ξυνοικῆσαι ἀνδράσιν· ἢν γὰρ κυήσωσιν, ὑγιέες γίνονται· εἰ δὲ μή, ἢ αὐτίκα ἅμα τῇ ἥβῃ ἢ ὀλίγον ὕστερον ἁλώσεται, εἴπερ μὴ ἑτέρῃ νούσῳ· τῶν δὲ ἠνδρωμένων γυναικῶν αἱ στεῖραι μᾶλλον ταῦτα πάσχουσιν.

3.6 Eight Month Child chs. 6–7

6 φασὶ γὰρ τοὺς ὀγδόους τῶν μηνῶν καὶ χαλεπώτατα φέρειν τὰς γαστέρας, ὀρθῶς λέγουσαι. ἔστι δὲ οὐ μοῦνον ὁ χρόνος οὗτος, ἀλλὰ καὶ ἡμέραι πρόσεισιν ἀπό τε τοῦ ἑβδόμου μηνὸς καί ἀπὸ τοῦ ἐνάτου. ἀλλὰ τὰς ἡμέρας οὐχ ὁμοίως οὔτε λέγουσιν οὔτε γινώσκουσιν αἱ γυναῖκες. πλανῶνται γὰρ διὰ τὸ μὴ κατὰ τὸ αὐτὸ γίνεσθαι, ἀλλὰ τὸ μὲν ἀπὸ τοῦ ἑβδόμου μηνὸς πλείονας ἡμέρας προσγενέσθαι ἐς τὰς τεσσαράκοντα, τὸ δὲ ἀπὸ τοῦ ἐνάτου.

7 Χρὴ δὲ οὐκ ἀπιστεῖν τῇσι γυναιξίν ἀμφὶ τῶν τόκων. λέγουσι γάρ, ἅπερ ἂν εἰδέωσι, καὶ αἰεὶ ἐρέουσιν. οὐ γὰρ ἂν πεισθείησαν οὔτ' ἔργῳ οὔτε λόγῳ ἄλλο τι γνῶναι ἢ τὸ ἐν τοῖσι σώμασιν αὐτέων γινόμενον. τοῖσι δὲ βουλομένοισιν ἄλλο τι λέγειν ἔξεστιν, αἱ δὲ κρίνουσαι καὶ τὰ νικητήρια διδοῦσαι περὶ τούτου τοῦ λόγου αἰεὶ ἐρέουσι καὶ φήσουσι τίκτειν καὶ ἑπτάμηνα καὶ ὀκτάμηνα καὶ ἐννάμηνα καὶ δεκάμηνα καὶ ἑνδεκάμηνα, καὶ τούτων τὰ ὀκτάμηνα οὐ περιγίνεσθαι, τὰ δ' ἄλλα περιγίνεσθαι.

3.7 On the Diseases of Women I ch. 62

καὶ ἔστιν ὅτε τῇσι μὴ γινωσκούσῃσιν ὑφ' ὅτευ νοσεῦσι φθάνει τὰ νοσήματα ἀνίητα γινόμενα, πρὶν ἂν διδαχθῆναι τὸν ἰητρὸν ὀρθῶς ὑπὸ τῆς νοσεούσης ὑφ' ὅτου νοσέει· καὶ γὰρ αἰδέονται φράζειν, κἢν εἰδῶσι, καί σφιν δοκέουσιν αἰσχρὸν εἶναι ὑπὸ ἀπειρίης καὶ ἀνεπιστημοσύνης. Ἅμα δὲ καὶ οἱ ἰητροὶ ἁμαρτάνουσιν, οὐκ ἀτρεκέως πυνθανόμενοι τὴν πρόφασιν τῆς νούσου, ἀλλ'

she utters fearful things. [The visions] command them to leap about, to fall into wells, to hang themselves, as though that were better and of any use at all. When there are no phantasms, there is a certain pleasure, from which the woman loves death as though it were some good. When the patient returns to her senses, women dedicate many other offerings to Artemis, and especially the most expensive women's robes: they do this on the orders of priests, though they are deceived. The recovery from this complaint comes when there is no blockage to the outflow of blood. For my part I order the young women, whenever they suffer from this, to have intercourse with a man as soon as possible. If they conceive, they become healthy. But if not, she will be seized by this disease either just when she reaches puberty or a little later, unless she is affected by some other disease. Among married women, the childless ones suffer from this more.

3.6 *Eight Month Child* chs. 6–7

The women who say they suffer most during the eighth month of pregnancy speak correctly, but the time involved is not only this one, but days also enter from the seventh month and from the ninth. Yet women do not speak of the days in the same manner, nor do they understand them. They are mistaken because it does not always happen in the same way: sometimes more days are added from the seventh month, sometimes from the ninth, to arrive at the forty days.

One must not doubt what women say about childbirth, for they say what they know and they will always say so. They could not be persuaded either by fact or by logical argument to know otherwise than what goes on in their own bodies. Some may wish to argue otherwise, but women who decide the contest and give the victory prize concerning this argument say and always will say that they bear seven and eight and nine and ten and eleven months' children, and that of these the eight months' children do not survive, but the others do.

3.7 *On the Diseases of Women* I ch. 62

Sometimes when the women do not recognize why they are sick, the diseases become incurable, before the doctor has been correctly instructed by the sick woman why she is sick. For they are ashamed to speak, even if they know, and they think that some shame has come on them, out of their inexperience and lack of understanding.

ὡς τὰ ἀνδρικὰ νοσήματα ἰώμενοι· καὶ πολλὰς εἶδον διεφθαρμένας ἤδη ὑπὸ τοιούτων παθημάτων. Ἀλλὰ χρὴ ἀνερωτᾶν αὐτίκα ἀτρεκέως τὸ αἴτιον· διαφέρει γὰρ ἡ ἴησις πολλῷ τῶν γυναικηΐων νοσημάτων καὶ τῶν ἀνδρώων.

3.8 Oath

Ὄμνυμι Ἀπόλλωνα ἰητρὸν καὶ Ἀσκληπιὸν καὶ Ὑγείαν καὶ Πανάκειαν καὶ θεοὺς πάντας τε καὶ πάσας, ἵστορας ποιεύμενος, ἐπιτελέα ποιήσειν κατὰ δύναμιν καὶ κρίσιν ἐμὴν ὅρκον τόνδε καὶ συγγραφὴν τήνδε· ἡγήσεσθαι μὲν τὸν διδάξαντά με τὴν τέχνην ταύτην ἴσα γενέτῃσιν ἐμοῖς, καὶ βίου κοινώσεσθαι, καὶ χρεῶν χρηΐζοντι μετάδοσιν ποιήσεσθαι, καὶ γένος τὸ ἐξ αὐτοῦ ἀδελφοῖς ἴσον ἐπικρινεῖν ἄρρεσι, καὶ διδάξειν τὴν τέχνην ταύτην, ἢν χρηΐζωσι μανθάνειν, ἄνευ μισθοῦ καὶ συγγραφῆς, παραγγελίης τε καὶ ἀκροήσιος καὶ τῆς λοίπης ἁπάσης μαθήσιος μετάδοσιν ποιήσεσθαι υἱοῖς τε ἐμοῖς καὶ τοῖς τοῦ ἐμὲ διδάξαντος, καὶ μαθητῇσι συγγεγραμμένοις τε καὶ ὡρκισμένοις νόμῳ ἰητρικῷ, ἄλλῳ δὲ οὐδενί. διαιτήμασί τε χρήσομαι ἐπ᾽ ὠφελείῃ καμνόντων κατὰ δύναμιν καὶ κρίσιν ἐμήν, ἐπὶ δηλήσει δὲ καὶ ἀδικίῃ εἴρξειν. οὐ δώσω δὲ οὐδὲ φάρμακον οὐδενὶ αἰτηθεὶς θανάσιμον, οὐδὲ ὑφηγήσομαι συμβουλίην τοιήνδε· ὁμοίως δὲ οὐδὲ γυναικὶ πεσσὸν φθόριον δώσω. ἁγνῶς δὲ καὶ ὁσίως διατηρήσω βίον τὸν ἐμὸν καὶ τέχνην τὴν ἐμήν. οὐ τεμέω δὲ οὐδὲ μὴν λιθιῶντας, ἐκχωρήσω δὲ ἐργάτῃσιν ἀνδράσι πρήξιος τῆσδε. ἐς οἰκίας δὲ ὁκόσας ἂν ἐσίω, ἐσελεύσομαι ἐπ᾽ ὠφελείῃ καμνόντων, ἐκτὸς ἐὼν πάσης ἀδικίης ἑκουσίης καὶ φθορίης, τῆς τε ἄλλης καὶ ἀφροδισίων ἔργων ἐπί τε γυναικείων σωμάτων καὶ ἀνδρώων, ἐλευθέρων τε καὶ δούλων. ἃ δ᾽ ἂν ἐν θεραπείῃ ἢ ἴδω ἢ ἀκούσω, ἢ καὶ ἄνευ θεραπείης κατὰ βίον ἀνθρώπων, ἃ μὴ χρή ποτε ἐκλαλεῖσθαι ἔξω, σιγήσομαι, ἄρρητα ἡγεύμενος εἶναι τὰ τοιαῦτα. ὅρκον μὲν οὖν μοι τόνδε ἐπιτελέα ποιέοντι, καὶ μὴ συγχέοντι, εἴη ἐπαύρασθαι καὶ βίου καὶ τέχνης δοξαζομένῳ παρὰ πᾶσιν ἀνθρώποις ἐς τὸν αἰεὶ χρόνον· παραβαίνοντι δὲ καὶ ἐπιορκέοντι, τἀναντία τούτων.

3.9 Law ch. 5

v Τὰ δὲ ἱερὰ ἐόντα πρήγματα ἱεροῖσιν ἀνθρώποισι δείκνυται· βεβήλοισι δὲ οὐ θέμις, πρὶν ἢ τελεσθῶσιν ὀργίοισιν ἐπιστήμης.

At the same time the doctors too make mistakes, by not ascertaining accurately the cause of the disease, but by proceeding to treatment as though they were dealing with men's diseases. I have seen many women perish already from such sufferings as these. But one must at the outset accurately inquire into the cause. For the cure of the diseases of women differs greatly from that of those of men.

3.8 Oath

I swear by Apollo Physician, by Asclepius, by Health, by Panacea and by all the gods and goddesses, making them my witnesses, that I will carry out, according to my ability and judgment, this oath and this indenture. To hold my teacher in this art equal to my own parents; to make him partner in my livelihood; when he is in need of money to share mine with him; to consider his family as my own brothers, and to teach them this art, if they want to learn it, without fee or indenture; to impart precept, oral instruction, and all other instruction to my own sons, the sons of my teacher, and to indentured pupils who have taken the physician's oath, but to nobody else. I will use treatment to help the sick according to my ability and judgment, but never with a view to injury and wrong-doing. Neither will I administer a poison to anybody when asked to do so, nor will I suggest such a course. Similarly I will not give to a woman a pessary to cause abortion. But I will keep pure and holy both my life and my art. I will not use the knife, not even, verily, on sufferers from stone, but I will give place to such as are craftsmen therein. Into whatsoever houses I enter, I will enter to help the sick, and I will abstain from all intentional wrong-doing and harm, especially from abusing the bodies of man or woman, bond or free. And whatsoever I shall see or hear in the course of my profession, as well as outside my profession in my intercourse with men, if it be what should not be published abroad, I will never divulge, holding such things to be holy secrets. Now if I carry out this oath, and break it not, may I gain for ever reputation among all men for my life and for my art; but if I transgress it and forswear myself, may the opposite befall me.

3.9 *Law* ch. 5

v Things however that are holy are revealed only to men who are holy. The profane may not learn them until they have been initiated into the mysteries of science.

3.10 Pindar, *Pythian* 3. 45–58

καί ῥά νιν Μάγνητι φέρων πόρε Κενταύρῳ διδάξαι
πολυπήμονας ἀνθρώποισιν ἰᾶσθαι νόσους.

τοὺς μὲν ὦν, ὅσσοι μόλον αὐτοφύτων
ἑλκέων ξυνάονες, ἢ πολιῷ χαλχῷ μέλη τετρωμένοι
ἢ χερμάδι τηλεβόλῳ,
ἢ θερινῷ πυρὶ περθόμενοι δέμας ἢ
χειμῶνι, λύσαις ἄλλον ἀλλοίων ἀχέων
ἔξαγεν, τοὺς μὲν μαλακαῖς ἐπαοιδαῖς ἀμφέπων,
τοὺς δὲ προσανέα πί-
νοντας, ἢ γυίοις περάπτων πάντοθεν
φάρμακα, τοὺς δὲ τομαῖς ἔστασεν ὀρθούς.

ἀλλὰ κέρδει καὶ σοφία δέδεται.
ἔτραπεν καὶ κεῖνον ἀγάνορι μισθῷ
χρυσὸς ἐν χερσὶν φανείς
ἄνδρ᾽ ἐκ θανάτου κομίσαι
ἤδη ἀλωκότα· χερσὶ δ᾽ ἄρα Κρονίων
ῥίψαις δι᾽ ἀμφοῖν ἀμπνοὰν στέρνων κάθελεν
ὠκέως, αἴθων δὲ κεραυνὸς ἐνέσκιμψεν μόρον.

3.11 Epidaurus Inscriptions, Stele B, 22, 23, 36

XXII | Ἕρμων Θ[άσιος. τοῦτο]ν τυφλὸν ἐόντα ἰάσατο· μετὰ δὲ τοῦτο τὰ ἴατρα οὐκ ἀ|πάγοντ[α ὁ θεός νιν] ἐπόησε τυφλὸν αὖθις· ἀφικόμενον δ᾽ αὐτον καὶ πάλιν | ἐγκαθε[ύδοντα ὑγι]ῆ κατέστασε. XXIII || Ἀριστα[γόρα Τροζ]ανία. αὕτα ἕλμιθα ἔχουσα ἐν τᾶι κοιλίαι ἐνεκάθευδε | ἐν Τροζ[ᾶνι ἐν τῶι] τοῦ Ἀσκλαπιοῦ τεμένει καὶ ἐνύπνιον εἶδε· ἐδόκει οὑ | τοὺς υἱ[οὺς τοῦ θ]εοῦ, οὐκ ἐπιδαμοῦντος αὐτοῦ, ἀλλ᾽ ἐν Ἐπιδαύρωι ἐόντος, | τὰγ κεφα[λὰν ἀπο]ταμεῖν, οὐ δυναμένους δ᾽ ἐπιθέμεν πάλιν πέμψαι τινὰ πο[ὶ] | τὸν Ἀσκλ[απιόν, ὅ]πως μόληι· μεταξὺ δὲ ἁμέρα ἐπικαταλαμβάνει καὶ ὁ ἰαρ||ρεὺς ὁρῆι [σάφα τ]ὰν κεφαλὰν ἀφαιρημέναν ἀπὸ τοῦ σώματος· τᾶς ἐφερπού|σας δὲ νυκτ[ὸς Ἀρ]ισταγόρα ὄψιν εἶδε· ἐδόκει οἱ ὁ θεὸς ἵκων ἐξ Ἐπιδαύρου | ἐπιθεὶς τ[ὰν κε]φαλὰν ἐπὶ [τὸ]ν τράχαλον, μετὰ ταῦτα ἀνσχίσσας τὰγ κοιλ[ί|α]ν τὰν αὐτ[ᾶς ἐξ]ελεῖν τὰν ἕ[λμ]ιθα καὶ συρράψαι πάλιν, καὶ ἐκ τούτου ὑγ[ι|ὴ]s ἐγένετ[ο.

3.10 Pindar, *Pythian* 3. 45–58

He took him and gave him to the Magnesian Centaur
for instruction in healing the diseases that plague men.

Now all who came to him afflicted with natural sores
or with limbs wounded by gray bronze
or by a far-flung stone,
or with bodies wracked by summer fever
    or winter chill, he relieved of their various ills and

restored them; some he tended with calming incantations
while others drank soothing potions,
    or he applied remedies to all parts
of their bodies; still others he raised up with surgery.

But even wisdom is enthralled to gain.
Gold appearing in his hands
    with its lordly wage
prompted even him to bring back from death a man
already carried off. But then, with a cast from his hands,
    Kronos' son took the breath from both men's breasts
in an instant; the flash of lightning hurled down doom.

3.11 Epidaurus Inscriptions, Stele B, 22, 23, 36

22. Hermon of Thasus. His blindness was cured by Asclepius. But, since afterwards he did not bring the thank-offerings, the god made him blind again. When he came back and slept again in the Temple, he [*sc.*, the god] made him well.

23. Aristagora of Troezen. She had a tapeworm in her belly, and she slept in the Temple of Asclepius at Troezen and saw a dream. It seemed to her that the sons of the god, while he was not present but away in Epidaurus, cut off her head, but, being unable to put it back again, they sent a messenger to Asclepius asking him to come. Meanwhile day breaks and the priest clearly sees her head cut off from the body. When night approached, Aristagora saw a vision. It seemed to her the god had come from Epidaurus and fastened her head on to her neck. Then he cut open her belly, took the tapeworm out, and stitched her up again. And after that she became well.

XXXVI Καφισί[ας – – – τὸμ πόδα. οὗτος τοῖς τοῦ Ἀσ] | κλαπιοῦ θεραπεύμασιν ἐπ[ιγελῶν "χωλούς," ἔφα, "ἰάσασθαι ὁ θεὸς ψεύ] | δεται λέγων· ὡς, εἰ δύναμιν ε[ῖχε, τί οὐ τὸν Ἄφαιστον ἰάσατο"; ὁ δὲ θεὸς] | τᾶς ὕβριος ποινὰς λαμβάνω[ν οὐκ ἔλαθε· ἱππεύων γὰρ ὁ Καφισίας ὑπὸ] | τοῦ βουκεφάλα ἐν τᾶι ἕδραι [γαργαλισθέντος ἐπλάγη ὥστε πηρωθῆ] ||μεν τὸμ πόδα παραχρῆμα καὶ [φοράδαν εἰς τὸ ἱαρὸν ἀγκομισθῆμεν.] | ὕ[σ]τερον δὲ πολλὰ καθικετεύ[σαντα αὐτὸν ὁ θεὸς ὑγιῆ ἐπόησε.]

3.12 *Regimen* IV. ch. 90

XC Προσημαίνει δὲ καὶ τάδε ἐς ὑγείην· τῶν ἐπὶ γῆς ὀξὺ ὁρῆν καὶ ὀξὺ ἀκούειν, ὁδοιπορεῖν τε ἀσφαλῶς καὶ τρέχειν ἀσφαλῶς καὶ ταχὺ ἄτερ φόβου, καὶ τὴν γῆν ὁρῆν λείην καὶ καλῶς εἰργασμένην, καὶ τὰ δένδρεα θαλέοντα καὶ πολύκαρπα καὶ ἥμερα, καὶ ποταμοὺς ῥέοντας κατὰ τρόπον καὶ ὕδατι καθαρῷ μήτε πλέονι μήτε ἐλάσσονι τοῦ προσήκοντος, καὶ τὰς κρήνας καὶ τὰ φρέατα ὡσαύτως. ταῦτα πάντα σημαίνει ὑγείην τῷ ἀνθρώπῳ, καὶ τὸ σῶμα κατὰ τρόπον πάσας τε τὰς περιόδους καὶ τὰς προσαγωγὰς καὶ τὰς ἀποκρίσεις εἶναι. εἰ δέ τι τούτων ὑπεναντίον ὁρῷτο, βλάβος σημαίνει τι ἐν τῷ σώματι· ὄψιος μὲν καὶ ἀκοῆς βλαπτομένων, περὶ τὴν κεφαλὴν νοῦσον σημαίνει· τοῖσιν οὖν ὀρθρίοισι περιπάτοισι καὶ τοῖσιν ἀπὸ δείπνου πλείοσι χρηστέον πρὸς τῇ προτέρῃ διαίτῃ. τῶν σκελέων δὲ βλαπτομένων, ἐμέτοισιν ἀντισπαστέον, καὶ τῇ παλῃ πλείονι χρηστέον πρὸς τῇ προτέρῃ διαίτῃ. γῆ δὲ τραχείη οὐ καθαρὴν τὴν σάρκα σημαίνει· τοῖσιν οὖν ἀπὸ τῶν γυμνασίων περιπάτοισι πλείοσι χρηστέον. δένδρων ἀκαρπία σπέρματος τοῦ ἀνθρωπίνου διαφθορὴν δηλοῖ· ἢν μὲν οὖν φυλλορροοῦντα ἢ τὰ δένδρα, ὑπὸ τῶν ὑγρῶν καὶ ψυχρῶν βλάπτεται· ἢν δὲ τεθήλῃ μέν, ἄκαρπα δὲ ᾖ, ὑπὸ τῶν θερμῶν καὶ ξηρῶν· τὰ μὲν οὖν θερμαίνειν καὶ ξηραίνειν τοῖσι διαιτήμασι χρή, τὰ δὲ ψύχειν τε καὶ ὑγραίνειν. ποταμοὶ δὲ κατὰ τρόπον μὴ γινόμενοι αἵματος περίοδον σημαίνουσι, πλέον μὲν ῥέοντες ὑπερβολήν, ἔλασσον δὲ ῥέοντες ἔλλειψιν· δεῖ δὲ τῇ διαίτῃ τὸ μὲν αὐξῆσαι, τὸ δὲ μειῶσαι. μὴ καθαρῷ δὲ ῥέοντες ταραχὴν σημαίνουσι· καθαίρεται δὲ ὑπὸ τῶν τρόχων καὶ τῶν περιπάτων πνεύματι πυκνῷ διακινεόμενα. κρῆναι καὶ φρέατα περὶ τὴν κύστιν τι σημαίνει· ἀλλὰ χρὴ τοῖσιν οὐρητικοῖσιν ἐκκαθαίρειν. θάλασσα δὲ ταρασσομένη κοιλίης νοῦσον σημαίνει· ἀλλὰ χρὴ τοῖσι διαχωρητικοῖσι καὶ κούφοισι καὶ μαλακοῖσιν ἐκκαθαίρειν. γῆ κινευμένη ἢ οἰκίη ὑγιαίνοντι μὲν ἀσθενείην

36. Cephisias ... with the foot. He laughed at the cures of Asclepius and said: 'If the god says he has healed lame people he is lying; for, if he had the power to do so, why has he not healed Hephaestus?' But the god did not conceal that he was inflicting penalty for the insolence. For Cephisias, when riding, was stricken by his bull-headed horse which had been tickled in the seat, so that instantly his foot was crippled and on a stretcher he was carried into the Temple. Later on, after he had entreated him earnestly, the god made him well.

3.12 *Regimen* IV. ch. 90

XC The following too are signs that foretell health. To see and hear clearly the things on the earth, to walk surely, to run surely, quickly and without fear, to see the earth level and well tilled, trees that are luxuriant, covered with fruit and cultivated, rivers flowing naturally, with water that is pure, and neither higher nor lower than it should be, and springs and wells that are similar. All these indicate health for the dreamer, and that the body with all its circuits, diet and secretions are proper and normal. But if anything be seen that is the reverse of these things, it indicates some harm in the body. If sight or hearing be impaired, it indicates disease in the region of the head. In addition to the preceding regimen the dreamer should take longer walks in the early morning and after dinner. If it be the legs that are injured, the revulsion should be made with emetics, and in addition to the preceding regimen there should be more wrestling. For the earth to be rough indicates that the flesh is impure. So the walks after exercises must be made longer. Fruitless trees signify corruption of the human seed. Now if the trees are shedding their leaves, the harm is caused by moist, cold influences; if leaves abound without any fruit, by hot, dry influences. In the former case regimen must be directed towards warming and drying; in the latter towards cooling and moistening. When rivers are abnormal they indicate a circulation of the blood; high water excess of blood, low water defect of blood. Regimen should be made to increase the latter and lessen the former. Impure streams indicate disturbance of the bowels. The impurities are removed by running on the round track and by walks, which stir them up by accelerated respiration. Springs and cisterns indicate some trouble of the bladder; it should be thoroughly purged by diuretics. A troubled sea indicates disease

σημαίνει, νοσέοντι δὲ ὑγείην καὶ μετακίνησιν τοῦ ὑπάρχοντος. τῷ μὲν οὖν ὑγιαίνοντι μεταστῆσαι τὴν δίαιταν συμφέρει· ἐμεσάτω δὲ πρῶτον, ἵνα προσδέξηται αὖτις κατὰ μικρόν· ἀπὸ γὰρ τῆς ὑπαρχούσης κινεῖται πᾶν τὸ σῶμα. τῷ δὲ ἀσθενέοντι συμφέρει χρῆσθαι τῇ αὐτῇ διαίτῃ· μεθίσταται γὰρ ἤδη τὸ σῶμα ἐκ τοῦ παρεόντος. κατακλυζομένην γῆν ἀπὸ ὕδατος ἢ θαλάσσης ὁρῆν νοῦσον σημαίνει, ὑγρασίης πολλῆς ἐνεούσης ἐν τῷ σώματι· ἀλλὰ χρὴ τοῖσιν ἐμέτοισι καὶ τῇσιν ἀναριστίῃσι καὶ τοῖσι πόνοισι καὶ τοῖσι διαιτήμασι ξηροῖσι· ἔπειτα προσάγειν ἐξ ὀλίγων καὶ ὀλίγοισιν. οὐδὲ μέλαιναν ὁρῆν τὴν γῆν οὐδὲ κατακεκαυμένην ἀγαθόν, ἀλλὰ κίνδυνος ἰσχυροῦ νοσήματος ἀντιτυχεῖν καὶ θανασίμου· ξηρασίης γὰρ ὑπερβολὴν σημαίνει ἐν τῇ σαρκί· ἀλλὰ χρὴ τούς τε πόνους ἀφελεῖν, τοῦ τε σίτου ὅσα τε ξηρὰ καὶ δριμέα καὶ οὐρητικά· διαιτῆσθαί τε τῆς τε πτισάνης καθέφθῳ τῷ χυλῷ, καὶ σίτοισι κούφοισιν ὀλίγοισι, ποτῷ δὲ πλέονι ὑδαρεῖ λευκῷ, λουτροῖσι πολλοῖσι· μὴ ἄσιτος λουέσθω, μαλακευνείτω, ῥαθυμείτω, ψῦχος καὶ ἥλιον φυλασσέσθω· εὔχεσθαι δὲ Γῇ καὶ Ἑρμῇ καὶ ἥρωσιν. εἰ δὲ κολυμβῆν ἐν λίμνῃ ἢ ἐν θαλάσσῃ ἢ ἐν ποταμοῖσι δοκεῖ, οὐκ ἀγαθόν· ὑπερβολὴν γὰρ ὑγρασίης σημαίνει· συμφέρει δὲ καὶ τούτῳ ξηραίνειν τῇ διαίτῃ, τοῖσί τε πόνοισι πλείοσι· πυρέσσοντι δὲ ἀγαθόν· σβέννυται γὰρ τὸ θερμὸν ὑπὸ τῶν ὑγρῶν.

3.13 Prognosis ch. 1

1 τὸν ἰητρὸν δοκεῖ μοι ἄριστον εἶναι πρόνοιαν ἐπιτηδεύειν· προγινώσκων γὰρ καὶ προλέγων παρὰ τοῖσι νοσέουσι τά τε παρεόντα καὶ τὰ προγεγονότα καὶ τὰ μέλλοντα ἔσεσθαι, ὁκόσα τε παραλείπουσιν οἱ ἀσθενέοντες ἐκδιηγεύμενος πιστεύοιτο ἂν μᾶλλον γινώσκειν τὰ τῶν νοσεύντων πρήγματα, ὥστε τολμᾶν ἐπιτρέπειν τοὺς ἀνθρώπους σφᾶς αὐτοὺς τῷ ἰητρῷ. τὴν δὲ θεραπείην ἄριστα ἂν ποιέοιτο προειδὼς τὰ ἐσόμενα ἐκ τῶν παρεόντων παθημάτων. ὑγιέας μὲν γὰρ ποιεῖν ἅπαντας τοὺς νοσέοντας ἀδύνατον· τοῦτο γὰρ καὶ τοῦ προγινώσκειν τὰ μέλλοντα ἀποβήσεσθαι κρέσσον ἂν ἦν· ἐπειδὴ δὲ οἱ ἄνθρωποι ἀποθνήσκουσιν, οἱ μὲν πρὶν ἢ καλέσαι τὸν ἰητρὸν ὑπὸ τῆς ἰσχύος τῆς νούσου, οἱ δὲ καὶ ἐσκαλεσάμενοι παραχρῆμα ἐτελεύτησαν, οἱ μὲν ἡμέρην μίαν ζήσαντες, οἱ δὲ ὀλίγῳ

of the belly; it should be thoroughly purged by light, soft aperients. Trembling of the earth or of a house indicates illness when the dreamer is in health, and a change from disease to health when he is sick. So it is beneficial to change the regimen of a healthy dreamer. Let him first take an emetic, that he may resume nourishment again little by little, for it is the present nourishment that is troubling all the body. A sick dreamer benefits by continuing the same regimen, for the body is already changing from its present condition. To see the earth flooded by water or sea signifies a disease, as there is much moisture in the body. What is necessary is to take emetics, to avoid luncheon, to exercise and to adopt a dry diet. Then there should be a gradual increase of food, little by little, and little to begin with. It is not good either to see the earth black or scorched, but there is a danger of catching a violent, or even a fatal disease, for it indicates excess of dryness in the flesh. What is necessary is to give up exercises and such food as is dry and acrid and diuretic. Regimen should consist of barley-water well boiled, light and scanty meals, copious white wine well diluted, and numerous baths. No bath should be taken on an empty stomach, the bed should be soft and rest abundant. Chill and the sun should be avoided. Pray to Earth, Hermes and the Heroes. If the dreamer thinks that he is diving in a lake, in the sea, or in a river, it is not a good sign, for it indicates excess of moisture. In this case also benefit comes from a drying regimen and increased exercises. But for a fever patient these dreams are a good sign, for the heat is being suppressed by the moisture.

3.13 *Prognosis* ch. 1

1 I hold that it is an excellent thing for a physician to practise forecasting. For if he discover and declare unaided by the side of his patients the present, the past and the future, and fill in the gaps in the account given by the sick, he will be the more believed to understand the cases, so that men will confidently entrust themselves to him for treatment. Furthermore, he will carry out the treatment best if he know beforehand from the present symptoms what will take place later. Now to restore every patient to health is impossible. To so do indeed would have been better even than forecasting the future. But as a matter of fact men do die, some owing to the severity of the disease before they summon the physician, others expiring immediately after calling him in—living one day or a little longer—

πλείονα χρόνον, πρὶν ἢ τὸν ἰητρὸν τῇ τέχνῃ πρὸς ἕκαστον νόσημα ἀνταγωνίσασθαι. γνῶναι οὖν χρὴ τῶν τοιούτων νοσημάτων τὰς φύσιας, ὁκόσον ὑπὲρ τὴν δύναμίν εἰσιν τῶν σωμάτων καὶ τούτων τὴν πρόνοιαν ἐκμανθάνειν. οὕτω γὰρ ἄν τις θαυμάζοιτο δικαίως καὶ ἰητρὸς ἀγαθὸς ἂν εἴη· καὶ γὰρ οὓς οἷόν τε περιγίνεσθαι ἔτι μᾶλλον ἂν δύναιτο διαφυλάσσειν ἐκ πλείονος χρόνου προβουλευόμενος πρὸς ἕκαστα, καὶ τοὺς ἀποθανευμένους τε καὶ σωθησομένους προγινώσκων τε καὶ προλέγων ἀναίτιος ἂν εἴη.

before the physician by his art can combat each disease. It is necessary, therefore, to learn the natures of such diseases, how much they exceed the strength of men's bodies, and to learn how to forecast them. For in this way you will justly win respect and be an able physician. For the longer time you plan to meet each emergency the greater your power to save those who have a chance of recovery, while you will be blameless if you learn and declare beforehand those who will die and those who will get better.

4
Tragedy

Many of the key themes of this book occur repeatedly throughout the corpus of Greek tragedy, causation and responsibility, good and evil, reality and appearances, authority and control. An entire volume could easily be devoted to those topics in Greek drama alone. We shall have to be more than usually selective, concentrating on just a handful of plays to study what they have to say about plagues, disease, madness, pollution, about foreknowledge and helplessness: who is sound, who ill, who is mad, who can tell, who save?

Sophocles is important for our purposes not just because his extant plays, the *Oedipus Tyrannus* especially, deal with such themes with such subtlety and depth, but also because of other facts we know about his life. His period of activity as a playwright began in 468 (the first time he competed) and ended, in a sense, only after his death (in 406) with the posthumous victory of the *Oedipus at Colonus* in 401. He lived through the terrible plague at Athens, that first struck in 430–429 and that was to play such an important role in the Peloponnesian War.

The question immediately arises as to whether the *Oedipus Tyrannus* itself reflects Sophocles' first-hand experience of that very real epidemic. Unfortunately we have no firm date for that play, which may have been written any time between 430 and 420. There is no need, to be sure, as Vidal-Naquet pointed out (Vernant and Vidal-Naquet 1988, 303–4), to see this play as a direct or even indirect response to the Athenian plague. We must remember that the theme of a plague striking a whole population at war was already etched on the Greek imagination by the first book of the *Iliad*. But some scholars (such as Knox 1964) believe that it is likely that the *Oedipus Tyrannus* was written after 429—in which case the audience present at its production cannot have failed to see the connection between the evils that afflict Thebes in the tragedy, and the actual disease that decimated their own contemporaries. At Athens, however, there was no Oedipus in control, whose self-blinding could, in a sense, bring the pollution to an end.

The second important fact of Sophocles' life is that he is reported to have been one of those responsible for the introduction of the cult of Asclepius at Athens around 420. Sophocles was as famous a member of the literate elite in Athens as anyone. His readiness to sponsor the cult of the healing hero is testimony to its popularity among that elite. Again there is no need to associate that sponsorship with the Athenian plague and see it as evidence of Sophocles' dissatisfaction with purely naturalistic methods of healing. Thucydides cannot have been the only person to have registered that both lay and religious healers were helpless confronted by the plague. Yet whatever Sophocles may have thought about the styles of medicine represented in the Hippocratic Corpus, it seems fair to infer that he did not exclude the idea that prayer to the gods might contribute to healing. He would hardly have sponsored Asclepius if he thought the whole idea of the gods being at work was nonsense. As for his plays, we should not attempt to draw conclusions about Sophocles' own religious beliefs on the basis of what he makes characters in the tragedy say and do. Rather, we should see them as evidence for, precisely, the Greek imagination, even while here, as so often elsewhere, the relationship between the real and the imaginary is complex.

The *Oedipus Tyrannus* is full of plagues and pollutions, prophecies, riddle-solving, ignorance, and self-knowledge. At the start of the play Oedipus who is king at Thebes believes himself to be the son of Polybus and Merope, king and queen of Corinth (774). Of course the audience knows that his real father and mother are Laius and Jocasta, who had tried to kill him by exposing him on the mountain, in order to escape, as they hoped, the prophecy they had been given, that their son would kill his father and marry his mother. But that attempt to do away with him is thwarted by the shepherd, who disobeyed his orders to kill the young baby and had pity on him, with the consequence that the boy survived to be brought up at Corinth by Polybus and Merope. But Oedipus had left Corinth on his receiving an oracle from Phoebus Apollo with precisely the same prediction, that he would marry his mother and kill his father (791 ff.). To avoid any possibility of that happening, Oedipus distances himself from the pair he believes to be his parents. On his way to Thebes he kills an old man (whom of course he does not recognize) who blocks his way with his chariot and companions. Oedipus thinks that he has killed them all (813), though one in fact escaped (118) later to play a crucial role in the identification of the dead old man as Laius. When Oedipus arrives at Thebes, he finds it suffering from the depredations of the monstrous Sphinx, whose riddle he alone is able to solve. What is the creature who goes two-footed, four-footed, three-footed? Answer a human being (there is an obvious aspect of self-revelation in this) as an adult, as a baby, and as an old man with a stick. A grateful populace of Thebes makes him king and he marries the previous king's widow, in other words his mother Jocasta.

All that happens before the action of the play begins—the information being introduced with the greatest skill and discretion during the course of the drama itself. But the action itself begins (like the *Iliad*) with the plague. Oedipus must once again come to the rescue (58 ff.) [T 4.1], 'Children, I pity you. I know, I am not ignorant of the desires with which you have come; yes, I know that you are all sick, and, sick as you are, none of you is as sick as I.' Of course that is true in a way he does not yet understand: for *he* is the source of the city's pollution. Yet he does not himself suffer from the plague. When he says he is sick, he just means sick at heart.

But in response to the city's sufferings, he takes the initiative: he has found the only remedy (*iasis*, 68) he could see, namely to send Creon (brother of Iocasta) to Apollo at Delphi to discover by what act or word he can protect the city. It is true to his proud character that he assumes that he will, once again, be the saviour of the city, and he commits himself to doing whatever the god suggests. Creon duly returns with the news that Apollo has ordered that they drive out of the land a pollution, *miasma*. With what purification (*katharmos*, 99) [T 4.2]? With banishment or death. The cause of the pollution is the killer of Laius, and so the investigation into his death, that will inexorably lead to the identification of Oedipus as the killer, begins.

In the process we have Oedipus first consulting Teiresias, but when Teiresias begins to point the finger at Oedipus himself, he explodes in indignation, calling Teiresias the worst of evils (334) and suspecting a plot hatched by Creon to remove him from the throne (380ff.) [T 4.3]. Creon has suborned this crafty *magos* ('magician'), this tricky *agurtes* (charlatan)—using two of the terms the Hippocratic treatise *On the Sacred Disease* also employs to characterize its opponents, the 'purifiers', as devious quacks. Oedipus reminds him that it was he himself who solved the riddle of the sphinx: where was Teiresias' famous prophetic skill on that occasion? Creon too, in turn, gets accused by Oedipus of disloyalty and much worse.

As the pieces of the jigsaw are gradually fitted together—Oedipus' father is *not* Polybus, the son whom Laius exposed was *not* killed, it was *not* a group that killed Laius, but just a single man, so the sole survivor reports, and he was *not* killed with the rest of Laius' entourage—so the sense of the need for that cleansing Apollo had demanded becomes overwhelming. 'Neither Ister nor Phasis could wash clean this house', the messenger says at 1228. Indeed the pollution goes back long before the deeds of Oedipus. The whole of the house of Pelops, from which Laius comes, was afflicted by pollution (Pelops' father, Tantalus, had killed his son and served him up as a dish for the gods: though he was later restored to life) and by curses (those of Pelops' father-in-law, Oenomaus, especially). Jocasta who realizes the truth some time before Oedipus spells it out, takes her own life. Oedipus bursts into the palace, discovers her dead (some *daimon* shows him the corpse, for none of the mortal attendants did) and blinds himself with one of the brooches from her dress.

From the first of the passages I cited down to the end of the play, the vocabulary of disease, *nosos, nosema, nosein,* is used both of the diseases that are described as afflicting the people of Thebes and of the state of Oedipus himself. When he is about to come back on stage after his blinding, the messenger says: 'his disease (*nosema*) is too great for him to bear' (1293). What is needed is a remedy, a cure (*iasis*), a cleansing (*katharmos*) for the pollution (*miasma*). The unfolding of the action leads to Oedipus' eventual self-knowledge. But who knows what, and on what basis, provide two of the chief articulating themes of the plot. Oracles have to be consulted—but can they be trusted? Prophets such as the blind Teiresias have a greater understanding of the truth—or do they? What about the political machinations that may be at work and the corruption that may be suspected? Of course the play is not about medicine, about medical diagnosis and treatment. But human misfortune is depicted, repeatedly, in terms of diseases. Who can tell when they will strike, and why? What was the cause, indeed what type of cause is at work? Who knows what to do, to bring about relief? The workings of the gods provide much of the answer that the text gives. But no one in the play, or watching it, can be sure.

Oedipus in the *Oedipus Tyrannus* is a pollution on Thebes that has to be removed from the plague-ridden city for it to be restored to health. In that role he has often been compared to a *pharmakos,* a scapegoat,[1] who has to be driven from the community to save it from its troubles. Yet the source of pollution may also be a source of salvation.

---

[1] The literature is very extensive, but see e.g. Knox 1964, 1998; Sabbatucci 1978; Burkert 1979, 59ff.; Segal 1981; Vegetti 1983 ch. 1; Girard 1986; Vernant and Vidal-Naquet 1988, 16ff., 128ff. It should be emphasized that while these scholars agree there is some link between the

That ambivalence comes out clearly in the other Oedipus play, the *Oedipus at Colonus*, produced after Sophocles' own death. Oedipus' two sons fight over who is to rule Thebes, and over who is to control Oedipus himself. Polyneices tries to force Oedipus to return with him to Thebes, for he senses that the old man holds the key to success. But Oedipus, accompanied by his daughters, seeks asylum in Athens, where they are received by king Theseus. At the end of the play the messenger reports the apotheosis of Oedipus (1586ff., 1595ff. [T 4.4]). After washing and bathing Oedipus tells his daughters to withdraw (1641) for they should not see what it is not right to see. The god had called him (1626). Only Theseus was to witness what happened next, and he had to shade his eyes from the sight he could not endure. When the rest of those there look round, Oedipus was no longer there—and yet no one could tell how he died. The burial of Oedipus in Attica was thereafter to ensure that all his powers for good would be devoted to the country that had given him refuge. The man becomes a hero in the Greek sense, between the gods and mere mortals. From being a source of pollution he turns into a source of protection: we are dealing with a notion of the sacred that spans both extraordinary evil and extraordinary good, both danger and salvation.

The sense that exceptional skill or exceptional character is both a source of great benefit and a danger comes out in a different context in the next play we should consider, the *Philoctetes*. Philoctetes had been abandoned on the way to Troy by the other Achaean heroes because of the terrible wound with which he is afflicted. But it turns out that to take Troy they need both him and his bow. He is the archer par excellence, and his bow is no good without him, nor he without his bow. This play is all about loyalty and betrayal, straight dealings and deceit. The wily Odysseus first persuades the young Neoptolemus to trick Philoctetes into parting with his bow—

figure of Oedipus and the institution of the *pharmakos*, quite what that connection is, how important it is for our understanding of the play, and what its wider significance is, are much disputed questions.

only for Neoptolemus later to realize that that is wrong, undergoing a veritable *rite de passage* in the process of this self-realization.[2] The resolution at the end of the play has to be brought about by the personal, divine, intervention of Heracles (1409 ff.). But Philoctetes is as ambivalent a figure as Oedipus. On the one hand, he stinks from his running sore: he still suffers from his unhealed wound (38 ff.) [T 4.5]. Only at the end does Heracles send Asclepius to heal him (1437). On the other, he holds the key to taking Troy. Those with exceptional skills are—we understand—to be revered, even to be feared. We recall that Empedocles had said he was greeted by his fellow citizens as a god. Yet that acclaim carries with it its own risks and dangers.

Tragedy is all about the gods and prophecies fulfilled in unexpected, or in all too expected, ways. No extant Greek play goes as far as Hesiod had done in stating as an unequivocal general thesis that god rewards justice with health and injustice with disease. Rather many individuals find themselves caught up in the doom of their families whose accursed misfortunes carry on from one generation to the next. But celebrations of human ability, human know-how, can also be found. Prometheus in the *Prometheus Vinctus* attributed to Aeschylus famously praises the skills he says come from the gift of fire that he stole from Zeus to give to humans. He taught men, he says at 436 ff., the skills of building houses, of how to tell the seasons by the stars, of number, and most marvellous of all, that of the remedies for diseases and a whole gamut of techniques of prophecy (476) [T 4.6]. He presides, of course, as his own name, Prometheus, indicates, over all manner of foresight. We may note in passing that this focuses attention on the *abilities*—of being able to bring about a cure, of knowing the future—even though, as we saw in the previous chapter, there was considerable disagreement among those who claimed to have those abilities about how precisely

---

[2] The suggestion that this self-realization may be connected with the institution of the *ephebeia* is proposed by Vidal-Naquet in Vernant and Vidal-Naquet 1988, ch. 7.

Tragedy 91

they were to be displayed. It is the success that Prometheus celebrates, and questions as to how it is to be achieved are not, of course, allowed to obtrude.

But a similar celebration, this time without reference to the divine provenance of human abilities, comes in the famous chorus of Sophocles' *Antigone* (332 ff.) [T 4.7]. 'Many things are formidable and none more formidable than humans.' He can cross the sea, till the soil, capture wild beasts and fish, tame the horse and bull. He has learnt speech and social life and architecture. He meets the future armed with resource against all eventualities. Death, Hades, alone is something from which he has no means of flight: but he has contrived escape from desperate maladies, diseases (*nosoi*).

Such a paean of praise for humankind and its skills seems extravagantly, almost foolishly, optimistic. It is as if no shadow from plagues real or imaginary is cast over this celebration. Medicine, it is claimed, has remedies even for terrible diseases and there is no suggestion here that these cures are only to be achieved with the help of the gods or of Asclepius. Yet restored in its context in the action of the play, this chorus can be seen in a very different light. This is a rare, indeed the only, moment of optimism, when somehow or other Polyneices' body has received its proper burial (though the chorus does not yet know how and by whom this was done)—despite Creon's command that it should lie unburied as punishment for his having dared to wage war against his brother, Eteocles, and against Thebes. Yet we should recognize that this optimism is short-lived. The very next chorus begins (582): 'happy are those whose lifespan is free from the taste of evils: but those whose house has been shaken by the gods have no end of destruction (*ate*) . . . There is no escape (597).' While one chorus trumpets the resourcefulness of humankind, the next suggests rather its helplessness. God's will is inescapable and his ways inscrutable.

The theme of evils as diseases, diseases as evils, has already appeared in Sophocles. That is given a new twist in one of Euripides' most powerful plays, the *Bacchae,* a sustained problematization of madness, what it consists in, why people are mad, what remedies are any use. Dionysus has come to Thebes accompanied by his Asiatic women devotees, the Bacchants, but king Pentheus rejects his worship, a rejection that eventually leads to his death at the hands of his own mother, Agave. She had gone with a band of Theban women to the mountains to celebrate the god. Pentheus, enticed by Dionysus to spy on the women, whom he suspects of lewd and drunken behaviour, is discovered by his mother, but she is out of her wits. She thinks he is a lion, and she slaughters him with her own hands. She re-enters Thebes carrying his head in her deluded triumph and is slowly led to a realization of what she has done.

We have encountered before the themes of the threatening nature of foreigners and of women. In this play the chorus, consisting of Bacchants, stress their Asiatic origin (64), while, when Dionysus talks of being worshipped by the barbarians, Pentheus contrasts this with the better sense that Greeks possess (483). But I am more concerned here with the discourse of madness, with accusations of madness by those who stress their own sound sense, with the accounts given of mad behaviour and with the confusion that these engender. Nearly all the characters in the play, the chorus, Agave and the Theban women, Pentheus, Teiresias and Cadmus, even Pentheus' servants, are implicated in one way or another.

The chorus itself speaks of the frenzy of their fellow-worshippers of Bacchus, the mad Satyrs *(mainomenoi saturoi,* 130) and of their own rapture (135ff.) [T 4.8]. As for the Theban women, led by Agave, their madness is sent by Dionysus, so he himself says (36) and Pentheus for once thinks the same, describing their madness as a 'new disease' (353–4). Cadmus in turn agrees (1295). When Agave finally comes to her senses, this is her returning to her right mind, becoming *eunous* again (1269ff.). But Pentheus, who prides himself on his good sense, is also said by Teiresias to be mad (359) because he rejects Dionysus. Seduced by Dionysus to spy on the Bacchants he is described as mad (999) even while

Dionysus says that even before that, he had 'no sound wits' (947–8). Even the servant, who brings in Dionysus bound and announces that the imprisoned Bacchants have escaped, is said by Pentheus to be mad (451). As for Teiresias and Cadmus, they, according to Pentheus, have taken leave of their senses, when they decide to join the God's devotees (252, 343 ff.)

The exchanges between Pentheus, Teiresias, and Cadmus, early in the play (215–369) [T 4.9, 4.10] are particularly striking. Pentheus sees nothing but an excuse for immoral behaviour in the Bacchants' rites (224) and says there is nothing healthy or sound (*hygies*) in them (262). To that Teiresias retorts that Pentheus may seem wise, but there is no sense (*phrenes*) in his words (266–9). He lectures Pentheus on Dionysus' miraculous birth and his gifts to humankind, wine, especially, that brings sleep (there is no other remedy, *pharmakon*, for sufferings, 283). The god is a prophet (298) [T 4.10]. Bacchic frenzy and madness (*to maniodes*) are full of prophecy (299) and he can be seen in action in battle, when panic seizes soldiers even before a blow is struck. That too is a madness that comes from Dionysus (305).

Teiresias goes on to warn Pentheus not to be arrogant, and not to think that it is just political might (*kratos*) that has power over humans (310). 'Nor, even if you think so—but your opinion is sick (*nosei*)—should you think you are wise (or sober, *phronein*).'[3] You should accept the god and welcome him. As for women, Dionysus does not compel them to be chaste: chaste behaviour is a matter of their inborn nature (*phusis*), but chastity will not be undone by Bacchic frenzy (317f.) Teiresias, for his part, together with Cadmus, will dance in celebration of the god, old as they are. 'You are most painfully mad,' he concludes to Pentheus (326), 'nor will you be cured by *pharmaka* (remedies, spells) nor are you ill without them.'

[3] Here and for verses 326 ff. I offer translations that, at the cost of some elegance, aim to keep as close as possible to the syntax and semantics of the Greek expressions.

Both the positive and the negative range of *pharmakon* are here dramatically juxtaposed—or rather they are indistinguishable. It is *pharmaka* that are responsible for his madness—nor can *pharmaka* cure him. Equally no wedge can be driven between *pharmaka* as spells, as drugs, or as remedies. Pentheus is convinced he is as right as rain. But Teiresias is sure that to reject the god is mad (whether or not that madness, like many others in the play, is Dionysus' own doing). As for Cadmus, he takes the politic line. Even if this god is no god, he says (333) you had better call him god.

Quite what Euripides himself believed about the gods is the subject of a famous scholarly controversy, with Verrall's disputes with his contemporaries finding echoes in modern writings. But that is beside the point. We have no need to enter that debate to register what the play tells us about the powers and dangers of the divine, about the perils of madness and its being confounded with good sense. Ordinary human responses to crises may be useless. You may think it is sensible to stick to what you are familiar with, avoiding trouble by not tangling with these strange practices from foreign parts. But what may look like prudent judgement may turn out to be madness. There is a wisdom that is no wisdom (395). But who is to know? Mere human judgement may be altogether inadequate to this vital task, and when it fails, what happens to the boundary between wisdom and folly, and between folly and madness? If someone represents themselves as particularly knowledgeable or wise—a seer or a king, maybe—who can verify whether they are right? Dionysus himself is on stage in this play and he speaks for himself—or does he? The 'I' who is the character Dionysus refers to Dionysus in the third person (517, 649, 849) as well as in the first (1340: both at once, for example at 498). Besides, we are in the theatre, are we not?[4]

The unpredictability of the gods, and the difficulty in keeping in with all of them, are the leading themes in the last play

---

[4] The themes of the mask of Dionysus, and his simultaneous presence on stage and in the theatre, are powerfully developed by Vernant in Vernant and Vidal-Naquet 1988 ch. 17.

I wish to comment on. This is Euripides' *Hippolytus*, which also picks up the topic of love or passion as disease. The action of the play is sandwiched between speeches by two goddesses: Aphrodite speaks the prologue and Artemis appears in the closing scene. Aphrodite has been slighted by Hippolytus, who worships the virgin goddess Artemis and will have nothing to do with the works of Aphrodite. But Aphrodite vows revenge. Phaedra, Hippolytus' step-mother, falls madly in love with Hippolytus, but, when repulsed by him, takes her own life and denounces Hippolytus to his father, Theseus. Theseus believes Phaedra, curses Hippolytus, driving him into exile. Hippolytus is killed when a thunderbolt from Zeus frightens the horses of his chariot team and a great wave overwhelms him. As we have learnt to expect, divine actions and motivations are interwoven with human and 'natural' ones. That Aphrodite starts the action in no way removes all responsibility from the shoulders of Phaedra, Hippolytus, Theseus, themselves.

But when Phaedra first conceives her passion for Hippolytus, her confidante, the Nurse, diagnoses disease. She invokes 'the troubles (evils) mortals have, the hateful illnesses (*nosoi*)' and addressing Phaedra asks 'what shall I do for you? What shall I not?' (177f.) [T 4.12]. 'Better it is to be sick', she claims (186) 'than to tend the sick.' The first is simple; the second involves both grief—mental pain—and hard work.

Phaedra's own opening speeches refer to her physical symptoms (we might say) as much as to her emotions. 'Raise up my body, hold my head erect. My limbs are unstrung. Take my fair arms, servants. It is a burden to have this headdress on my head. Take it off, spread my tresses on my shoulders.' The Nurse's response is to try to encourage her to be calm. 'You will endure your sickness (*nosos*) more easily with calm and nobility of heart. Mortals must endure trouble' (203ff.). She should not speak such wild words, born of madness (*mania*, 214, cf. 232, 238), in public! After plenty of further exchanges, the Nurse remains baffled: she later says she is no prophet able to recognize clearly what is hidden, 346.

Finally Phaedra confesses she is in love. It is the Nurse who, registering Phaedra's reaction to the mention of his name, identifies Hippolytus as the object of her passion, only for her to become distraught herself.

Phaedra herself has said, according to the Nurse (279), that she is not ill. As Phaedra herself puts it (317) her mind has a pollution (*miasma*). But she presents with all the signs of sickness. In such straits it is natural for a woman to confide in another woman. Indeed we saw in the last chapter that, faced with their women patients, the male doctors represented in the Hippocratic Corpus were often rather at a loss, not clear whether to trust what they were told, and yet recognizing that women thought they knew well enough what was going on in their bodies, at least where childbirth was concerned. Euripides' depiction of the exchanges between Phaedra and the Nurse exploits the idea that a woman will talk more easily to another woman about love and disease, but it also confirms that the line between those two is a fine one. Rather, there is no fundamental distinction between the two, for love, in the final analysis, is an affliction.

Works of high literature, let me say again, are bound to pose a particular challenge to interpretation. But from the point of view of what these plays assume their audience will understand and respond to, they can be used for the light they throw on the Greek imagination. Whether or not that audience believed in the Olympian gods and the other agencies put on stage is immaterial: they certainly accepted the actions as real. They certainly recognized the playing out of the drama as being 'true to life'. Who knows what the future holds? Who can tell what misfortunes may strike and why? When experts diagnose the problems and offer remedies, can they be trusted? Those problems, those ills, those diseases, where do they come from, and how should they be responded to or remedied? The plague of a population, the wound of an individual, lovesickness, mark calamity, whether heaven-sent or not: but those marked out may be as much objects to revere as to pity. The gods often achieve their ends—obscure as they are—

through disease. Humans may try to understand, diagnose, cure: but their helplessness is evident.

Yet it is not that the inevitable-seeming unfolding of the action absolves humans from having to decide what to do. 'Alas, what shall I do?' is a refrain that haunts Greek tragedy, from Orestes in Aeschylus *Choephoroi* (899) to the Nurse in Euripides' *Hippolytus*. Though so often in the dark, at a loss to know whether the gods have taken offence and if so, why, and how to go about placating them, or what to do in general, humans have nevertheless to strain every nerve to get the answers right—except that their efforts so often come to nothing (as was the fate, as we saw, of Greek doctors of every description in their attempts to understand and to cure). To seem pious, or wise, or even good, offered no immunity to calamity, indeed no immunity was to be had, any more than there was for disease. Its sudden onset, often unexplained, often inexplicable, maybe irremediable, captures, in so many respects, the very essence of the human predicament, serving as not merely analogous to, but itself a key example of, human vulnerability. So at least the Greek tragedians—and indeed their audiences—evidently believed.

CHAPTER 4 TEXTS

4.1 Sophocles, *Oedipus Tyrannus* 58–72

Οι. ὦ παιδες οἰκτροί, γνωτὰ κοὐκ ἄγνωτά μοι
προσήλθεθ' ἱμείροντες, εὖ γὰρ οἶδ' ὅτι
νοςεῖτε πάντες· καὶ νοςοῦντες, ὡς ἐγὼ 60
οὐκ ἔςτιν ὑμῶν ὅςτις ἐξ ἴςου νοςεῖ.
τὸ μὲν γὰρ ὑμῶν ἄλγος εἰς ἕν' ἔρχεται
μόνον καθ' αὑτόν, κοὐδέν' ἄλλον, ἡ δ' ἐμὴ
ψυχὴ πόλιν τε κἀμὲ καὶ ς' ὁμοῦ ςτένει.
ὥςτ' οὐχ ὕπνῳ γ' εὕδοντά μ' ἐξεγείρετε, 65
ἀλλ' ἴςτε πολλὰ μέν με δακρύςαντα δή,
πολλὰς δ' ὁδοὺς ἐλθόντα φροντίδος πλάνοις.
ἣν δ' εὖ ςκοπῶν ηὕριςκον ἴαςιν μόνην,
ταύτην ἔπραξα· παῖδα γὰρ Μενοικέως
Κρέοντ', ἐμαυτοῦ γαμβρόν, ἐς τὰ Πυθικὰ 70
ἔπεμψα Φοίβου δώμαθ', ὡς πύθοιθ' ὅ τι
δρῶν ἢ τί φωνῶν τήνδ' ἐρυςαίμην πόλιν.

4.2 Sophocles, *Oedipus Tyrannus* 95–104

Κρ. λέγοιμ' ἂν οἷ' ἤκουςα τοῦ θεοῦ πάρα. 95
ἄνωγεν ἡμᾶς Φοῖβος ἐμφανῶς, ἄναξ,
μίαςμα χώρας, ὡς τεθραμμένον χθονὶ
ἐν τῇδ', ἐλαύνειν μηδ' ἀνήκεςτον τρέφειν.
Οι. ποίῳ καθαρμῷ; τίς ὁ τρόπος τῆς ξυμφορᾶς;
Κρ. ἀνδρηλατοῦντας, ἢ φόνῳ φόνον πάλιν 100
λύοντας, ὡς τόδ' αἷμα χειμάζον πόλιν.
Οι. ποίου γὰρ ἀνδρὸς τήνδε μηνύει τύχην;
Κρ. ἦν ἡμίν, ὦναξ, Λάιός ποθ' ἡγεμὼν
γῆς τῆςδε, πρὶν ςὲ τήνδ' ἀπευθύνειν πόλιν.

4.3 Sophocles, *Oedipus Tyrannus* 380–403

Οι. ὦ πλοῦτε καὶ τυραννὶ καὶ τέχνη τέχνης 380
ὑπερφέρουςα τῷ πολυζήλῳ βίῳ,
ὅςος παρ' ὑμῖν ὁ φθόνος φυλάςςεται,
εἰ τῆςδέ γ' ἀρχῆς οὕνεχ', ἣν ἐμοὶ πόλις
δωρητόν, οὐκ αἰτητόν, εἰςεχείριςεν,
ταύτης Κρέων ὁ πιςτός, οὑξ ἀρχῆς φίλος, 385

CHAPTER 4 TEXTS

4.1 Sophocles, *Oedipus Tyrannus* 58–72

OEDIPUS: Children, I pity you! I know, I am not ignorant of the desires with which you have come; yes, I know that you are all sick, and, sick as you are, none of you is as sick as I. Your pain comes upon each by himself and upon no other; but my soul mourns equally for the city and for myself and for you. And so you are not waking me from sleep, but know that I have shed many a tear, and have travelled many roads in the wanderings of reflection. The only remedy which, by careful thought, I have found I have applied; I have sent Creon, son of Menoeceus, my wife's brother, to the Pythian halls of Phoebus, so that he may learn by what deed or word I may protect this city.

4.2 Sophocles, *Oedipus Tyrannus* 95–104

CREON: I will tell you what I heard from the god. The lord Phoebus orders us plainly to drive out from the land a pollution, one that has been nourished in this country, and not to nourish it till it cannot be cured.
OEDIPUS: With what means of purifying? what is the nature of the trouble?
CREON: By banishment, or by repaying killing with killing, since it is this bloodshed that has brought the storm upon the city.
OEDIPUS: And who is the man whose fate he is revealing?
CREON: King, Laius was once lord of this land, before you guided it.

4.3 Sophocles, *Oedipus Tyrannus* 380–403

OEDIPUS: O riches and kingship and skill surpassing skill in a life much-envied, how great is the hatred that you store up, if it is for the sake of this royal power, which the city placed in my hands as a gift, though I had not asked it, that Creon the trusty, my friend from the first, has crept up to me and longs to throw me out, setting upon me this wizard hatcher of plots, this crafty beggar, who

λάθρᾳ μ' ὑπελθὼν ἐκβαλεῖν ἱμείρεται,
ὑφεὶς μάγον τοιόνδε μηχανορράφον,
δόλιον ἀγύρτην, ὅςτις ἐν τοῖς κέρδεςιν
μόνον δέδορκε, τὴν τέχνην δ' ἔφυ τυφλός.
ἐπεὶ φέρ' εἰπέ, ποῦ cὺ μάντις εἶ cαφής; 390
πῶς οὐχ, ὅθ' ἡ ῥαψῳδὸς ἐνθάδ' ἦν κύων,
ηὔδας τι τοῖςδ' ἀςτοῖςιν ἐκλυτήριον;
καίτοι τό γ' αἴνιγμ' οὐχὶ τοὐπιόντος ἦν
ἀνδρὸς διειπεῖν, ἀλλὰ μαντείας ἔδει·
ἣν οὔτ' ἀπ' οἰωνῶν cὺ προὐφάνης ἔχων 395
οὔτ' ἐκ θεῶν του γνωτόν· ἀλλ' ἐγὼ μολών,
ὁ μηδὲν εἰδὼς Οἰδίπους, ἔπαυcά νιν,
γνώμῃ κυρήcας οὐδ' ἀπ' οἰωνῶν μαθών·
ὃν δὴ cὺ πειρᾷς ἐκβαλεῖν, δοκῶν θρόνοις
παραστατήςειν τοῖς Κρεοντείοις πέλας. 400
κλαίων δοκεῖς μοι καὶ cὺ χὼ cυνθεὶς τάδε
ἀγηλατήςειν· εἰ δὲ μὴ 'δόκεις γέρων
εἶναι, παθὼν ἔγνως ἂν οἷά περ φρονεῖς.

4.4 Sophocles, *Oedipus at Colonus* 1595–607, 1620–57

Αγ. ἀφ' οὗ μέcος cτὰς τοῦ τε Θορικίου πέτρου 1595
κοίλης τ' ἀχέρδου κἀπὶ λαΐνου τάφου
καθέζετ'· εἶτ' ἔλυcε δυςπινεῖς cτολάς.
κἄπειτ' αὔcας παῖδας ἠνώγει ῥυτῶν
ὑδάτων ἐνεγκεῖν λουτρὰ καὶ χοάς ποθεν·
τὼ δ' εὐχλόου Δήμητρος εἰς προcόψιον 1600
πάγον μολούcα τάcδ' ἐπιστολὰς πατρὶ
ταχεῖ 'πόρευcαν ξὺν χρόνῳ, λουτροῖς τέ νιν
ἐcθῆτί τ' ἐξήcκηcαν ᾗ νομίζεται.
ἐπεὶ δὲ πᾶcαν ἔcχε δρῶντος ἡδονὴν
κοὐκ ἦν ἔτ' ἀργὸν οὐδὲν ὧν ἐφίετο, 1605
κτύπηcε μὲν Ζεὺς χθόνιος, αἱ δὲ παρθένοι
ῥίγηcαν, ὡς ἤκουcαν·

τοιαῦτ' ἐπ' ἀλλήλοιcιν ἀμφικείμενοι 1620
λύγδην ἔκλαιον πάντες. ὡς δὲ πρὸς τέλος
γόων ἀφίκοντ' οὐδ' ἔτ' ὠρώρει βοή,
ἦν μὲν cιωπή, φθέγμα δ' ἐξαίφνης τινος
θώϋξεν αὐτόν, ὥcτε πάντας ὀρθίας
cτῆcαι φόβῳ δείcαντας εὐθέως τρίχας· 1625

has sight only when it comes to profit, but in his art is blind! Why, come, tell me, how can you be a true prophet? Why when the versifying hound was here did not you speak some word that could release the citizens? Indeed, her riddle was not one for the first comer to explain! It required prophetic skill, and you were exposed as having no knowledge from the birds or from the gods. No, it was I that came, Oedipus who knew nothing, and put a stop to her; I hit the mark by native wit, not by what I learned from birds. And it is I that you are trying to throw out, thinking that you will stand close to the throne of Creon. Both you and he who hatched this plan will regret, I think, your attempt to drive out the curse; and if you did not seem to be old, you would learn by suffering how dangerous are your thoughts.

4.4 Sophocles, *Oedipus at Colonus* 1595–607, 1620–57

MESSENGER: Between this and the Thorician rock he took his stand, and sat down by the hollow pear tree and the tomb of stone; then he undid his filthy garments. Next he called upon his daughters, telling them to bring water for washing and libation from a running stream somewhere. And they went to the hill of verdant Demeter that was in view and discharged these duties swiftly for their father, and gave him the bath and the raiment this is customary. But when he had got all the pleasure belonging to a doer, and none of his commands had been left unfulfilled, Zeus of the earth thundered, and the maidens shuddered when they heard it.

Thus, clinging closely to each other, all of them sobbed; but when they came to the end of their lamenting, and no sound still rose up, there was silence, and suddenly the voice of someone hailed him, so that the hair of all stood upright suddenly in terror. For the god called him often and from many places: 'You there, Oedipus, why do we wait to go? You have delayed too long!' But

καλεῖ γὰρ αὐτὸν πολλὰ πολλαχῇ θεός·
"ὦ οὗτος οὗτος, Οἰδίπους, τί μέλλομεν
χωρεῖν; πάλαι δὴ τἀπὸ coῦ βραδύνεται."
ὁ δ' ὡc ἐπῄcθετ' ἐκ θεοῦ καλούμενος,
αὐδᾷ μολεῖν οἱ γῆc ἄνακτα Θηcέα. 1630
κἀπεὶ προcῆλθεν, εἶπεν, "ὦ φίλον κάρα,
δόc μοι χερὸc cῆc πίcτιν ἀρχαίαν τέκνοιc,
ὑμεῖc τε, παῖδεc, τῷδε· καὶ καταίνεcον
μήποτε προδώcειν τάcδ' ἑκών, τελεῖν δ' ὅc' ἂν
μέλλῃc φρονῶν εὖ ξυμφέροντ' αὐταῖc ἀεί." 1635
ὁ δ', ὡc ἀνὴρ γενναῖοc, οὐκ οἴκτου μέτα
κατῄνεcεν τάδ' ὅρκιοc δράcειν ξένῳ.
ὅπωc δὲ ταῦτ' ἔδραcεν, εὐθὺc Οἰδίπουc
ψαύcαc ἀμαυραῖc χερcὶν ὧν παίδων λέγει,
"ὦ παῖδε, τλάcαc χρὴ †τὸ γενναῖον φέρειν† 1640
χωρεῖν τόπων ἐκ τῶνδε, μηδ' ἃ μὴ θέμιc
λεύccειν δικαιοῦν, μηδὲ φωνούντων κλύειν.
ἀλλ' ἔρπεθ' ὡc τάχιcτα· πλὴν ὁ κύριοc
Θηcεὺc παρέcτω μανθάνειν τὰ δρώμενα."
τοcαῦτα φωνήcαντοc εἰcηκούcαμεν 1645
ξύμπαντεc· ἀcτακτεὶ δὲ cὺν ταῖc παρθένοιc
cτένοντεc ὡμαρτοῦμεν. ὡc δ' ἀπήλθομεν,
χρόνῳ βραχεῖ cτραφέντεc, ἐξαπείδομεν
τὸν ἄνδρα τὸν μὲν οὐδαμοῦ παρόντ' ἔτι,
ἄνακτα δ' αὐτὸν ὀμμάτων ἐπίcκιον 1650
χεῖρ' ἀντέχοντα κρατόc, ὡc δεινοῦ τινοc
φόβου φανέντοc οὐδ' ἀναcχετοῦ βλέπειν.
ἔπειτα μέντοι βαιὸν οὐδὲ cὺν λόγῳ
ὁρῶμεν αὐτὸν γῆν τε προcκυνοῦνθ' ἅμα
καὶ τὸν θεῶν Ὄλυμπον ἐν ταὐτῷ χρόνῳ. 1655
μόρῳ δ' ὁποίῳ κεῖνοc ὤλετ' οὐδ' ἂν εἷc
θνητῶν φράcειε πλὴν τὸ Θηcέωc κάρα.

4.5 Sophocles, *Philoctetes* 38–47

Νε. ἰοὺ ἰού· καὶ ταῦτά γ' ἄλλα θάλπεται
ῥάκη, βαρείαc του νοcηλείαc πλέα.
Οδ. ἀνὴρ κατοικεῖ τούcδε τοὺc τόπουc cαφῶc, 40
κἄcτ' οὐχ ἑκάc που. πῶc γὰρ ἂν νοcῶν ἀνὴρ
κῶλον παλαιᾷ κηρὶ προcτείχοι μακράν;
ἀλλ' ἢ 'πὶ φορβῆc μαcτὺν ἐξελήλυθεν

when he realized that the god was calling him, he told the king of the country, Theseus, to come to him. And when he had approached, he said, 'My dear friend, pray give the ancient pledge of a handclasp to my children, and do you daughters, give the same to him! And promise that you will never willingly betray them, and that you will always accomplish kindly all that will do them good.'

And he like a noble man, without lamenting promised upon oath that he would do this for the stranger. And when he had done this, at once Oedipus laid his feeble hands upon his children and said, 'Daughters, you must bear this with a noble mind and depart from these regions, and not claim to look upon what may not be seen, or to hear such speech. Come, go with all speed! Only let him who is responsible, Theseus, be here to learn what is being done.'

We all heard him speak these words; and we accompanied the maidens, with floods of tears. And when we had departed, after a short time we turned around, and could see that the man was no longer there, and the king was holding his hand before his face to shade his eyes, as though some terrifying sight, which he could not bear to look on, had been presented. But then after a moment, with no word spoken, we saw him salute the earth and the sky, home of the gods, at the same moment. But by what death that man perished none among mortals could tell but Theseus.

4.5 Sophocles, *Philoctetes* 38–47

NEOPTOLEMUS: Ah, ah! Here is something else, rags drying in the sun, stained with matter from some grievous sore!

ODYSSEUS: Clearly this is the place where the man lives, and he must be not far off; for how could a man whose leg is stricken with an ancient affliction travel far? But either he has gone off to look for food, or perhaps he knows some healing herb. So send the man

ἢ φύλλον εἴ τι νώδυνον κάτοιδέ που.
τὸν οὖν παρόντα πέμψον ἐς κατασκοπήν, 45
μὴ καὶ λάθῃ με προσπεσών· ὡς μᾶλλον ἂν
ἕλοιτ' ἔμ' ἢ τοὺς πάντας Ἀργείους λαβεῖν.

4.6 Aeschylus, *Prometheus Vinctus* 476–500

Πρ. τὰ λοιπά μου κλύουσα θαυμάσῃι πλέον,
οἴας τέχνας τε καὶ πόρους ἐμησάμην·
τὸ μὲν μέγιστον, εἴ τις ἐς νόσον πέσοι,
οὐκ ἦν ἀλέξημ' οὐδέν, οὔτε βρώσιμον
οὐ χριστὸν οὐδὲ πιστόν, ἀλλὰ φαρμάκων 480
χρείαι κατεσκέλλοντο, πρίν γ' ἐγώ σφισιν
ἔδειξα κράσεις ἠπίων ἀκεσμάτων,
αἷς τὰς ἁπάσας ἐξαμύνονται νόσους·
τρόπους τε πολλοὺς μαντικῆς ἐστοίχισα,
κἄκρινα πρῶτος ἐξ ὀνειράτων ἃ χρὴ 485
ὕπαρ γενέσθαι, κληδόνας τε δυσκρίτους
ἐγνώρισ' αὐτοῖς ἐνοδίους τε συμβόλους,
γαμψωνύχων τε πτῆσιν οἰωνῶν σκεθρῶς
διώρισ', οἵτινές τε δεξιοὶ φύσιν
εὐωνύμους τε, καὶ δίαιταν ἥντινα 490
ἔχουσ' ἕκαστοι καὶ πρὸς ἀλλήλους τίνες
ἔχθραι τε καὶ στέργηθρα καὶ συνεδρίαι·
σπλάγχνων τε λειότητα, καὶ χροιὰν τίνα
ἔχουσ' ἂν εἴη δαίμοσιν πρὸς ἡδονὴν
χολή, λοβοῦ τε ποικίλην εὐμορφίαν· 495
κνίσῃ τε κῶλα συγκαλυπτὰ καὶ μακρὰν
ὀσφῦν πυρώσας δυστέκμαρτον εἰς τέχνην
ὥδωσα θνητούς, καὶ φλογωπὰ σήματα
ἐξωμμάτωσα πρόσθεν ὄντ' ἐπάργεμα.
τοιαῦτα μὲν δὴ ταῦτ'· 500

4.7 Sophocles, *Antigone* 332–64

Χο. πολλὰ τὰ δεινὰ κοὐδὲν ἀνθρώπου δεινότερον πέλει·
τοῦτο καὶ πολιοῦ πέραν
πόντου χειμερίῳ νότῳ 335
χωρεῖ, περιβρυχίοισιν
περῶν ὑπ' οἴδμασιν, θεῶν
τε τὰν ὑπερτάταν, Γᾶν

you have with you to look out, in case he should suddenly fall upon me. How much rather he would take me than all the other Argives!

4.6 Aeschylus, *Prometheus Vinctus* 476–500

PROMETHEUS: Hear but the rest and thou shalt wonder the more at the arts and resources I devised. This first and foremost: if ever man fell ill, there was no defence—no healing food, no ointment, nor any draught—but for lack of medicine they wasted away, until I showed them how to mix soothing remedies wherewith they now ward off all their disorders. And I marked out many ways whereby they might read the future, and among dreams I first discerned which are destined to come true; and voices baffling interpretation I explained to them, and signs from meetings by the way. The flight of crook-taloned birds I distinguished clearly—which by nature are auspicious, which sinister—their various modes of life, their mutual feuds and loves, and their consortings; and the smoothness of their entrails, and what colour the gall must have to please the gods, and the speckled symmetry of the liver-lobe; and the thigh-bones, enwrapped in fat, and the long chine I burned and initiated mankind into an occult art. Also I cleared their vision to discern signs from flames, erstwhile obscure. So much then touching these arts.

4.7 Sophocles, *Antigone* 332–64

CHORUS: Many things are formidable, and none more formidable than humans. He crosses the gray sea beneath the winter wind, passing beneath the surges that surround him; and he wears away the highest of the gods, Earth, immortal and unwearying, as his ploughs go back and forth from year to year, turning the soil with the aid of the breed of horses.

And he captures the tribe of thoughtless birds and the races of

ἄφθιτον, ἀκαμάταν ἀποτρύεται
ἰλλομένων ἀρότρων ἔτοc εἰc ἔτοc, 340
ἱππείῳ γένει πολεύων.

κουφονόων τε φῦλον ὀρ-
νίθων ἀμφιβαλὼν ἄγει
καὶ θηρῶν ἀγρίων ἔθνη
πόντου τ' εἰναλίαν φύcιν 345
cπείραιcι δικτυοκλώcτοιc,
περιφραδὴc ἀνήρ· κρατεῖ
δὲ μηχαναῖc ἀγραύλου
θηρὸc ὀρεccιβάτα, λαcιαύχενά θ' 350
ἵππον ὀχμάζεται ἀμφὶ λόφον ζυγῷ
οὔρειόν τ' ἀκμῆτα ταῦρον.

καὶ φθέγμα καὶ ἀνεμόεν φρόνημα καὶ ἀcτυνόμουc 355
ὀργὰc ἐδιδάξατο καὶ δυcαύλων
πάγων ὑπαίθρεια καὶ
δύcομβρα φεύγειν βέλη
παντοπόροc· ἄποροc ἐπ' οὐδὲν ἔρχεται 360
τὸ μέλλον· Ἅιδα μόνον
φεῦξιν οὐκ ἐπάξεται·
νόcων δ' ἀμηχάνων φυγὰc
ξυμπέφραcται. 364

4.8 Euripides, *The Bacchae* 135–67

Χο. ἡδὺς ἐν ὄρεσιν, ὅταν ἐκ θιάσων δρομαί- 135
  ων πέσῃ πεδόσε, νε-
  βρίδος ἔχων ἱερὸν ἐνδυτόν, ἀγρεύων
αἷμα τραγοκτόνον, ὠμοφάγον χάριν, ἱέμε-
νος ἐς ὄρεα Φρύγια, Λύδι', ὁ δ' ἔξαρχος Βρόμιος, 140
  εὐοῖ.
ῥεῖ δὲ γάλακτι πέδον, ῥεῖ δ' οἴνῳ, ῥεῖ δὲ μελισσᾶν
  νέκταρι.
  Συρίας δ' ὡς λιβάνου κα-
  πνὸν ὁ Βακχεὺς ἀνέχων
  πυρσώδη φλόγα πεύκας 145
  ἐκ νάρθηκος ἀίσσει
  δρόμῳ καὶ χοροῖσιν
  πλανάτας ἐρεθίζων
  ἰαχαῖς τ' ἀναπάλλων,

wild beasts and the watery brood of the sea, catching them in the woven coils of nets, man the skilful. And he contrives to overcome the beast that roams the mountain, and tames the shaggy-maned horse and the untiring mountain bull, putting a yoke about their necks.

And he has learned speech and wind-swift thought and the temper that rules cities, and how to escape the exposure of the inhospitable hills and the sharp arrows of the rain, all-resourceful; he meets nothing in the future without resource; only from Hades shall he apply no means of flight; and he has contrived escape from desperate maladies.

4.8 Euripides, *The Bacchae* 135–67

CHORUS: O what delight is in the mountains!
   There the celebrant, wrapped in his sacred fawnskin,
   Flings himself on the ground surrendered,
   While the swift-footed company streams on;
   There he hunts for blood, and rapturously
   Eats the raw flesh of the slaughtered goat,
   Hurrying on to the Phrygian or Lydian mountain heights.
   Possessed, ecstatic, he leads their happy cries;
   The earth flows with milk, flows with wine,
   Flows with nectar of bees;
   The air is thick with a scent of Syrian myrrh.
   The celebrant runs entranced, whirling the torch
   That blazes red from the fennel-wand in his grasp,
   And with shouts he rouses the scattered bands,
   Sets their feet dancing,

τρυφερόν ⟨τε⟩ πλόκαμον εἰς αἰθέρα ῥίπτων. 150
ἅμα δ' εὐάσμασι τοιάδ' ἐπιβρέμει·
Ὦ ἴτε βάκχαι,
[ὦ] ἴτε βάκχαι,
Τμώλου χρυσορόου χλιδᾷ
μέλπετε τὸν Διόνυσον 155
βαρυβρόμων ὑπὸ τυμπάνων,
εὔια τὸν εὔιον ἀγαλλόμεναι θεὸν
ἐν Φρυγίαισι βοαῖς ἐνοπαῖσί τε,
λωτὸς ὅταν εὐκέλαδος 160
ἱερὸς ἱερὰ παίγματα βρέμῃ, σύνοχα
φοιτάσιν εἰς ὄρος εἰς ὄρος· ἡδομέ- 165
να δ' ἄρα, πῶλος ὅπως ἅμα ματέρι
φορβάδι, κῶλον ἄγει ταχύπουν σκιρτήμασι βάκχα.

4.9 Euripides, *The Bacchae* 215–25, 248–62

Πεν. ἔκδημος ὢν μὲν τῆσδ' ἐτύγχανον χθονός, 215
κλύω δὲ νεοχμὰ τήνδ' ἀνὰ πτόλιν κακά,
γυναῖκας ἡμῖν δώματ' ἐκλελοιπέναι
πλασταῖσι βακχείαισιν, ἐν δὲ δασκίοις
ὄρεσι θοάζειν, τὸν νεωστὶ δαίμονα
Διόνυσον, ὅστις ἔστι, τιμώσας χοροῖς· 220
πλήρεις δὲ θιάσοις ἐν μέσοισιν ἑστάναι
κρατῆρας, ἄλλην δ' ἄλλοσ' εἰς ἐρημίαν
πτώσσουσαν εὐναῖς ἀρσένων ὑπηρετεῖν,
πρόφασιν μὲν ὡς δὴ μαινάδας θυοσκόους,
τὴν δ' Ἀφροδίτην πρόσθ' ἄγειν τοῦ Βακχίου. 225

ἀτὰρ τόδ' ἄλλο θαῦμα, τὸν τερασκόπον
ἐν ποικίλαισι νεβρίσι Τειρεσίαν ὁρῶ
πατέρα τε μητρὸς τῆς ἐμῆς—πολὺν γέλων— 250
νάρθηκι βακχεύοντ'· ἀναίνομαι, πάτερ,
τὸ γῆρας ὑμῶν εἰσορῶν νοῦν οὐκ ἔχον.
οὐκ ἀποτινάξεις κισσόν; οὐκ ἐλευθέραν
θύρσου μεθήσεις χεῖρ', ἐμῆς μητρὸς πάτερ;
σὺ ταῦτ' ἔπεισας, Τειρεσία· τόνδ' αὖ θέλεις 255
τὸν δαίμον' ἀνθρώποισιν ἐσφέρων νέον
σκοπεῖν πτερωτοὺς κἀμπύρων μισθοὺς φέρειν.
εἰ μή σε γῆρας πολιὸν ἐξερρύετο,
καθῆσ' ἂν ἐν βάκχαισι δέσμιος μέσαις,

As he shakes his delicate locks to the wild wind.
And amidst the frenzy of song he shouts like thunder:
'On, on! Run, dance, delirious, possessed!
You, the beauty and grace of golden Tmolus,
Sing to the rattle of thunderous drums,
Sing for joy,
Praise Dionysus, god of joy!
Shout like Phrygians, sing out the tunes you know,
While the sacred pure-toned flute
Vibrates the air with holy merriment,
In time with the pulse of the feet that flock
To the mountains, to the mountains!'
And, like a foal with its mother at pasture,
Runs and leaps for joy every daughter of Bacchus.

4.9 Euripides, *The Bacchae* 215–25, 248–62

PENTHEUS: I've been away from Thebes, as it happens; but I've heard the news—this extraordinary scandal in the city. Our women, I discover, have abandoned their homes on some pretence of Bacchic worship, and go gadding about in the woods on the mountain side, dancing in honour of this upstart god Dionysus, whoever he may be. They tell me, in the midst of each group of revellers stands a bowl full of wine; and the women go creeping off this way and that to lonely places and there give themselves to lecherous men, under the excuse that they are Maenad priestesses; though in their ritual Aphrodite comes before Bacchus.

He turns to go, and sees CADMUS *and* TEIRESIAS.
Why, look! another miracle! Here's the prophet Teiresias, and my mother's father, playing the Bacchant, in dappled fawnskin and carrying fennel-wands! Well, there's a sight for laughter! (*But he is raging, not laughing.*] Sir, I am ashamed to see two men of your age with so little sense of decency. Come, you are my grandfather: throw away your garland, get rid of that thyrsus. *You* persuaded him into this, Teiresias. No doubt you hope that, when you have introduced this new god to the people, you will be his appointed seer, you will collect the fees for sacrifices. Your grey hairs are your protection; otherwise you should sit with all these crazy females in prison, for encouraging such pernicious performances.

τελετὰς πονηρὰς εἰσάγων· γυναιξὶ γὰρ 260
ὅπου βότρυος ἐν δαιτὶ γίγνεται γάνος,
οὐχ ὑγιὲς οὐδὲν ἔτι λέγω τῶν ὀργίων.

4.10 Euripides, *The Bacchae* 298–305, 309–27

Τειρ.   μάντις δ' ὁ δαίμων ὅδε· τὸ γὰρ βακχεύσιμον
καὶ τὸ μανιῶδες μαντικὴν πολλὴν ἔχει·
ὅταν γὰρ ὁ θεὸς ἐς τὸ σῶμ' ἔλθῃ πολύς, 300
λέγειν τὸ μέλλον τοὺς μεμηνότας ποιεῖ.
Ἄρεώς τε μοῖραν μεταλαβὼν ἔχει τινά·
στρατὸν γὰρ ἐν ὅπλοις ὄντα κἀπὶ τάξεσιν
φόβος διεπτόησε πρὶν λόγχης θιγεῖν.
μανία δὲ καὶ τοῦτ' ἐστὶ Διονύσου πάρα. 305

  ἀλλ' ἐμοί, Πενθεῦ, πιθοῦ·
μὴ τὸ κράτος αὔχει δύναμιν ἀνθρώποις ἔχειν, 310
μηδ', ἢν δοκῇς μέν, ἡ δὲ δόξα σου νοσῇ,
φρονεῖν δόκει τι· τὸν θεὸν δ' ἐς γῆν δέχου
καὶ σπένδε καὶ βάκχευε καὶ στέφου κάρα.
οὐχ ὁ Διόνυσος σωφρονεῖν ἀναγκάσει
γυναῖκας ἐς τὴν Κύπριν, ἀλλ' ἐν τῇ φύσει 315
[τὸ σωφρονεῖν ἔνεστιν εἰς τὰ πάντ' ἀεί]
τοῦτο σκοπεῖν χρή· καὶ γὰρ ἐν βακχεύμασιν
οὖσ' ἥ γε σώφρων οὐ διαφθαρήσεται.
ὁρᾷς, σὺ χαίρεις, ὅταν ἐφεστῶσιν πύλαις
πολλοί, τὸ Πενθέως δ' ὄνομα μεγαλύνῃ πόλις· 320
κἀκεῖνος, οἶμαι, τέρπεται τιμώμενος.
ἐγὼ μὲν οὖν καὶ Κάδμος, ὃν σὺ διαγελᾷς,
κισσῷ τ' ἐρεψόμεσθα καὶ χορεύσομεν,
πολιὰ ξυνωρίς, ἀλλ' ὅμως χορευτέον,
κοὐ θεομαχήσω σῶν λόγων πεισθεὶς ὕπο. 325
μαίνῃ γὰρ ὡς ἄλγιστα, κοὔτε φαρμάκοις
ἄκη λάβοις ἂν οὔτ' ἄνευ τούτων νοσεῖς.

4.11 Euripides, *Hippolytus* 176–214

Τρ.   ὦ κακὰ θνητῶν στυγεραί τε νόσοι·
τί σ' ἐγὼ δράσω, τί δὲ μὴ δράσω;
τόδε σοι φέγγος, λαμπρὸς ὅδ' αἰθήρ,
ἔξω δὲ δόμων ἤδη νοσερᾶς
δέμνια κοίτης. 180

As for women, my opinion is this: when the sparkle of sweet wine appears at their feasts, no good can be expected from their ceremonies.

4.10 Euripides, *The Bacchae* 298–305, 309–27

TEIRESIAS: The god is a prophet: for Bacchic ecstasy and madness are full of prophecy When the god enters the body in strength, he makes those possessed speak the future. He shares too a part of Ares: fear has sometimes scattered an army, ready armed and in battle formation, before a spear has been brandished. This madness too is from Dionysus.

Come, Pentheus, listen to me: do not boast that force has power over humans: nor, even if you think so—but your opinion is sick—should you think you are wise. Receive the god into the country and pour libations to him and celebrate his rites and garland your head. Dionysus will not compel women to be temperate where love is concerned: that lies in their nature. But you must consider this. A chaste woman will not be corrupted in the Bacchic rites. See: you are pleased when many stand before the gates, and the city glorifies the name of Pentheus. So too he, I think, takes delight in being honoured. So then I and Cadmus, whom you make fun of, will wear the ivy-wreath and will dance, grey-haired both of us and yet we must dance. And I shall never fight against the gods, persuaded by arguments of yours. For you are most painfully mad: nor will you be cured by spells—and nor are you ill without them.

4.11 Euripides, *Hippolytus* 176–214

NURSE: Oh, the troubles mortals have, the hateful illnesses! What shall I do for you? What shall I not? Here is daylight and here the bright sky, and your sickbed stands now outside the house. For to come out here was all you talked of. But soon you will hurry back into your chamber, for you soon slip from contentment and find

δεῦρο γὰρ ἐλθεῖν πᾶν ἔπος ἦν coι,
τάχα δ' ἐc θαλάμουc cπεύcειc τὸ πάλιν.
ταχὺ γὰρ cφάλληι κοὐδενὶ χαίρειc,
οὐδέ c' ἀρέcκει τὸ παρόν, τὸ δ' ἀπὸν
φίλτερον ἡγῆι.   185
κρεῖccον δὲ νοcεῖν ἢ θεραπεύειν·
τὸ μέν ἐcτιν ἁπλοῦν, τῶι δὲ cυνάπτει
λύπη τε φρενῶν χερcίν τε πόνοc.
πᾶc δ' ὀδυνηρὸc βίοc ἀνθρώπων
κοὐκ ἔcτι πόνων ἀνάπαυcιc.   190
ἀλλ' ὅτι τοῦ ζῆν φίλτερον ἄλλο
cκότοc ἀμπίcχων κρύπτει νεφέλαιc.
δυcέρωτεc δὴ φαινόμεθ' ὄντεc
τοῦδ' ὅτι τοῦτο cτίλβει κατὰ γῆν
δι' ἀπειροcύνην ἄλλου βιότου   195
κοὐκ ἀπόδειξιν τῶν ὑπὸ γαίαc,
μύθοιc δ' ἄλλωc φερόμεcθα.
Φα.   αἴρετέ μου δέμαc, ὀρθοῦτε κάρα·
λέλυμαι μελέων cύνδεcμα φίλων.
λάβετ' εὐπήχειc χεῖραc, πρόπολοι.   200
βαρύ μοι κεφαλῆc ἐπίκρανον ἔχειν·
ἄφελ', ἀμπέταcον βόcτρυχον ὤμοιc.
Τρ.   θάρcει, τέκνον, καὶ μὴ χαλεπῶc
μετάβαλλε δέμαc·
ῥᾶιον δὲ νόcον μετά θ' ἡcυχίαc   205
καὶ γενναίου λήματοc οἴcειc.
μοχθεῖν δὲ βροτοῖcιν ἀνάγκη.
Φα.   αἰαῖ.
πῶc ἂν δροcερᾶc ἀπὸ κρηνῖδοc
καθαρῶν ὑδάτων πῶμ' ἀρυcαίμαν,
ὑπό τ' αἰγείροιc ἔν τε κομήτηι   210
λειμῶνι κλιθεῖc' ἀναπαυcαίμαν;
Τρ.   ὦ παῖ, τί θροεῖc·
οὐ μὴ παρ' ὄχλωι τάδε γηρύcηι,
μανίαc ἔποχον ῥίπτουcα λόγον;

joy in nothing, taking no pleasure in what is at hand but loving instead what you do not have. Better it is to be sick than to tend the sick. The first is a single thing, while the second joins grief of heart to toil of hand. But the life of mortals is wholly trouble, and there is no rest from toil. Anything we might love more than life is hid in a surrounding cloud of darkness, and we show ourselves unhappy lovers of whatever light there is that shines on earth because we are ignorant of another life and the world below is not revealed to us. We are aimlessly borne along by mere tales.

PHAEDRA: Raise up my body, hold my head erect! My limbs are unstrung! Take my fair arms, servants! It is a burden to have this headdress on my head. Take it off, spread my tresses on my shoulders!

NURSE: Courage, my child! Do not shift your body so violently. You will endure your sickness more easily with calm and nobility of heart. Mortals must endure trouble.

PHAEDRA: Oh, oh! How I long to draw a drink of pure water from a dewy spring and to take my rest lying under the poplar trees and in the uncut meadow!

NURSE: My child, what are these words of yours? Stop saying such things before the crowd, hurling wild words that are borne on madness!

5
The Historians

We can talk of historiography being invented in Greece in the work first of Herodotus and then of Thucydides in this sense, that their claim to attention and to prestige took a different form from that of any earlier writers. That claim was based on being able to give a true account of what happened, in Herodotus' case in the Persian Wars, in Thucydides' in the Peloponnesian War. Herodotus reconstructs the past, Thucydides deals with contemporary events. But both distance themselves from works that we should call fiction, the telling of stories that had nothing to do with real events, however much verisimilitude they could command. True, the connection and the distinction between 'myth' and 'logos' were, and remained, problematic, for 'myth' could cover any narrative account, fictional or not, and 'logos' equally could be used of any story, true or false. Nevertheless both Herodotus and Thucydides are at pains to justify their claim to record what actually happened. In neither case are their histories limited to mere descriptions of how it was. Both memorialize the past. Both have lessons to convey about what can be learned from it, and about human nature generally.

In a sense the claim to deliver the truth antedates Herodotus. This is not just a matter of Hesiod saying, in the *Theogony,* 26 ff., that the Muses, his inspiration, know, when they wish, how to speak the truth—for as he also says they can speak falsehoods that resemble the truth (Pucci 1977). But one of the earliest Greek prose-writers, Hecataeus, opened his work on *Genealogies* by contrasting what he has to say— which is true—with the many and absurd tales of the Greeks.

The Historians

That work, so far as we can judge from the fragments of it that have survived, adopts a rationalizing approach to myths and legends. But it did not attempt a narrative account of events over a period of time. Meanwhile the other lost work of Hecataeus we know about was more of a geographical account of the Mediterranean world than a historical survey. True, much of the earlier part of Herodotus' work is also 'geographical' (to use our category), especially his accounts of Egypt and Scythia. But they provide the background to the story of the Persians' attempt to conquer Greece.

It is not that the recording of events in Herodotus and Thucydides meets all or only the criteria that we might associate with modern historiography. The boundaries between genres in the ancient world scarcely ever coincide with ours. As Nicole Loraux put it, Thucydides is no colleague. But their claims include that of narrating what happened—as well as spelling out its significance. However, Herodotus also engages in aetiological explanations (for example of the Nile's flooding) that are similar to those we find in the Presocratic philosophers. Moreover both he and Thucydides have, as we shall see, a good deal to say about disease. There is, in both cases, an important overlap between their interests and those of the doctors we studied in Chapter 3.

Herodotus prides himself on the research, *historie*, he has undertaken, collecting and sifting stories about past events from a variety of witnesses. He contrasts occasions when he can speak confidently from personal experience, telling us what he has himself seen, with those where he is only reporting what he has been told (Hartog 1988). He often gives several different accounts of the same episode, specifying his sources and usually giving his own verdict in conclusion. We are to have confidence in him (so we are to understand) because he has done his homework and our confidence may be increased insofar as he tells us frankly about the limits of what he is sure about and where he has to admit he is baffled. We may note, in passing, that this parallels what happens in several of the Hippocratic treatises, where the authors freely confess their own ignorance of their patients' complaints and even their own inability to treat them (see above Ch. 3 n. 7).

We often find Herodotus casting doubt on tall stories, tales of humans with goats' feet (4. 25), Scythian stories about werewolves (4. 105), what the Egyptians say about the phoenix (2. 73). Sometimes he offers a rationalization of a mythical story, as when he glosses the popular belief that the vale of Tempe was the work of Poseidon by suggesting that it was brought about by an earthquake: so given that Poseidon is the earthshaker, that idea is reasonable (7. 129). Under the rules of double determination, those accounts are, of course, perfectly compatible, for the God can work *through* earthquakes.

A belief that wicked acts eventually get to be punished underlies many particular stories and in a sense is implied by the whole history. The overweening arrogance of the Persians in general and of Xerxes in particular gets its just deserts when they are defeated by the Greeks at Salamis and Plataea. One way in which Herodotus is half inclined to believe that god's retribution works is through disease. At 4. 202–5 [T 5.1] he recounts the fate of Pheretime who had punished the people of Barce for the murder of Arcesilaus by cutting off the breasts of the women and impaling the men on stakes round the city wall. Pheretime herself comes to a sticky end: she dies a horrible death 'her body seething with worms while she was still alive'. That elicits the comment from Herodotus that excessive retribution exacted by humans is hateful in the eyes of the gods.

Elsewhere too, when discussing the way the Agyllaeans were affected by crippling diseases (1. 167) or Pheros went blind (2. 111) or why the Enarieis in Scythia suffer from the 'female sickness' (1. 105) [T 5.2], he is inclined to see heaven at work. Thus the Agyllaeans had stoned the Phoceans to death, and when they consulted the oracle at Delphi as to why they and their animals were crippled, they were told to institute rites in honour of the Phoceans to make amends (here we have an aetiological element at work, for Herodotus says that those rites are still carried out). Pheros' blindness is connected with his having insulted the river Nile. However, that story is given in oratio obliqua, as something that has been reported to Herodotus, and it does not get his explicit endorsement.

The Enarieis case is particularly interesting as it can be compared with another account of what seems precisely the same affliction in the Hippocratic treatise *On Airs Waters Places* (ch. 22, *CMG* I 1 2, 72. 10ff. [T 5.3]) though there the writer calls them Anarieis. The Hippocratic author says that the impotence that affects these people comes from horseback-riding, which leads to varicose veins, which the Scythians treat by cutting the vein that runs behind the ear. But those veins (he believes) are linked to the seminal vessels, and cutting them causes impotence. He is clear, however, that the disease has nothing to do with gods.

Herodotus first says that the Scythians who robbed the temple of Heavenly Aphrodite at Ascalon were punished by the goddess with the female sickness and adds that their descendants still suffer from it. This is the reason the Scythians themselves give for their mysterious complaint and those who go to their country can see what it is like. True, Herodotus just tells this story as he says he has it from the Scythians, without giving his own view on the subject. Yet the contrast with the Hippocratic author is striking, for he goes out of his way to deny that the gods were involved. Like the author of *On the Sacred Disease* he asserts that this disease is no more of divine origin than any other. 'Each of them has a nature of its own, and none arises without its natural cause'—and this peculiar affliction of the Scythians is no exception.

A number of more complex cases allow us to see the tension, in Herodotus, between acceptance of traditional accounts and the rationalization of them, between theodicy and naturalism. The accounts of the madness of Cambyses and of Cleomenes illustrate how he hedges his bets. Cambyses' behaviour, in attempting to kill the calf sacred to Apis (3. 28–30) [T 5.4], was enough to label him mad, and the

Egyptians were convinced, so Herodotus tells us, that it was because of that sacrilegious act that he went mad. Various other extravagant acts follow, including against his own kin, ending with him kicking his pregnant sister (whom he had married) and causing her to miscarry. Herodotus then comments (3. 33): 'These were the acts of a madman, whether or not his madness was due to his treatment of Apis' (in fact Herodotus had said that even before that, Cambyses was far from sound in mind). 'It may indeed have been the result of any one of the evils that affect humans, and there is a story that he had suffered from childbirth from the serious disease that some call sacred. There would then be nothing strange in the fact that since a serious disease affected his body, so too he was not well in his mind.' On the one hand, the order in which these stories are presented may favour the view that Herodotus' own conclusion was that Cambyses' complaint had a natural cause. On the other, it is clear that this does not exonerate him, in Herodotus' eyes, for his acts of savagery are still *his* work.

The case of Cleomenes, king of Sparta, is obviously closer to home and Herodotus' account (6. 75) [T 5.5] is appreciably more complex. As evidence that he was mad Herodotus first cites his striking a Spartan and then his self-mutilation, ending in his death. Most Greeks, he continues, thought that this grizzly end was due to his having suborned the Pythian priestess to get her to deny that Demaratus was the son of Ariston. That denial contributed to Demaratus being deposed as king—as Herodotus had just recounted (6. 65 ff). But both the Athenians and the Argives had a different explanation. The Athenians said it was because Cleomenes had destroyed the precinct of Demeter and Persephone when he invaded Eleusis, and the Argives that it was punishment for the acts of treachery and sacrilege he had committed when he killed those who had taken refuge in the temple of Argos, after a battle, and had burnt the temple down. That prompts Herodotus to give us the whole of that story, after which he returns to the explanation of Cleomenes' madness that the

Spartans gave (6. 84) [T 5.6]. They deny that that was a punishment from heaven. Rather it came from his habit of drinking his wine neat—a custom he had picked up from associating with Scythians. The Spartans' view is the only entirely naturalistic one mentioned. Moreover Herodotus concludes his whole account by giving his own opinion on the matter, namely that 'Cleomenes came to grief as a punishment for what he did to Demaratus'. That is not the precise wording of what he had said 'many of the Greeks' believed, but it certainly supports the view that his madness was a result of divine retribution.

Herodotus is evidently inclined, on occasion, to endorse the traditional belief that being afflicted with disease—physical or mental—may be the gods' doing, the retribution they exact for some offence to them or other wrongdoing. The Cleomenes story shows both how widespread some such idea was—at least according to Herodotus' report of what the Athenians and Argives and other Greeks believed—and also that there was frequent disagreement about particular cases. Even if a lot of Greeks diagnosed divine punishment, they certainly did not agree about what that punishment was for exactly. Herodotus himself sees heaven at work in the unfolding of events and gives a moral twist to particular stories when he can.

At the same time he sets himself up as critic and judge of other people's stories, playing them off against one another on some occasions, often expressing his doubts on the grounds of their implausibility, or the unreliability of those who recounted them. That includes criticizing some of the ideas that his predecessor Hecataeus had put forward. He is probably in mind when Herodotus criticizes as ridiculous those who give accounts of circuits of the earth in which the earth is round, as if drawn by compasses, with Europe and Asia of the same size (4. 36, cf. 42). Yet when Herodotus himself discusses the source of the Nile, he too thinks it plausible to assume a certain symmetry between the great river Ister (Danube) running across Europe and the Nile across Africa—

allowing the inference that the great river reported in West Africa (the Niger) was in fact the upper reaches of the Nile. Here is yet another example of rivalry between competing Masters of Truth. Herodotus' claim to superiority rests on his insistence on the comprehensiveness of his research and the soundness of his judgement. But where disease is concerned, we have seen what a wide range of opinions would have been entertained by members of his audience on their provenance and causation, as well as how diverse were the views of Herodotus himself on the subject. It is clear that his tactic is to keep his options open, giving naturalistic explanations on occasion, but being ready to invoke the hand of heaven where that seemed compatible with his understanding of the possibilities of divine retribution.

Yet Herodotus, while not named, is in turn implicitly criticized by his successor, Thucydides, where the topics of health and disease take on a particular resonance and where we can detect further rivalries, not just with other historiographers, but with the naturalistic doctors represented in our Hippocratic texts. Just as the Hippocratic *Epidemics* contain, in addition to individual case histories, accounts of epidemic diseases that struck whole communities on particular occasions associated with certain climatic and other circumstances, so too we have a full description of the plague that struck Athens, first in Thucydides 2. 47–54, and then more briefly in 3. 87.

Of course this was a significant factor in the war, both because of the loss of life at Athens and because of the effects the plague had on Athenian morale. So Thucydides was in duty bound to include some discussion. Yet he does so, as we shall see, for more than just those circumstantial reasons. His description invites comparison—and contrast—with those in the *Epidemics*. In the background we should never forget that a Greek reader will be thinking of that other emblematic account of the plague, in the first book of the *Iliad*. Moreover the plague plays an important role in the justification of Thucydides' historiography itself. Just as diseases can be diagnosed and recognized when they come again, so political ills have their objective causes. Since human nature remains broadly the same, learning the lessons of the past is important for future conduct. The role of the historian is thus to provide a 'possession for always' (1. 22) [T 5.7].

No less than four considerations, then, lead to Thucydides giving the plague such prominence. First it was an important factor in the war, which led, secondly, to moral degradation and depression. Thirdly it gives Thucydides a chance to show that he knows as much about this as any doctor. Fourthly and most importantly, it provides him with a model for objective —'scientific'—historiography, for history (broadly) repeats itself (as human nature remains the same) just as diseases do.

Thucydides tells us that he himself suffered from the disease and saw others who did so. Anyone, he says (2. 48) [T 5.8], whether doctor or lay person, may, according to their own opinions, say what the origin of it is likely to have been and what causes they think had the power to bring about so great a change. We may note in passing that change is often mentioned among the causes of diseases in Hippocratic treatises.[1] So as one who survived the plague, Thucydides presents himself as a reliable witness to it, just as much an authority on the subject as the doctors who, as he goes on to explain, were quite at a loss as to how to treat it.

But that is not the only point. He gives us an explicit reason for his account. 'I shall give a statement of what it was like, which people can study in case it should ever attack again, to equip themselves with foreknowledge so that they shall not fail to recognize it' (2. 48) [T 5.8]. If we turn to some of the

[1] Changes in the seasons are associated with the onset of diseases in such Hippocratic texts as *Aphorisms* III 1, L IV 486. 4 ff. (cf. 2–23), *On Airs Waters Places* ch. 11 *CMG* I 1 2, 52. 15 ff. (cf. chs. 1, 24. 3 ff., and 10, 46. 16 ff.), and changes in the wind in particular are held responsible for certain complaints in *On the Sacred Disease* ch. 13 Littré VI 384. 4 ff., ch. 16 Jones (cf. *On Airs Waters Places* ch. 5, *CMG* I 1 2, 32. 6 ff.). In the treatise *On Humours* ch. 17, L V 498. 7 ff., it is suggested that one can infer not only likely diseases from changes in the weather, but also in certain circumstances changes in the weather from diseases.

passages in which he speaks about the motives for his own history, we can see the parallelism. His history, unlike that of others that were produced as much for entertainment as for enlightenment, is a 'possession for always'. Why? Because it reveals the motives at work in human behaviour, the consequences of human ambition and greed, for instance, the dire effects of war itself on morality and morale. In book 3. 82 [T 5.9] when he talks of the degrading effects of civil war, *stasis*, he spells the point out. Such grave sufferings come upon cities because of their internal strife, sufferings such as happen and always will happen 'as long as human nature is the same', though they will be more or less severe according to the circumstances of each case. His whole history is, one may say, an account of human political misfortunes that will enable anyone to diagnose and anticipate them when they recur—just as his description of the plague will enable diagnosis and prognosis of that disease to be made. In this context the detailed description of the plague stands as a model for what he claims for his whole work. Both are validated on the assumption that they deal with *natures*—with the regularities of physical diseases mirrored in the regularities of political troubles that are the consequence of human nature being the same.

Although the point should not be exaggerated, the locations of the two main references to the plague in his history give them added dramatic force. At 2. 35 ff. we are given the funeral speech which Pericles pronounces over those who died in battle during the previous year. Nothing could be more poignant than the juxtaposition between Pericles' great paean of praise for Athens—the educator of Greece, the shining example of successful democracy, gloriously combining freedom and responsibility—and the paragraph that follows at 2. 47 [T 5.8] which speaks of the Spartan invasion of Attica and the first onslaught of the plague. It was said to have broken out previously, in Lemnos and elsewhere—but nowhere on the scale on which it affected Athens. The doctors were unable out of ignorance to treat the disease (and they themselves especially died from the disease as they were particularly exposed to it) nor was any other human art of any use. As for those who made supplication at the sanctuaries or resorted to divination and so on, that was all completely futile, and at the end people gave up all such recourses, being overwhelmed by the disaster.

The first account of the plague gains added significance by the contrast with Pericles' optimism. The second at 3. 87 follows Thucydides' account of the moral degradation that was one of the effects of the war, the passage I cited before. Here the stark juxtaposition between moral and physical calamities gives added resonance to both. The moral degradation is like a plague: the plague is one aspect of the *total* degradation that afflicted those who were caught up in the war.

By telling us straight away that the doctors could not cope, and then that he himself suffered from the disease, Thucydides stakes his claim to talk about it. Whether or not he was familiar with the type of description we find in the Hippocratic *Epidemics*, that we mentioned before, he gives us his account as though it was just as worthy of attention as theirs. The similarities and the differences between what we read in Thucydides and in those Hippocratic texts, which have been studied by Parry 1969 especially, are striking. In the background we may recall other occasions when Masters of Truth and others offered their own diagnoses of diseases and plagues, not just the rival views of maladies we have just been considering from Herodotus, but those both real and imaginary that have punctuated our account in each of the preceding chapters. But the implicit rivalry between Thucydides and the Hippocratics is particularly striking since their approaches had so much in common.

First Thucydides' description resembles one of the so-called constitutions in the *Epidemics* that set out the general state of health in the year in question. 'It was universally agreed that this particular year was exceptionally free from disease as far as other afflictions were concerned' (2. 49). Then there is a search for the external or triggering cause, the *prophasis*. Sometimes, for no apparent *prophasis*, suddenly people who had been in good health were seized by fever, redness and inflammation of the eyes, and so on. The parallels here include several Hippocratic cases where the presence or absence of a *prophasis* is noted.[2] We should also recall that *prophasis* is the term contrasted with *aitia* when Thucydides speaks of the causes of the outbreak of hostilities between Athens and the Peloponnesians in 1. 23. There he contrasts the truest *prophasis*, the real underlying factor, with the alleged reasons, the *aitiai*.

The absence of a *prophasis* is noted, but this leads into a full account of the signs and symptoms of an attack. Much of the vocabulary is familiar from our Hippocratic texts, heat or fever (here *thermai*: i.e. a high temperature), redness of the eyes (*eruthemata*) and their inflammation *(phlogosis)*, the throat and tongue becoming bloody, the breath fetid, sneezing, hoarseness, and coughing. When the disease got down to the stomach, Thucydides continues, there was 'every kind of evacuation of bile named by doctors'—which we may see as a dig at excessive elaboration of humoral theories and nomenclature. Convulsions follow, the colour of the body is noted (not pale, but reddish, livid) and its breaking out in small blisters and sores. As in many case histories in the *Epidemics* psychological factors are noted. Thucydides remarks on loss of memory (2. 49) and especially despondency (51).

He even goes along with the significance of what the Hippocratics called critical days. There are many rival theories of such periodicities in different Hippocratic works, some associating crises and exacerbations or remissions with particular sequences of odd-numbered or even-numbered days (counting from the onset of the disease), others offering other patterns (Lloyd 1991, ch. 9, 214–16), and many of the individual case histories record quite complex patterns of such crises, as they set out the progress of each patient's condition

---

[2] One instance from the *Epidemics* case histories where a particular *prophasis*, ('a grief with a reason for it') is noted at the outset of a complaint, is case 11 of the second series in *Epidemics* III, L III 134. 1 ff. Rawlings 1975 discusses the range of the use of this term in Hippocratic and other texts.

day by day. But Thucydides mentions that most died on the seventh or ninth day (49).

However what quite definitely marks out Thucydides' account from any that we find in our Hippocratic writers is first and foremost his dwelling on the reaction to the experience of the plague as a whole. This is not just a matter of the despondency that affected many patients (which can, as noted, be paralleled in the Hippocratics[3]). Thucydides says that as soon as anyone became aware that they were affected they gave themselves up for lost (2. 51). Then he tells us that those who recovered from the plague recognized that they would not be again affected by it—and promptly thought of themselves as invulnerable to every kind of disease. But he especially underlines the lawlessness, *anomia*, and disregard for all decency, that followed the plague. People buried their dead any way they could (52), ignoring what was right and proper, even putting their dead on someone else's funeral pyre. This sudden change of fortune led them to abandon all sense of moderation and shame. They lived for the pleasures of the moment, unrestrained by fear of gods or the laws of humans. Seeing that everyone suffered alike, they judged that it made no difference whether one was pious or not, as all alike could be seen dying. No one expected to live long enough, to be called to account or to pay the penalty for their misdeeds.

Once again the parallel with Thucydides' comments in book 3 is suggestive. There we learn that moral degradation stems from political factionalism. Here in the account of the plague we are told that immorality of a different type can be a reaction to the awful sufferings of epidemic disease. There in book 3 he claims to have uncovered what will be true so long as human nature remains the same. In book 2 he makes the assumption that the plague may well recur. As noted, he claims his account is useful to enable people to recognize it should it recur.

[3] Despondency is noted, but rather as a symptom than as a reaction to disease, in such Hippocratic case histories as case 6 of the first series, and cases 11 and 15 of the second in *Epidemics* III, L III 5. 28, 134. 4, 146. 4.

Thucydides is the diagnostician of natural ills and moral ones, the diagnostician, even if he is in no position to produce the remedies for either type of misfortune, and in that respect is as helpless as the doctors facing the plague. Yet one final point of difference separates him from the authors of the constitutions in the *Epidemics*. While they often give highly differentiated diagnoses, identifying different types of complaint affecting different groups of patients (the young, for example, rather than the old, or males rather than females, or the bilious rather than the phlegmatic), Thucydides' assumption is that the plague has a *single* general pathology. He speaks of *the* disease, *nosos* at 2. 47 and 50, *nosema* at 51, *nosos* again when the plague returns at 3. 87. True, he notes that different people's reactions differed—some after all survived while many succumbed. But he writes as if he were dealing with *one* disease.

We can see why. It is only if there is a single determinate syndrome to which the various complex signs and symptoms can be related that his claim to provide useful information, to be able later to recognize its recurrence, can be sustained. We can surely not fail to be struck by the similarity, and again the difference, between that claim and those made by priests and prophets and others who have figured in our story so far, from Calchas in the *Iliad* to Teiresias in the *Oedipus Tyrannus*. They had a special reputation for superior wisdom, for knowing more than others, for being able to say why the plague had struck, and what was to be done about it. But their causal accounts related to gods and their treatments to ritual purification. Thucydides likewise knows as much as anyone about the Athenian plague, and describes it in detail and with care, concentrating, indeed, on description, rather than attempting to identify the cause or causes as such. Yet he does so in a totally naturalistic vein, even while he discounts the efforts that both supernaturalistic and naturalist healers offered. The only help that can be offered is the knowledge that will enable the plague to be recognized again. But then foreknowledge is itself valuable, not just in the domain of physical sickness, but in that of the moral degradation that can infect social and political life through and through. And that, after all, provides one of the main reasons why he wrote his history.

CHAPTER 5 TEXTS

5.1 Herodotus 4. 202–3. 1, 205

202 τοὺς μὲν νυν αἰτιωτάτους τῶν Βαρκαίων ἡ Φερετίμη, ἐπείτε οἱ ἐκ τῶν Περσέων παρεδόθησαν, ἀνεσκολόπισε κύκλῳ τοῦ τείχεος, τῶν δέ σφι γυναικῶν τοὺς μαζοὺς ἀποταμοῦσα περιέστιξε καὶ τούτοισι τὸ τεῖχος·
2 τοὺς δὲ λοιποὺς τῶν Βαρκαίων ληίην ἐκέλευσε θέσθαι τοὺς Πέρσας, πλὴν ὅσοι αὐτῶν ἦσαν Βαττιάδαι τε καὶ τοῦ φόνου οὐ μεταίτιοι· τούτοισι δὲ τὴν
203 πόλιν ἐπέτρεψε ἡ Φερετίμη. τοὺς ὦν δὴ λοιποὺς τῶν Βαρκαίων οἱ Πέρσαι ἀνδραποδισάμενοι ἀπήισαν ὀπίσω.

205 Οὐ μὲν οὐδὲ ἡ Φερετίμη εὖ τὴν ζόην κατέπλεξε. ὡς γὰρ δὴ τάχιστα ἐκ τῆς Λιβύης τεισαμένη τοὺς Βαρκαίους ἀπενόστησε ἐς τὴν Αἴγυπτον, ἀπέθανε κακῶς· ζῶσα γὰρ εὐλέων ἐξέζεσε, ὡς ἄρα ἀνθρώποισι αἱ λίην ἰσχυραὶ τιμωρίαι πρὸς θεῶν ἐπίφθονοι γίνονται. ἡ μὲν δὴ Φερετίμης τῆς Βάττου τοιαύτη τε καὶ τοσαύτη τιμωρίη ἐγένετο ἐς Βαρκαίους.

5.2 Herodotus 1. 105. 4

105 4 τοῖσι δὲ τῶν Σκυθέων συλήσασι τὸ ἱρὸν τὸ ἐν Ἀσκάλωνι καὶ τοῖσι τούτων αἰεὶ ἐκγόνοισι ἐνέσκηψε ἡ θεὸς θήλεαν νοῦσον· ὥστε ἅμα λέγουσί τε οἱ Σκύθαι διὰ τοῦτό σφεας νοσέειν, καὶ ὁρᾶν παρ' ἑωυτοῖσι τοὺς ἀπικνεομένους ἐς τὴν Σκυθικὴν χώρην ὡς διακέαται τοὺς καλέουσι ἐνάρεας οἱ Σκύθαι.

5.3 Airs, Waters, Places ch. 22

XXII Ἔτι τε πρὸς τούτοισιν εὐνουχίαι γίνονται οἱ πλεῖστοι ἐν Σκύθῃσι καὶ γυναικεῖα ἐργάζονται καὶ ὡς αἱ γυναῖκες διαιτεῦνται διαλέγονταί τε ὁμοίως· καλεῦνταί τε οἱ τοιοῦτοι Ἀναριεῖς. οἱ μὲν οὖν ἐπιχώριοι τὴν αἰτίην προστιθέασι θεῷ καὶ σέβονται τούτους τοὺς ἀνθρώπους καὶ προσκυνέουσι, δεδοικότες περὶ ἑωυτῶν ἕκαστοι. ἐμοὶ δὲ καὶ αὐτῷ δοκεῖ ταῦτα τὰ πάθεα θεῖα εἶναι καὶ τἆλλα πάντα καὶ οὐδὲν ἕτερον ἑτέρου θειότερον οὐδὲ ἀνθρωπινώτερον, ἀλλὰ πάντα ὁμοῖα καὶ πάντα θεῖα. ἕκαστον δὲ αὐτῶν ἔχει φύσιν τὴν ἑωυτοῦ καὶ οὐδὲν ἄνευ φύσιος γίνεται. καὶ τοῦτο τὸ πάθος ὥς

CHAPTER 5 TEXTS

5.1 Herodotus 4. 202–3. 1, 205

The men of Barca who were most deeply involved in the murder of Arcesilaus were delivered up by the Persians to Pheretima, who impaled them on stakes all round the city wall. She also cut off their wives' breasts, and stuck those up, too, in the same position. The rest of the people she gave over to the Persian soldiery to pillage, with the exception of those who belonged to the house of Battus and were not implicated in the murder. To these last she gave control of the town. Everyone else the Persians reduced to slavery, and then started on their march for home.

A fitting conclusion to this story is the manner of Pheretima's death—for the web of her life was not woven happily to the end. No sooner had she returned to Egypt after her revenge upon the people of Barca, than she died a horrible death, her body seething with worms while she was still alive. Thus this daughter of Battus, by the nature and severity of her punishment of the Barcaeans, showed how true it is that all excess in such things draws down upon men the anger of the gods.

5.2 Herodotus 1. 105. 4

The Scythians who robbed the temple at Ascalon were punished by the goddess with the infliction of what is called the 'female disease', and their descendants still suffer from it. This is the reason the Scythians give for this mysterious complaint, and travellers to the country can see what it is like. The Scythians call those who suffer from it 'Enarees'.

5.3 *Airs, Waters, Places* ch. 22

Moreover, the great majority among the Scythians become impotent, do women's work, live like women and converse accordingly. Such men they call Anaries. Now the natives put the blame on to Heaven, and respect and worship these creatures, each fearing for himself. I too think that these diseases are divine, and so are all others, no one being more divine or more human than any other; all are alike, and all divine. Each of them has a nature of its own, and none arises without its natural cause. How, in my opinion, this disease arises I will explain. The habit of riding causes swellings at

μοι δοκεῖ γίνεσθαι φράσω· ὑπὸ τῆς ἱππασίης αὐτοὺς κέδματα λαμβάνει, ἅτε αἰεὶ κρεμαμένων ἀπὸ τῶν ἵππων τοῖς ποσίν· ἔπειτα ἀποχωλοῦνται καὶ ἑλκοῦνται τὰ ἰσχία, οἳ ἂν σφόδρα νοσήσωσιν. ἰῶνται δὲ σφᾶς αὐτοὺς τρόπῳ τοιῷδε. ὁκόταν γὰρ ἄρχηται ἡ νοῦσος, ὄπισθεν τοῦ ὠτὸς ἑκατέρου φλέβα τάμνουσιν. ὁκόταν δὲ ἀπορρυῇ τὸ αἷμα, ὕπνος ὑπολαμβάνει ὑπὸ ἀσθενείης καὶ καθεύδουσιν. ἔπειτα ἀνεγείρονται, οἱ μέν τινες ὑγιέες ἐόντες, οἱ δ' οὔ. ἐμοὶ μὲν οὖν δοκεῖ ἐν ταύτῃ τῇ ἰήσει διαφθείρεσθαι ὁ γόνος. εἰσὶ γὰρ παρὰ τὰ ὦτα φλέβες, ἃς ἐάν τις ἐπιτάμῃ, ἄγονοι γίνονται οἱ ἐπιτμηθέντες. ταύτας τοίνυν μοι δοκέουσι τὰς φλέβας ἐπιτάμνειν. οἱ δὲ μετὰ ταῦτα ἐπειδὰν ἀφίκωνται παρὰ γυναῖκας καὶ μὴ οἷοί τ' ἔωσι χρῆσθαί σφισιν, τὸ πρῶτον οὐκ ἐνθυμεῦνται, ἀλλ' ἡσυχίην ἔχουσι. ὁκόταν δὲ δὶς καὶ τρὶς καὶ πλεονάκις αὐτοῖσι πειρωμένοισι μηδὲν ἀλλοιότερον ἀποβαίνῃ, νομίσαντές τι ἡμαρτηκέναι τῷ θεῷ, ὃν ἐπαιτιῶνται, ἐνδύονται στολὴν γυναικείην καταγνόντες ἑωυτῶν ἀνανδρείην. γυναικίζουσί τε καὶ ἐργάζονται μετὰ τῶν γυναικῶν ἃ καὶ ἐκεῖναι.

Τοῦτο δὲ πάσχουσι Σκυθέων οἱ πλούσιοι, οὐχ οἱ κάκιστοι ἀλλ' οἱ εὐγενέστατοι καὶ ἰσχὺν πλείστην κεκτημένοι, διὰ τὴν ἱππασίην, οἱ δὲ πένητες ἧσσον· οὐ γὰρ ἱππάζονται. καίτοι ἐχρῆν, ἐπεὶ θειότερον τοῦτο τὸ νόσευμα τῶν λοιπῶν ἐστιν, οὐ τοῖς γενναιοτάτοις τῶν Σκυθέων καὶ τοῖς πλουσιωτάτοις προσπίπτειν μούνοις, ἀλλὰ τοῖς ἅπασιν ὁμοίως, καὶ μᾶλλον τοῖσιν ὀλίγα κεκτημένοισιν, εἰ δὴ τιμώμενοι χαίρουσιν οἱ θεοὶ καὶ θαυμαζόμενοι ὑπ' ἀνθρώπων καὶ ἀντὶ τούτων χάριτας ἀποδιδόασιν. εἰκὸς γὰρ τοὺς μὲν πλουσίους θύειν πολλὰ τοῖς θεοῖς καὶ ἀνατιθέναι ἀναθήματα ἐόντων χρημάτων πολλῶν καὶ τιμᾶν, τοὺς δὲ πένητας ἧσσον διὰ τὸ μὴ ἔχειν, ἔπειτα καὶ ἐπιμεμφομένους ὅτι οὐ διδόασι χρήματα αὐτοῖσιν, ὥστε τῶν τοιούτων ἁμαρτιῶν τὰς ζημίας τοὺς ὀλίγα κεκτημένους φέρειν μᾶλλον ἢ τοὺς πλουσίους. ἀλλὰ γάρ, ὥσπερ καὶ πρότερον ἔλεξα, θεῖα μὲν καὶ ταῦτά ἐστιν ὁμοίως τοῖς ἄλλοις· γίνεται δὲ κατὰ φύσιν ἕκαστα.

5.4 Herodotus 3. 28. 2–30. 1

28 ὁ δὲ Ἆπις οὗτος ὁ Ἔπαφος γίνεται μόσχος ἐκ βοὸς ἥτις οὐκέτι οἵη τε γίνεται ἐς γαστέρα ἄλλον βάλλεσθαι γόνον. Αἰγύπτιοι δὲ λέγουσι σέλας ἐκ τοῦ οὐρανοῦ ἐπὶ τὴν βοῦν κατίσχειν καί μιν ἐκ τούτου τίκτειν τὸν Ἆπιν.

3 ἔχει δὲ ὁ μόσχος οὗτος ὁ Ἆπις καλεόμενος σημήια τοιάδε, ἐὼν μέλας ἐπὶ μὲν τῷ μετώπῳ λευκὸν τετράγωνον, ἐπὶ δὲ τοῦ νώτου αἰετὸν εἰκασμένον,

29 ἐν δὲ τῇ οὐρῇ τὰς τρίχας διπλάς, ὑπὸ δὲ τῇ γλώσσῃ κάνθαρον. ὡς δὲ

the joints, because they are always astride their horses; in severe cases follow lameness and sores on the hips. They cure themselves in the following way. At the beginning of the disease they cut the vein behind each ear. When the blood has ceasd to flow faintness comes over them and they sleep. Afterwards they get up, some cured and some not. Now, in my opinion, by this treatment the seed is destroyed. For by the side of the ear are veins, to cut which causes impotence, and I believe that these are the veins which they cut. After this treatment, when the Scythians approach a woman but cannot have intercourse, at first they take no notice and think no more about it. But when two, three or even more attempts are attended with no better success, thinking that they have sinned against Heaven they attribute thereto the cause, and put on women's clothes, holding that they have lost their manhood. So they play the woman, and with the women do the same work as women do.

This affliction affects the rich Scythians because of their riding, not the lower classes but the upper, who possess the most strength; the poor, who do not ride, suffer less. But, if we suppose this disease to be more divine than any other, it ought to have attacked, not the highest and richest classes only of the Scythians, but all classes equally—or rather the poor especially, if indeed the gods are pleased to receive from men respect and worship, and repay these with favours. For naturally the rich, having great wealth, make many sacrifices to the gods, and offer many votive offerings, and honour them, all of which things the poor, owing to their poverty, are less able to do; besides, they blame the gods for not giving them wealth, so that the penalties for such sins are likely to be paid by the poor rather than by the rich. But the truth is, as I said above, these affections are neither more nor less divine than any others, and all and each are natural.

5.4 Herodotus 3. 28. 2–30. 1

This Apis—or Epaphus—is the calf of a cow which is never afterwards able to have another. The Egyptian belief is that a flash of light descends upon the cow from heaven, and this causes her to conceive Apis. The Apis-calf has distinctive marks: it is black, with a white diamond on its forehead, the image of an eagle on its back, the hairs on its tail double, and a scarab under its tongue. The priests brought the animal and Cambyses, half mad as he was, drew his

ἤγαγον τὸν Ἆπιν οἱ ἱρέες, ὁ Καμβύσης, οἷα ἐὼν ὑπομαργότερος, σπασάμενος τὸ ἐγχειρίδιον, θέλων τύψαι τὴν γαστέρα τοῦ Ἄπιος παίει τὸν
2 μηρόν· γελάσας δὲ εἶπε πρὸς τοὺς ἱρέας· Ὦ κακαὶ κεφαλαί, τοιοῦτοι θεοὶ γίνονται, ἔναιμοί τε καὶ σαρκώδεες καὶ ἐπαΐοντες σιδηρίων; ἄξιος μέν γε Αἰγυπτίων οὗτός γε ὁ θεός· ἀτάρ τοι ὑμεῖς γε οὐ χαίροντες γέλωτα ἐμὲ θήσεσθε. ταῦτα εἴπας ἐνετείλατο τοῖσι ταῦτα πρήσσουσι τοὺς μὲν ἱρέας ἀπομαστιγῶσαι, Αἰγυπτίων δὲ τῶν ἄλλων τὸν ἂν λάβωσι ὁρτάζοντα
3 κτείνειν. ⟨ἡ⟩ ὁρτὴ μὲν δὴ διελέλυτο Αἰγυπτίοισι, οἱ δὲ ἱρέες ἐδικαιεῦντο, ὁ δὲ Ἆπις πεπληγμένος τὸν μηρὸν ἔφθινε ἐν τῷ ἱρῷ κατακείμενος. καὶ τὸν μὲν τελευτήσαντα ἐκ τοῦ τρώματος ἔθαψαν οἱ ἱρέες λάθρῃ Καμβύσεω.
30 Καμβύσης δέ, ὡς λέγουσι Αἰγύπτιοι, αὐτίκα διὰ τοῦτο τὸ ἀδίκημα ἐμάνη, ἐὼν οὐδὲ πρότερον φρενήρης.

5.5 Herodotus 6.75

75 μαθόντες δὲ Κλεομένεα Λακεδαιμόνιοι ταῦτα πρήσσοντα κατῆγον αὐτὸν δείσαντες ἐπὶ τοῖσι αὐτοῖσι [ἐς Σπάρτην] τοῖσι καὶ πρότερον ἦρχε. κατελθόντα δὲ [αὐτὸν] αὐτίκα ὑπέλαβε μανίη νοῦσος, ἐόντα καὶ πρότερον ὑπομαργότερον· ὅκως γάρ τεῳ ἐντύχοι Σπαρτιητέων, ἐνέχραυε ἐς τὸ
2 πρόσωπον τὸ σκῆπτρον. ποιέοντα δὲ αὐτὸν ταῦτα καὶ παραφρονήσαντα ἔδησαν οἱ προσήκοντες ἐν ξύλῳ· ὁ δὲ δεθεὶς τὸν φύλακον μουνωθέντα ἰδὼν τῶν ἄλλων αἰτέει μάχαιραν· οὐ βουλομένου δὲ τὰ πρῶτα [τοῦ φυλάκου] διδόναι ἀπείλεε τά μιν λυθεὶς ποιήσει, ἐς ὃ δείσας τὰς ἀπειλὰς ὁ φύλακος
3 (ἦν γὰρ τῶν τις εἱλωτέων) διδοῖ οἱ μάχαιραν. Κλεομένης δὲ παραλαβὼν τὸν σίδηρον ἄρχετο ἐκ τῶν κνημέων ἑωυτὸν λωβώμενος· ἐπιτάμνων γὰρ κατὰ μῆκος τὰς σάρκας προέβαινε ἐκ τῶν κνημέων ἐς τοὺς μηρούς, ἐκ δὲ τῶν μηρῶν ἔς τε τὰ ἰσχία καὶ τὰς λαπάρας, ἐς ὃ ἐς τὴν γαστέρα ἀπίκετο καὶ ταύτην καταχορδεύων ἀπέθανε τρόπῳ τοιούτῳ, ὡς μὲν οἱ πολλοὶ λέγουσι Ἑλλήνων, ὅτι τὴν Πυθίην ἀνέγνωσε τὰ περὶ Δημαρήτου [γενόμενα] λέγειν, ὡς δὲ Ἀθηναῖοι [μοῦνοι] λέγουσι, διότι ἐς Ἐλευσῖνα ἐσβαλὼν ἔκειρε τὸ τέμενος τῶν θεῶν, ὡς δὲ Ἀργεῖοι, ὅτι ἐξ ἱροῦ αὐτῶν τοῦ Ἄργου Ἀργείων τοὺς καταφυγόντας ἐκ τῆς μάχης καταγινέων κατέκοπτε καὶ αὐτὸ τὸ ἄλσος ἐν ἀλογίῃ ἔχων ἐνέπρησε.

dagger, aimed a blow at its belly, but missed and struck its thigh. Then he laughed, and said to the priests: 'Do you call that a god, you poor blockheads? Are your gods flesh and blood? Do they feel the prick of steel? No doubt a god like that is good enough for the Egyptians; but you won't get away with trying to make a fool of me.' He then ordered the priests to be whipped by the men whose business it was to carry out such punishments, and any Egyptian who was found still keeping holiday to be put to death. In this way the festival was broken up, the priests punished, and Apis, who lay in the temple for a time wasting away from the wound in his thigh, finally died and was buried by the priests without the knowledge of Cambyses.

Even before this Cambyses had been far from sound in his mind; but the Egyptians are convinced that the complete loss of his reason was the direct result of this crime.

5.5 Herodotus 6.75

The Spartans, alarmed by the news of Cleomenes' proceedings in Arcadia, brought him home and restored him to the same power as he had before possessed. He had always been a little queer in the head, but no sooner had he returned to Sparta than he lost his wits completely, and began poking his staff into the face of everyone he met. As a result of this lunatic behaviour his relatives put him in the stocks. As he was lying there, fast bound, he noticed that all his guards had left him except one. He asked this man, who was a serf, to give him a knife. At first the fellow refused, but Cleomenes, by threats of what he would do to him when he recovered his liberty, so frightened him that he at last consented. As soon as the knife was in his hands, Cleomenes began to mutilate himself, beginning on his shins. He sliced his flesh into strips, working upwards to his thighs, and from them to his hips and sides, until he reached his belly, which he chopped into mincemeat. This finished him, and most people in Greece think that his unpleasant death was due to the fact that he corrupted the Priestess at Delphi and induced her to say what she did say about Demaratus; the Athenians, however, put it down to his destruction of the sacred precinct of Demeter and Persephone, on the occasion of his invasion of Eleusis; while the Argives maintain that it was a punishment for the acts of treachery and sacrilege he committed when, after a battle, he fetched the Argive fugitives from the temple of Argos, where they were taking shelter, and cut them to pieces, and then showed such contempt for the grove itself where the temple stood that he burned it down.

Chapter 5 Texts

5.6 Herodotus 6. 84. 1 and 84. 3

84 Ἀργεῖοι μέν νυν διὰ ταῦτα Κλεομένεά φασι μανέντα ἀπολέσθαι κακῶς, αὐτοὶ δὲ Σπαρτιῆταί φασι ἐκ δαιμονίου μὲν οὐδενὸς μανῆναι Κλεομένεα, Σκύθῃσι δὲ ὁμιλήσαντά μιν ἀκρητοπότην γενέσθαι καὶ ἐκ τούτου μανῆναι.

3 Κλεομένεα δὲ λέγουσι ἡκόντων τῶν Σκυθέων ἐπὶ ταῦτα ὁμιλέειν σφι μεζόνως, ὁμιλέοντα δὲ μᾶλλον τοῦ ἱκνεομένου μαθεῖν τὴν ἀκρητοποσίην παρ' αὐτῶν· ἐκ τούτου δὲ μανῆναί μιν νομίζουσι Σπαρτιῆται. ἔκ τε τόσου, ὡς αὐτοὶ λέγουσι, ἐπεὰν ζωρότερον βούλωνται πιεῖν, Ἐπισκύθισον λέγουσι. οὕτω δὴ Σπαρτιῆται τὰ περὶ Κλεομένεα λέγουσι· ἐμοὶ δὲ δοκέει τίσιν ταύτην ὁ Κλεομένης Δημαρήτῳ ἐκτεῖσαι.

5.7 Thucydides 1. 22

2 τὰ δ' ἔργα τῶν πραχθέντων ἐν τῷ πολέμῳ οὐκ ἐκ τοῦ παρατυχόντος πυνθανόμενος ἠξίωσα γράφειν, οὐδ' ὡς ἐμοὶ ἐδόκει, ἀλλ' οἷς τε αὐτὸς παρῆν καὶ παρὰ τῶν ἄλλων ὅσον δυνατὸν ἀκριβείᾳ περὶ ἑκάστου ἐπεξ-
3 ελθών. ἐπιπόνως δὲ ηὑρίσκετο, διότι οἱ παρόντες τοῖς ἔργοις ἑκάστοις οὐ ταὐτὰ περὶ τῶν αὐτῶν ἔλεγον, ἀλλ' ὡς ἑκατέρων τις εὐνοίας ἢ μνήμης
4 ἔχοι. καὶ ἐς μὲν ἀκρόασιν ἴσως τὸ μὴ μυθῶδες αὐτῶν ἀτερπέστερον φανεῖται· ὅσοι δὲ βουλήσονται τῶν τε γενομένων τὸ σαφὲς σκοπεῖν καὶ τῶν μελλόντων ποτὲ αὖθις κατὰ τὸ ἀνθρώπινον τοιούτων καὶ παραπλησίων ἔσεσθαι, ὠφέλιμα κρίνειν αὐτὰ ἀρκούντως ἕξει. κτῆμά τε ἐς αἰεὶ μᾶλλον ἢ ἀγώνισμα ἐς τὸ παραχρῆμα ἀκούειν ξύγκειται.

5.8 Thucydides 2. 47. 1–49. 6, 51. 2–4, 51. 6, 53. 1–4

47 Τοιόσδε μὲν ὁ τάφος ἐγένετο ἐν τῷ χειμῶνι τούτῳ. καὶ διελθόντος
2 αὐτοῦ πρῶτον ἔτος τοῦ πολέμου τοῦδε ἐτελεύτα. τοῦ δὲ θέρους εὐθὺς

Chapter 5 Texts

5.6 Herodotus 6. 84. 1 and 84. 3

Cleomenes' behaviour in this episode was, according to the Argives, the cause of his subsequent madness and miserable death. His own countrymen, however, deny that his madness was a punishment from heaven; they are convinced, on the contrary, that he lost his wits because, in his association with the Scythians, he had acquired the habit of drinking his wine neat.

The story is, that when the Scythian representatives came to discuss this scheme, Cleomenes spent more time with them than he need have done, or than was strictly appropriate, and during that time acquired the habit of taking wine without water—and went off his head in consequence. The Spartans tell us that ever since then they have used the phrase 'Scythian fashion' when they want a stronger drink than usual.

There, then, is the Spartan story for what it is worth; my own opinion is that Cleomenes came to grief as a punishment for what he did to Demaratus.

5.7 Thucydides 1. 22

But as to the facts of what occurred in the war, I thought it right to write them down not from what I learned from any chance informant, nor as seemed to me to be probable, but after going through each event—both those at which I was present and with regard to those where I learned from others—with as much accuracy as possible. The investigation was laborious, because those present at the several events did not give the same stories about them, but each according to their own conception and recollection. And the lack of the mythical may make my account less agreeable to listen to. But as for anyone who wishes to have a clear view both of the events that happened and those that will happen in such, or a similar, way in future according to human probability, if they deem my account to be of use, that is sufficient for me. Indeed it has been composed as a possession for always, rather than as a competition piece for the moment.

5.8 Thucydides 2. 47. 1–49. 6, 51. 2–4, 51. 6, 53. 1–4

47 Such was the funeral in this winter. When that was over, the first year of this war came to an end.

At the very beginning of summer, the Peloponnesians and their

Chapter 5 Texts

ἀρχομένου Πελοποννήσιοι καὶ οἱ ξύμμαχοι τὰ δύο μέρη ὥσπερ καὶ τὸ πρῶτον ἐσέβαλον ἐς τὴν Ἀττικήν (ἡγεῖτο δὲ Ἀρχίδαμος ὁ Ζευξιδάμου
3 Λακεδαιμονίων βασιλεύς), καὶ καθεζόμενοι ἐδῄουν τὴν γῆν. καὶ ὄντων αὐτῶν οὐ πολλάς πω ἡμέρας ἐν τῇ Ἀττικῇ ἡ νόσος πρῶτον ἤρξατο γενέσθαι τοῖς Ἀθηναίοις, λεγόμενον μὲν καὶ πρότερον πολλαχόσε ἐγκατασκῆψαι καὶ περὶ Λῆμνον καὶ ἐν ἄλλοις χωρίοις, οὐ μέντοι τοσοῦτός γε
4 λοιμὸς οὐδὲ φθορὰ οὕτως ἀνθρώπων οὐδαμοῦ ἐμνημονεύετο γενέσθαι. οὔτε γὰρ ἰατροὶ ἤρκουν τὸ πρῶτον θεραπεύοντες ἀγνοίᾳ, ἀλλ' αὐτοὶ μάλιστα ἔθνῃσκον ὅσῳ καὶ μάλιστα προσῇσαν, οὔτε ἄλλη ἀνθρωπεία τέχνη οὐδεμία· ὅσα τε πρὸς ἱεροῖς ἱκέτευσαν ἢ μαντείοις καὶ τοῖς τοιούτοις ἐχρήσαντο, πάντα ἀνωφελῆ ἦν, τελευτῶντές τε αὐτῶν ἀπέστησαν ὑπὸ τοῦ
48 κακοῦ νικώμενοι. ἤρξατο δὲ τὸ μὲν πρῶτον, ὡς λέγεται, ἐξ Αἰθιοπίας τῆς ὑπὲρ Αἰγύπτου, ἔπειτα δὲ καὶ ἐς Αἴγυπτον καὶ Λιβύην κατέβη καὶ ἐς τὴν
2 βασιλέως γῆν τὴν πολλήν. ἐς δὲ τὴν Ἀθηναίων πόλιν ἐξαπιναίως ἐσέπεσε, καὶ τὸ πρῶτον ἐν τῷ Πειραιεῖ ἥψατο τῶν ἀνθρώπων, ὥστε καὶ ἐλέχθη ὑπ' αὐτῶν ὡς οἱ Πελοποννήσιοι φάρμακα ἐσβεβλήκοιεν ἐς τὰ φρέατα· κρῆναι γὰρ οὔπω ἦσαν αὐτόθι. ὕστερον δὲ καὶ ἐς τὴν ἄνω πόλιν ἀφίκετο, καὶ
3 ἔθνῃσκον πολλῷ μᾶλλον ἤδη. λεγέτω μὲν οὖν περὶ αὐτοῦ ὡς ἕκαστος γιγνώσκει καὶ ἰατρὸς καὶ ἰδιώτης, ἀφ' ὅτου εἰκὸς ἦν γενέσθαι αὐτό, καὶ τὰς αἰτίας ἅστινας νομίζει τοσαύτης μεταβολῆς ἱκανὰς εἶναι δύναμιν ἐς τὸ μεταστῆσαι σχεῖν· ἐγὼ δὲ οἷόν τε ἐγίγνετο λέξω, καὶ ἀφ' ὧν ἄν τις σκοπῶν, εἴ ποτε καὶ αὖθις ἐπιπέσοι, μάλιστ' ἂν ἔχοι τι προειδὼς μὴ ἀγνοεῖν, ταῦτα δηλώσω αὐτός τε νοσήσας καὶ αὐτὸς ἰδὼν ἄλλους πάσχοντας.

49 Τὸ μὲν γὰρ ἔτος, ὡς ὡμολογεῖτο, ἐκ πάντων μάλιστα δὴ ἐκεῖνο ἄνοσον ἐς τὰς ἄλλας ἀσθενείας ἐτύγχανεν ὄν· εἰ δέ τις καὶ προύκαμνέ τι, ἐς τοῦτο
2 πάντα ἀπεκρίθη. τοὺς δὲ ἄλλους ἀπ' οὐδεμιᾶς προφάσεως, ἀλλ' ἐξαίφνης ὑγιεῖς ὄντας πρῶτον μὲν τῆς κεφαλῆς θέρμαι ἰσχυραὶ καὶ τῶν ὀφθαλμῶν ἐρυθήματα καὶ φλόγωσις ἐλάμβανε, καὶ τὰ ἐντός, ἥ τε φάρυγξ καὶ ἡ
3 γλῶσσα, εὐθὺς αἱματώδη ἦν καὶ πνεῦμα ἄτοπον καὶ δυσῶδες ἠφίει· ἔπειτα ἐξ αὐτῶν πταρμὸς καὶ βράγχος ἐπεγίγνετο, καὶ ἐν οὐ πολλῷ χρόνῳ κατέβαινεν ἐς τὰ στήθη ὁ πόνος μετὰ βηχὸς ἰσχυροῦ· καὶ ὁπότε ἐς τὴν καρδίαν στηρίξειεν, ἀνέστρεφέ τε αὐτὴν καὶ ἀποκαθάρσεις χολῆς πᾶσαι ὅσαι ὑπὸ ἰατρῶν ὠνομασμέναι εἰσὶν ἐπῇσαν, καὶ αὗται μετὰ ταλαιπωρίας
4 μεγάλης. λύγξ τε τοῖς πλέοσιν ἐνέπιπτε κενή, σπασμὸν ἐνδιδοῦσα ἰσχυρόν,
5 τοῖς μὲν μετὰ ταῦτα λωφήσαντα, τοῖς δὲ καὶ πολλῷ ὕστερον. καὶ τὸ μὲν ἔξωθεν ἁπτομένῳ σῶμα οὔτ' ἄγαν θερμὸν ἦν οὔτε χλωρόν, ἀλλ'

Chapter 5 Texts

allies invaded Attica, with a two-thirds force as on the first occasion, under the command of Archidamus, son of Zeuxidamus, king of Sparta. They established themselves and began to ravage the land.

They had not yet spent many days in Attica when the plague first struck the Athenians. It is said to have broken out previously in many other places, in the region of Lemnos and elsewhere, but there was no previous record of so great a pestilence and destruction of human life. The doctors were unable to cope, since they were treating the disease for the first time and in ignorance: indeed, the more they came into contact with sufferers the more liable they were to lose their own lives. No other device of men was any help. Moreover, supplication at sanctuaries, resort to divination and the like were all unavailing. In the end people were overwhelmed by the disaster and abandoned their efforts against it.

48 The plague is said to have come first of all from Ethiopia beyond Egypt; and from there it fell on Egypt and Libya and on much of the King's land. It struck the city of Athens suddenly. People in the Piraeus caught it first, and so, since there were not yet any fountains there, they actually alleged that the Peloponnesians had put poison in the wells. Afterwards it arrived in the upper city too, and then deaths started to occur on a much larger scale. Everyone, whether doctor or layman, may say from his own experience what the origin of it is likely to have been, and what causes he thinks had the power to bring about so great a change. I shall give a statement of what it was like, which people can study in case it should ever attack again, to equip themselves with foreknowledge so that they shall not fail to recognize it. I can give this account because I both suffered from the disease myself and saw other victims of it.

49 It was universally agreed that this particular year was exceptionally free from disease as far as other afflictions were concerned. If people did first suffer from other illnesses, all ended in this. Others were afflicted with no apparent antecedent cause, but suddenly, when they were in good health. The disease began with a strong fever in the head, and redness and inflammation in the eyes; the first internal symptoms were that the throat and tongue became bloody and the breath unnatural and malodorous. This was followed by sneezing and hoarseness, and in a short time the affliction descended to the chest, producing violent coughing. When it became established in the stomach, it convulsed that and produced every kind of evacuation of bile named by the doctors, accompanied

ὑπέρυθρον, πελιτνόν, φλυκταίναις μικραῖς καὶ ἕλκεσιν ἐξηνθηκός· τὰ δὲ ἐντὸς οὕτως ἐκάετο ὥστε μήτε τῶν πάνυ λεπτῶν ἱματίων καὶ σινδόνων τὰς ἐπιβολὰς μηδ᾽ ἄλλο τι ἢ γυμνοὶ ἀνέχεσθαι, ἥδιστά τε ἂν ἐς ὕδωρ ψυχρὸν σφᾶς αὐτοὺς ῥίπτειν. καὶ πολλοὶ τοῦτο τῶν ἠμελημένων ἀνθρώπων καὶ ἔδρασαν ἐς φρέατα, τῇ δίψῃ ἀπαύστῳ ξυνεχόμενοι· καὶ ἐν τῷ ὁμοίῳ

6 καθειστήκει τό τε πλέον καὶ ἔλασσον ποτόν. καὶ ἡ ἀπορία τοῦ μὴ ἡσυχάζειν καὶ ἡ ἀγρυπνία ἐπέκειτο διὰ παντός. καὶ τὸ σῶμα, ὅσονπερ χρόνον καὶ ἡ νόσος ἀκμάζοι, οὐκ ἐμαραίνετο, ἀλλ᾽ ἀντεῖχε παρὰ δόξαν τῇ ταλαιπωρίᾳ, ὥστε ἢ διεφθείροντο οἱ πλεῖστοι ἐναταῖοι καὶ ἑβδομαῖοι ὑπὸ τοῦ ἐντὸς καύματος, ἔτι ἔχοντές τι δυνάμεως, ἢ εἰ διαφύγοιεν, ἐπικατιόντος τοῦ νοσήματος ἐς τὴν κοιλίαν καὶ ἑλκώσεώς τε αὐτῇ ἰσχυρᾶς ἐγγιγνομένης καὶ διαρροίας ἅμα ἀκράτου ἐπιπιπτούσης οἱ πολλοὶ ὕστερον δι᾽ αὐτὴν ἀσθενείᾳ διεφθείροντο.

51 2 ἔθνησκον δὲ οἱ μὲν ἀμελείᾳ, οἱ δὲ καὶ πάνυ θεραπευόμενοι. ἕν τε οὐδὲ ἓν κατέστη ἴαμα ὡς εἰπεῖν ὅτι χρῆν προσφέροντας ὠφελεῖν· τὸ γάρ τῳ
3 ξυνενεγκὸν ἄλλον τοῦτο ἔβλαπτεν. σῶμά τε αὔταρκες ὂν οὐδὲν διεφάνη πρὸς αὐτὸ ἰσχύος πέρι ἢ ἀσθενείας, ἀλλὰ πάντα ξυνῄρει καὶ τὰ πάσῃ διαίτῃ
4 θεραπευόμενα. δεινότατον δὲ παντὸς ἦν τοῦ κακοῦ ἥ τε ἀθυμία ὁπότε τις αἴσθοιτο κάμνων (πρὸς γὰρ τὸ ἀνέλπιστον εὐθὺς τραπόμενοι τῇ γνώμῃ πολλῷ μᾶλλον προΐεντο σφᾶς αὐτοὺς καὶ οὐκ ἀντεῖχον), καὶ ὅτι ἕτερος ἀφ᾽ ἑτέρου θεραπείας ἀναπιμπλάμενοι ὥσπερ τὰ πρόβατα ἔθνησκον· καὶ τὸν πλεῖστον φθόρον τοῦτο ἐνεποίει.

6 ἐπὶ πλέον δ᾽ ὅμως οἱ διαπεφευγότες τόν τε θνῄσκοντα καὶ τὸν πονούμενον ᾠκτίζοντο διὰ τὸ προειδέναι τε καὶ αὐτοὶ ἤδη ἐν τῷ θαρσαλέῳ εἶναι· δὶς γὰρ τὸν αὐτόν, ὥστε καὶ κτείνειν, οὐκ ἐπελάμβανεν. καὶ ἐμακαρίζοντό τε ὑπὸ τῶν ἄλλων, καὶ αὐτοὶ τῷ παραχρῆμα περιχαρεῖ καὶ ἐς τὸν ἔπειτα χρόνον ἐλπίδος τι εἶχον κούφης μηδ᾽ ἂν ὑπ᾽ ἄλλου νοσήματός ποτε ἔτι διαφθαρῆναι.

by great discomfort. Most victims then suffered from empty retching, which induced violent convulsions: they abated after this for some sufferers, but only much later for others. The exterior of the body was not particularly hot to the touch or yellow, but was reddish, livid and burst out in small blisters and sores. But inside the burning was so strong that the victims could not bear to put on even the lightest clothes and linens, but had to go naked, and gained the greatest relief by plunging into cold water. Many who had no one to keep watch on them even plunged into wells, under the pressure of insatiable thirst; but it made no difference whether they drank a large quantity or a small. Throughout the course of the disease people suffered from sleeplessness and inability to rest. For as long as the disease was raging, the body did not waste away, but held out unexpectedly against its suffering. Most died about the seventh or the ninth day from the beginning of the internal burning, while they still had some strength. If they escaped then, the disease descended to the bowels: there violent ulceration and totally fluid diarrhoea occurred, and most people then died from the weakness caused by that.

51. 2 Some victims were neglected and died; others died despite a great deal of care. There was not a single remedy, you might say, which ought to be applied to give relief, for what helped one sufferer harmed another. No kind of constitution, whether strong or weak, proved sufficient against the plague, but it killed off all, whatever regime was used to care for them. The most terrifying aspect of the whole affliction was the despondency that resulted when someone realised that he had the disease: people immediately lost hope, and so through their attitude of mind were much more likely to let themselves go and not hold out. In addition, one person caught the disease through caring for another, and so they died like sheep: this was the greatest cause of loss of life.

51. 6 Those who had come through the disease had the greatest pity for the suffering and the dying, since they had previous experience of it and were now feeling confident for themselves, as the disease did not attack the same person a second time, or at any rate not fatally. Those who recovered were congratulated by the others, and in their immediate elation cherished the vain hope that for the future they would be immune to death from any other disease.

53 Πρῶτόν τε ἦρξε καὶ ἐς τἆλλα τῇ πόλει ἐπὶ πλέον ἀνομίας τὸ νόσημα. ῥᾷον γὰρ ἐτόλμα τις ἃ πρότερον ἀπεκρύπτετο μὴ καθ' ἡδονὴν ποιεῖν, ἀγχίστροφον τὴν μεταβολὴν ὁρῶντες τῶν τε εὐδαιμόνων καὶ αἰφνιδίως θνῃσκόντων καὶ τῶν οὐδὲν πρότερον κεκτημένων, εὐθὺς δὲ τἀκείνων
2 ἐχόντων. ὥστε ταχείας τὰς ἐπαυρέσεις καὶ πρὸς τὸ τερπνὸν ἠξίουν
3 ποιεῖσθαι, ἐφήμερα τά τε σώματα καὶ τὰ χρήματα ὁμοίως ἡγούμενοι. καὶ τὸ μὲν προσταλαιπωρεῖν τῷ δόξαντι καλῷ οὐδεὶς πρόθυμος ἦν, ἄδηλον νομίζων εἰ πρὶν ἐπ' αὐτὸ ἐλθεῖν διαφθαρήσεται· ὅτι δὲ ἤδη τε ἡδὺ πανταχόθεν τε ἐς αὐτὸ κερδαλέον, τοῦτο καὶ καλὸν καὶ χρήσιμον κατέστη.
4 θεῶν δὲ φόβος ἢ ἀνθρώπων νόμος οὐδεὶς ἀπεῖργε, τὸ μὲν κρίνοντες ἐν ὁμοίῳ καὶ σέβειν καὶ μὴ ἐκ τοῦ πάντας ὁρᾶν ἐν ἴσῳ ἀπολλυμένους, τῶν δὲ ἁμαρτημάτων οὐδεὶς ἐλπίζων μέχρι τοῦ δίκην γενέσθαι βιοὺς ἂν τὴν τιμωρίαν ἀντιδοῦναι, πολὺ δὲ μείζω τὴν ἤδη κατεψηφισμένην σφῶν ἐπικρεμασθῆναι, ἣν πρὶν ἐμπεσεῖν εἰκὸς εἶναι τοῦ βίου τι ἀπολαῦσαι.

5.9 Thucydides 3. 82

82 Οὕτως ὠμὴ ⟨ἡ⟩ στάσις προυχώρησε, καὶ ἔδοξε μᾶλλον, διότι ἐν τοῖς πρώτη ἐγένετο, ἐπεὶ ὕστερόν γε καὶ πᾶν ὡς εἰπεῖν τὸ Ἑλληνικὸν ἐκινήθη, διαφορῶν οὐσῶν ἑκασταχοῦ τοῖς τε τῶν δήμων προστάταις τοὺς Ἀθηναίους ἐπάγεσθαι καὶ τοῖς ὀλίγοις τοὺς Λακεδαιμονίους. καὶ ἐν μὲν εἰρήνῃ οὐκ ἂν ἐχόντων πρόφασιν οὐδ' ἑτοίμων παρακαλεῖν αὐτούς, πολεμουμένων δὲ καὶ ξυμμαχίας ἅμα ἑκατέροις τῇ τῶν ἐναντίων κακώσει καὶ σφίσιν αὐτοῖς ἐκ τοῦ αὐτοῦ προσποιήσει ῥᾳδίως αἱ ἐπαγωγαὶ τοῖς νεωτερίζειν τι
2 βουλομένοις ἐπορίζοντο. καὶ ἐπέπεσε πολλὰ καὶ χαλεπὰ κατὰ στάσιν ταῖς πόλεσι, γιγνόμενα μὲν καὶ αἰεὶ ἐσόμενα, ἕως ἂν ἡ αὐτὴ φύσις ἀνθρώπων ᾖ, μᾶλλον δὲ καὶ ἡσυχαίτερα καὶ τοῖς εἴδεσι διηλλαγμένα, ὡς ἂν ἕκασται αἱ μεταβολαὶ τῶν ξυντυχιῶν ἐφιστῶνται. ἐν μὲν γὰρ εἰρήνῃ καὶ ἀγαθοῖς πράγμασιν αἵ τε πόλεις καὶ οἱ ἰδιῶται ἀμείνους τὰς γνώμας ἔχουσι διὰ τὸ μὴ ἐς ἀκουσίους ἀνάγκας πίπτειν· ὁ δὲ πόλεμος ὑφελὼν τὴν εὐπορίαν τοῦ καθ' ἡμέραν βίαιος διδάσκαλος καὶ πρὸς τὰ παρόντα τὰς ὀργὰς τῶν πολλῶν ὁμοιοῖ.

53   In other respects too the plague marked the beginning of a decline to greater lawlessness in the city. People were more willing to dare to do things which they would not previously have admitted to enjoying, when they saw the sudden changes of fortune, as some who were prosperous suddenly died, and their property was immediately acquired by others who had previously been destitute. So they thought it reasonable to concentrate on immediate profit and pleasure, believing that their bodies and their possessions alike would be short-lived. No one was willing to persevere in struggling for what was considered an honourable result, since he could not be sure he would not perish before he achieved it. What was pleasant in the short term, and what was in any way conducive to that, came to be accepted as honourable and useful. No fear of the gods or law of men had any restraining power, since it was judged to make no difference whether one was pious or not, as all alike could be seen dying. No one expected to live long enough to have to pay the penalty for his misdeeds: people tended much more to think that a sentence already decided was hanging over them, and that before it was executed they might reasonably get some enjoyment out of life.

5.9   Thucydides 3. 82

That is how savage the course of the civil war became, and it seemed even worse than it was because it was the first of all. Later indeed one might say that the whole Greek world was turned upside-down, as grievances in different places prompted the democratic leaders to call in the Athenians and the oligarchs to call in the Spartans. In peace they would not have had the excuse or the willingness to issue the invitation; but when they were at war, and there was an alliance available to each side to harm their opponents and at the same time strengthen themselves, it was easy for those who wanted to bring about a revolution to call in outsiders. Many grave sufferings attacked the cities through civil war, of the kind that continue to happen and always will happen as long as human nature remains the same, but more or less severe, and varying in form, as imposed by the changes of circumstances in individual cases. In peace and in favourable conditions both cities and individuals pursue better policies because they are not caught by unwanted constraints; but war, which takes away the ready supply of one's daily needs, is a violent teacher and brings the passions of the majority to the same level as their circumstances.

6
Plato

It may seem extraordinary to some students of ancient philosophy to find a whole chapter devoted to Plato in a book on disease and the Greek imagination. Yet we can study four different aspects of his thought where the notion of disease plays an important role, first in his psychology, then relatedly in his theory of justice—both in the individual and in the state—and thirdly in his views on authority and insistence on the need for experts, not least in the moral and political domains. Finally there is his own extended discussion of diseases both of the body and of the soul in the *Timaeus*—clear recognition, surely, of his sense of the importance of the topic, even though why he should have considered it so important, and decided to devote so many pages to it in his cosmological work, are questions we shall have to tackle and try to resolve at the end of this chapter.

One recurrent theme that serves to link Plato's ideas in the physical, to the psychological, social, moral, and even cosmological domains, relates to his notion of what the good order of composite wholes consists in. Within the body, between the body and the soul, within the soul, within the state, he speaks of good relations in terms of harmony, health, justice, and of bad ones, conversely, in terms of discord, disease, injustice.

Even before he developed his theory of the three parts, or faculties, of the soul (reasoning, spirit, and appetite), he presented certain analogies between the body and the soul. In the *Gorgias* he talks of the three kinds of evils (*poneriai*) that affect wealth, the body, and the soul, namely poverty, disease, and injustice (477c). Just as anyone would want to be rid of disease in the body, so similarly they will surely wish to be relieved of injustice in the soul, namely by receiving due punishment (477aff.). This is in an argument that it is better for the wrongdoer to be punished than to escape punishment. While the best state for the body is not to be sick at all, if it does suffer from disease it is far better to be treated than not. So in the analogous situation in the soul, we need treatment to rid us of wickedness. The courts make us more just, acting in the same way as medicine (*iatrike*) does to relieve us of the sickness of the body (477e) [T 6.1]. Of course many kinds of medical treatment for the body, cautery, surgery, are painful. Punishment of the soul too is painful, but it secures the desirable end that we no longer have a soul that is unhealthy, corrupt, unjust, and unholy (479bc).

The analogy is developed further at *Gorgias* 504bff., 505aff. [T 6.2]. Regularity (*taxis*) and order (*kosmos*) in the body are called health and strength, and the people who can bring such order into the body are trainers and doctors. So too the orderly and regular states of the soul are lawfulness and produce justice and temperance. This then is what the good orator will aim to bring about. Just as the doctor will not allow the patient to do just what he or she likes, so where the soul is concerned, it should be restrained in its desires when it is in a depraved state (505b). So the conclusion follows (though Callicles will not accept it) that it is better for the soul to be punished than to live a life of uncorrected licence.

The two key themes thus introduced are first that the soul can be as disordered and as sick as the body, and secondly that just as there are doctors who know what to do in the case of physical diseases, so there are people who will be able to say how the soul is to be treated and cured of its injustice. The terms 'just' and 'unjust' in the arguments we have considered apply in the first instance to the individual person, but of course they also have general political relevance. Justice in the individual is good order within the soul: but analogously justice in the state is a matter of good order and lawfulness there.

In the *Republic* Socrates and his interlocutors investigate both these manifestations of justice, and discuss the state to see justice writ large, before turning to the individual to identify justice there. The assumption is that justice will exhibit the same structure in both parts of the comparison. Both types of justice, in Plato's view, exemplify the single Form of Justice.

When they first set out in *Republic* 2 to construct the ideal state by considering what functions are absolutely necessary (the skill to procure food and shelter, principally) the account they arrive at is rejected by Glaucon as a 'city of pigs'. It is unbearably primitive, even though it is described as the *healthy* city (*hygies, hygiene*, 372e, 373b) [T 6.3]. When they introduce such luxuries as tables and chairs, and dancing girls, the healthy state of the city with its healthy diet is compromised and it becomes the 'fevered' one *(phlegmainousan,* 372e), that they nevertheless take as the subject for their analysis of the ideal state and the place of justice in it. Certainly once they leave behind the healthy city, they will need doctors (373d) to look after all the complaints that will arise from the more complicated diet.

As in the *Gorgias*, health in the body is the analogue of health in the soul at *Republic* 444cff. [T 6.4]. Both excellences (*aretai*: in the moral context the word is often translated virtue) depend on good order, the correct relationship between the elements that should rule and those that should be ruled. Just as healthy and sick practices produce health and disease in the body, so just and unjust acts instil justice and injustice in the soul. Once again the argument is used to show that it is better for the unjust to be punished than to escape (445aff.). What good order in the soul, and in the state, amounts to is spelled out in terms of the due relationship between the three parts he identifies in each. In the state it is the guardians who should be in control over the other two elements, the helpers and the money-makers, though each part has its own particular function to fulfil (434c). So similarly in the individual soul, reason should be in charge over spirit and appetite. But when in either case it comes to *ensuring* that order is maintained, severe measures may be necessary.

Here too the analogy with health and medicine is made to do important work. At 459c [T 6.5] we are told that when health can be secured by regimen (diet and exercise) and drugs (*pharmaka*) are not needed, an ordinary doctor will be up to the job. But when the complaints are more severe, then a courageous doctor is needed and drugs prescribed. So the philosopher-kings will need 'noble lies' to win the people round, including for example the myth of the metals to persuade them that there are fundamental differences between those who are pure gold and those who are made of baser metals, silver, or iron or brass (414b, 415a). Somehow or other they have got to agree that there are human natures of different kinds, with different values. What the philosopher-kings use to secure consent is recognized to be falsehoods (*pseudos*) but described as *pharmaka* (459c2).

Plato there exploits not just the analogy between the statesman and the doctor, but also the semantic range of *pharmaka* drugs, remedies, spells. Already at 389b Socrates says that truth is to be valued highly, but nevertheless lies may have to be used by human beings, in the form of a *pharmakon* (here primarily with the sense of remedy in general). But if so, that is the job of the doctor, not just of any lay person. The rulers (cast in the role of the doctor) are allowed to lie for the benefit of the state. But no one else is permitted to do so: that would be as bad, or worse, than a patient not telling his doctor or trainer about his bodily condition. At 414b, as we have seen, the myth of the metals is a falsehood the rulers use to justify keeping the sections of the state apart and insisting that there should be no cross-breeding between them. At 459c d again securing good order depends on control of procreation, and again the doctor's use of his kind of *pharmaka* is cited in justification for the type of *pharmakon* the ruler must use. Falsehood can prove useful: it can be a cure or remedy for the ills that affect the state. This is no actual physical drug, of course, but rather a spell or a charm. But the controversy surrounding Greek doctors' actual remedies is not allowed to obtrude, nor their doubtful efficacy, nor the association, indeed, between *pharmakon* as drug, at one end of the spectrum, and *pharmakon* as poison, at the other.

Starting from the idea that the body's disorder is manifest in disease, we have a first extension to the idea of the disorder/disease of the soul, namely injustice. That yields a characterization of the unjust person, where disorder reflects a failure of reason to control spirit and appetite. The second extension takes us to injustice in the state, arising from a disruption to the proper relations between its parts. The diseases of states—political ones—become a recurrent theme in the account given in the later books of the decline from the ideal constitution they have described. Thus tyranny, the worst kind of state of all, is said to come about when the same disease (*nosema*) that destroys oligarchy infects democracy in turn and enslaves it (563e) [T 6.6]. Excess, Socrates goes on, is likely to bring about the same type of change in seasons, in plants, in bodies, and not least in political constitutions. Too much freedom leads to slavery both in the individual and in the state. The diagnosis of the infection of political constitutions is then given. Idle good-for-nothings, like drones, some sting-less but some (the leaders) equipped with stings, arise and they produce disturbances in any state just as phlegm and bile do in the body. Just as you need a good doctor to be on the look-out for and to treat the latter, so you need a good law-giver to do the same in the state.

That theme recurs in the *Sophist* 227c ff. [T 6.7], where two kinds of evil, needing two kinds of purging or cleansing, are identified. We need a *katharsis* of the body, to rid it of its disease, but also one (also called a *katharmos*, 227d6, d10) for the soul, to rid it of *its* disease, namely faction, *stasis*. Disease and discord or faction (*stasis*) are, in a way, the same (228a): wickedness is the *stasis* and sickness (*nosos*) of the soul (228b). What is popularly called wickedness is most certainly a disease of the soul (228d), though in addition to the vice of cowardice, injustice and so on, there is a second kind of evil affection (*pathos*) namely ignorance. Once again the appropriate remedies are spelt out, punishment for injustice and education for ignorance.

We should pause for a moment to reflect on this whole complex of ideas, and first from the point of view of logical analysis. Sometimes we are given explicit analogies or comparisons. In many such cases the analogies are justified because both items compared exhibit the same general structure and exemplify the same general rule. But the terminology of disease, health, cure, remedy is also often applied directly to both the soul and the state. When in *Republic* 372e the true city is a kind of healthy one (*hygies tis*), the addition of the *tis* indicates some recognition of the extension of the term. But often there is no such qualification.

Some may wish to diagnose some of these uses as metaphorical. But the problem of so doing is the one I mentioned at the outset, namely the difficulty in giving any clear delineation of precisely what the literal applications cover. *Pharmaka,* in particular, come in many shapes and forms, and it is arbitrary to privilege physical drugs or poisons over other modes of remedy. The same can be said of purifications or *katharseis*. It is both less tendentious and more accurate to acknowledge, throughout, considerable semantic stretch. Plato himself evidently often felt no need to apologize for speaking of the health and disease of the city and for the soul's need for purging.

Then from the point of view of the substantive content of the ideas Plato puts forward, the two most striking theses he presents are first the claim that injustice in the soul and the state are objectively verifiable conditions, and secondly the idea that experts can be found both to diagnose, and to cure, them. Physical disease, it is assumed, is unproblematic, though in fact the Hippocratic doctors disagreed not just on whether apparently healthy people were really so, but even on what health itself consisted in, let alone on the principal causes of diseases. Certainly, however, physical disease is generally unproblematically bad. No one except the most deranged would want to suffer from illness. In the moral and political sphere that translates into the idea that we should naturally shun injustice and prefer to be punished for what we do wrong rather than escape punishment.

If so, then the lay person will no more be in a position to challenge what is prescribed in the injustice case than in the physical sickness one. There are experts, Plato claims, in diagnosing the state of the soul, in determining the health or sickness of the body politic, and their word must be accepted, even when they prescribe drastic remedies, getting rid of deviants and purging the city of what pollutes it in just the way the doctor uses cautery, surgery, or drugs to get rid of the pathogens in the body.

Those themes receive some of their most powerful expression in the *Laws*, which lays down severe penalties for those who disagree with the rulers, including on such matters as religious belief. Those who do not believe in the benevolent gods that govern the cosmos are punished first with imprisonment, but then if on release they do not recant, with death. Those who suffer from folly are to be given another chance, but for the hardened atheists, when they die, their bodies are to be taken from the country and refused burial (907e ff.). The whole topic of political purgation (*katharmos, kathairein*) is developed with medical analogies at 735b ff. [T 6.8]. 'The best purge is painful, like all medicines (*pharmaka*) of a drastic nature.' That combines punishment with vengeance, where the penalty is death or exile. 'It, as a rule, clears out the greatest criminals when they are incurable (*aniatoi*) and cause serious damage to the state.' Even the lesser, so-called milder, purges involve exiling the guilty, though their evacuation is to be given the euphemistic label of 'emigration'.

Yet there is first a philosophical difficulty in Plato's position and then a paradox. The difficulty, which has been explored in studies by Renford Bambrough (1967*a* and 1967*b*), relates to the disanalogies between medicine and politics. The doctor does not (usually) decide on goals, only on the means to them, whereas the statesman settles on ends that may be disagreed and controversial, as well as having to chart the manner of attaining them. Some defence can be offered on Plato's behalf, though the chief one that has been attempted (namely that health, the goal for medicine, may not be so unlike political ideals, after all, in that it is *not* unanimously agreed) is not one that Plato would approve, since it saves the analogy only at the risk of destroying his whole point, which was that in both cases there is a determinate objective truth that justifies the claim to authority by those who have it.

The paradox is this. Plato uses the model of the doctor to construct his image of the expert in moral and political matters. Yet the real-live doctors of Plato's day were—to judge from the evidence in the Hippocratic Corpus—far from being all the confident authorities that Plato's ideal would have us believe. Quite the reverse, in certain cases. We noted a whole range of Hippocratic texts where the writers confess that they were at a loss, unable to alleviate their patients' sufferings, let alone to cure them, uncertain as to the causes of their complaints as well as about what to do, responsible themselves even sometimes for treatment that they recognized, with the benefit of hindsight, to have been mistaken. The admiration we may feel for these writers' honesty is one side of the coin, but the other is the impression they give of their own helplessness when faced with difficult cases.

As we shall see at the end of this chapter, Plato evidently knew a lot about contemporary medicine: we shall be outlining later his own account of diseases, discussing its sources and asking why he wrote at such length on the subject. But medicine plays such a crucial role in his moral and political arguments that he seems to elide most of the difficulties in the application of the analogy. True, this is *ideal* medicine, and these are paragons of doctors who have secured that knowledge of objective causes and cures. Plato knew well enough, to be sure, that ordinary doctors fell far short. Yet for the sake of the construction of the ideal philosopher-king, he evidently thought that the authority of doctors was sufficiently impressive for them to serve as paradigms for that. This was true, even though his doctors were not represented as basing their practice on knowledge of the Forms. Indeed the fact that they did not (and it would have been very implausible to suggest that they did) makes his analogy all the more useful to him, as reaching to a wider audience than just those who accepted his particular metaphysical tenets. From that point of view, the great advantage of medicine was that it offered a case where many would agree that it dealt with objective cause–effect relations whether or not they were prepared to accept the further claim that the ultimate basis of the philosophers' authority was the theory of Forms.

Before we turn to what Plato has to say about disease in the *Timaeus* there is a further foray into the themes of disease and disorder that we should consider in the account of madness in the *Phaedrus*. The *Republic* insisted that reason must rule. The *Phaedrus* allows us to see that in a different light, and shows that Plato recognized that there are positive aspects to madness itself, what Dodds called 'the blessings of madness' (Dodds 1951, ch. 3). Socrates is led to recant the speech he had made that argued that the beloved should favour the non-lover over the lover, on the grounds that the lover is mad (shades of Phaedra in the *Hippolytus* if not also Sappho herself, though this time the lover and beloved are, of course, male). Madness is not a simple evil (244a) [T 6.9]. Indeed the greatest blessings come to us by way of madness when it is sent as a divine gift. Four illustrations are given, the last of which is the subject that concerns Socrates particularly, namely love itself.

The first three, expressed in some of the most convoluted language in Plato, relate to (1) prophecy, (2) purifications, and (3) the gift of poetry. As to (1) there is some typically playful etymologizing on the connection between *mania* (madness) and *mantike* (prophecy), but the passage ends by praising prophecy above augury (*oionistike*). The former is as far superior to the latter as madness when it comes from the gods is to mere human prudence. As to (2) Socrates speaks obscurely of the diseases and great sufferings that come on families from some ancient sin or guilt (*menimata*)—where purifications (*katharmoi*) with the help of prayers to the gods can procure relief. The interpretation of what precisely Plato has in mind here is disputed, but one possibility is the release from pollution attained at the end of Aeschylus' *Oresteia* when Orestes is purified and discharged of the pollution that followed from his killing his mother Clytaemnestra. As to (3) the third type, poetry, we are told that he who comes to the doors of poetry without the madness of the Muses has no chance of being a good poet. In *each* case we should note that it is when the madness in question is *under the protection of the gods* that it can produce the benefits of which Socrates speaks. It is far from being the case that madness as such is a good. Rather it would be more accurate to see Plato's position as echoing the ambivalence we noted in the presentation of such figures as Oedipus and Philoctetes.

However in the sequel in the *Phaedrus*, the relations within the soul are pictured with the image of a chariot team. The charioteer corresponds fairly obviously to the reasoning element in the soul, and his two horses, one good, one bad, to spirit and to appetite respectively. But as Ferrari in particular has shown (Ferrari 1987, 185ff.), the language in which the charioteer's control is described contains some striking and unexpected features. When the charioteer beholds the beloved (253e) [T 6. 10], the obedient horse is self-controlled. But the other, the horse that corresponds to appetite, is all for leaping upon the beloved.

This provokes what can only be described as a pretty violent response from the charioteer. The bad horse does not heed the goad or the whip of the charioteer, who later when he recalls true beauty is described as having to pull back on the reins with such force that the horses are brought down on their haunches. When this happens again, the charioteer pulls the bit in the mouth of the unruly horse, spattering his tongue and jaws with blood, and bringing him to the ground. When we reflect that the charioteer represents reason, the violence of his reaction to the sight of the beloved is remarkable and is testimony, of course, to the threat that the lower parts of the soul, appetite especially, pose to its rule. It is obviously not enough for the rational part to use mere argument in the circumstances described in the image. The violence of the horses is met with a violent—even horse-like[1] reaction on the part of the charioteer. If we transfer some of the lessons of the struggle within the soul here in the *Phaedrus* to the picture of reason and good rule we are given in the *Republic*, we can see that to attain justice and equilibrium may involve considerable turmoil. Disorder, or the threat of it, are the antecedents of establishing order. The control that reason has to exercise is indeed a control over scarcely controllable elements.

We come now to the account that Plato himself offers of diseases in the *Timaeus*. It was presumably not just to seem learned, or to encourage his readers to take a broad interest in a wide range of subjects, that he included this. Though we certainly hear, from Aristotle for example (*Politics* 1282^{a}3 ff.), of people who studied medicine not to practise it, but for the sake of their general education, medicine as such was not an obligatory part of what any cultivated individual needed to know. Again, while some earlier cosmologies included medical theorizing, the model they provided will not serve as the whole explanation for what Plato sought to do in the *Timaeus*.

We should begin by noting that the theories of disease it contains were taken sufficiently seriously by the author of *Anonymus Londinensis*, the history of medicine that draws on the work of Aristotle's pupil, Meno, for them to be given more space in that account, as we have it, than those of any other theorist, Hippocrates included. Of course Plato was a name to conjure with, but again that does not give the whole story. We might think it absurd to treat him as an authority on medical theory and practice. After all he never had any experience as a doctor himself. But first it is worth recalling that some of the

[1] Ferrari 1987, p. 189 and nn. 67–8 thus glosses the term *anepesen* used of the charioteer 'rearing back' when he sees the beloved at 254b8 and again at 254e1–2 with the addition of a reference to the starting-line of a race.

treatises in the Hippocratic Corpus, especially the general lectures or *epideixeis*, may well have been the work of writers who were not themselves practitioners. The gap between the doctor and the lay person was, in any case, far narrower in the ancient world, where the former had no legally recognized qualifications they could cite to justify their right to practise, and where we have already seen a lay person such as Thucydides prepared to give his account of the causes of the plague. If Plato felt he could, in some respects, vie with, in others (as we shall see) even outdo, the theories of the doctors on diseases, that is not so surprising in an ancient context as it would be in a modern one, where we certainly do not expect philosophers to claim competence to speak on medicine, not unless they also happen to be medically qualified.

Those remarks are based on the assumption that what we are given in the *Timaeus* is *Plato's* views, not just those he has copied from one or more earlier medical writer. That point has been disputed, because some have seen the cosmology in the *Timaeus* as a whole as just an amalgam of the ideas of other theorists (Taylor 1928). In the case of the passage on medicine, the preferred sources are Philistion and Philolaus, for example. Yet first the account of diseases in the *Timaeus* was accepted as Plato's in the history of medicine I have just mentioned. Indeed *Anonymus Londinensis* clearly distinguishes Plato's views from those of both Philistion and Philolaus in particular. Secondly, if it is puzzling that Plato gave such a detailed account of his own ideas on diseases, that puzzle is in no way alleviated by saying that what he was doing was just repeating what others had proposed. Of course he drew on others' views. But it is what he does with them, for *his* purposes, that is so intriguing and that enables us to appreciate his reasons for including disease so prominently in his cosmological account.

The discussion of diseases stretches from *Timaeus* 81e to 87b, with a continuation on health and therapy down to 90d. It opens with a rhetorical flourish. 'As regards diseases, how they originate, is clear in a way (*pou*) to everyone.' Elsewhere in the dialogue other theoretical discussions are similarly introduced as 'clear', for example that the four simple bodies, including fire and air, are bodies, *somata* (53c). But this time, with diseases, we cannot help feeling that Plato is about to skate over some of the difficulties and controversies. Three different sources of physical disease are then distinguished. First they arise from disorder in the simple bodies (which are themselves constituted by elementary triangles), then there are those that affect secondary structures (the homoeomerous compounds such as bone and flesh), and thirdly there are those that arise from air, phlegm, and bile. In each case Plato varies ideas that we can parallel in our more strictly medical writers, and in each instance the new twist he gives to those ideas has moral or political resonance. Just as the *Republic* and other dialogues describe the state's disorders in bodily terms, so conversely, we may say, the *Timaeus* describes the body's disorders partly in political terms.

The first origin of diseases is due to excess and deficiency. The terms often used in Hippocratic texts for those or cognate ideas are *plerosis* and *kenosis* (repletion and depletion).[2] But Plato uses *pleonexia* and *endeia* (excess and deficiency) (82a) [T 6.11]. The latter is a general word for lack or need, but the former has particular associations with greed, or wanting to have more than your fair share. The full range of applications of the term, from bodily diseases, through excesses in the weather, to political excesses and injustice, is exploited in the *Laws* at 906a–c. Here in the *Timaeus* (82a6) what excess and deficiency bring about in the body is said to be not just diseases (*nosoi*) but also *staseis*, the word used for political factions and disorder.[3] It is what oversteps the mark that

---

[2] e.g. *On Ancient Medicine* chs. 9 and 10 (*CMG* I 1, 41. 17ff., 42. 11ff.), cf. *On the Nature of Man* ch. 9 (*CMG* I 1 3, 188. 3ff. *plesmone* and *kenosis*), *On Diseases* IV chs. 32 and 33 (L VII 542. 12ff., 544. 14ff., referring to what is in excess or in default in the body), *On the Places in Man* ch. 42 (L VI 334. 1ff.).

[3] *On Breaths* ch. 7 (*CMG* I 1, 95. 6), for instance, uses the verb *stasiazein* of the interaction between unlikes in the body.

produces alterations, diseases and destructions, of a great variety of types.

The second main category of diseases continues to exploit moral and political terminology, even while the disorders in question affect such physical compounds in the body as flesh. When the substances interact and generate one another as they should, health is the result, but when not, diseases arise. When the material becomes 'reversed and corrupted' (82e f.) [T 6.12], then the substances no longer maintain their natural order (*taxis*) but 'being at enmity with themselves (*echthra*) they have no enjoyment of themselves, and being at war (*polemia*) with the established and regular constitution of the body, they destroy and dissolve it' (83a). So order in the body is contrasted with hostility and warfare. Once again the idea of warfare in the body can be found in Hippocratic texts, and already Alcmaeon had described the true balance of the elements in it as *isonomia*, equality, and their imbalance as 'monarchy'.[4] Plato was evidently not the first—nor would he be the last—writer to picture warfare within the body. But such an image was, evidently, particularly well suited to one of his important underlying messages.

The third variety of disease comes from air, phlegm, and bile. At 85b he takes a swipe at those who would deny the sacred character of the sacred disease. It is justly so called, but then Plato's rationalization of that is to say that it attacks the most sacred part of the body, the head, or more strictly its 'divine revolutions'. In this section order (*taxis*) and proportion (*summetria*) are the norm and their disturbance is disease (85c). When these are disrupted, the result is disorder (*ataxia*, 85e4) [T 6.13]. If we are in any doubt about the political overtones, these are made clear when the purgation of bile from the body is compared to the exiling of someone from a city in a state of faction or strife (*stasiazein*, 85e10).

Those are all diseases that affect the body, but the *Timaeus*

---

[4] Alcmaeon, Fr. 4. *On Breaths* ch. 6 (*CMG* I 1, 94. 21) spoke of factors that are *polemia*, hostile, to human nature.

also offers an account of those that affect the soul through the body, where disease takes the form of folly or mindlessness (*anoia*, 86b) [T 6.14]. There are two varieties of this, madness and ignorance. In a twist to the usual Socratic dictum or paradox that no one does wrong willingly, we are here told that no one is voluntarily wicked, since it is rather the case that they are diseased (86d). This springs in part from the effects of the humours running amok, though there is also a reference to the fact that political circumstances may contribute to these evils (87ab). The remedy for mental, as for bodily, disease, is to restore harmony or proportion (*summetria*) especially that between the body and the soul themselves.

Given that one of the most common Greek ideas of disease, found in many different versions in the Hippocratic writers and elsewhere, was that they arise from the interaction of opposite factors in the body, Plato's association of the causes of some diseases with the hostility between elements in the body is certainly not unprecedented. But we can see that he has selected and modified those common Greek themes that suit his underlying moral. The *Timaeus* is all about the work of the Demiurge, the divine Craftsman responsible for the order in the universe, and about the way that reason persuades necessity to bring about the best results. The description of the proper, natural state of the body in health as orderly and of its disruption as disorder is consonant with that cosmic message and fits those traditional Greek beliefs well enough. But Plato carries the politicization of the body much further than most, maybe than any, extant Greek medical theorist. His notions of order, proportion, harmony *span* the fields of politics, morality, 'physics' (the nature of things), and the body in particular. We should not say that those ideas arise in *one* of those fields, then to be applied to others. Rather, their power and relevance in each field get to be strengthened and confirmed by their use in others.

The *Republic* and the *Laws* insist on order in the state and order in the individual's psyche, and they associate the opposite, disorder, in each case, with what no one would desire, namely disease. But conversely, when it comes to an account of health and disease themselves, we find that they are described in terms that draw heavily on the political sphere. Goodness or virtue or excellence in every important domain turns out to be a matter of good order between potentially hostile elements (cf. *Timaeus* 87c4) [T 6.15]. Any disorder must be remedied by cures, purges, purifications, to restore, as far as possible, the original ideal balance.

The converse of the medicalizing of the city is the politicization of the body. While no doctor himself, Plato lays claim to knowing about diseases both of the body and of the soul. The conception of expert authority is one on which so much depends in his account of the ideal state, for the philosopher-kings must be people who know what is right and whose word should accordingly be accepted. But it is not just that political ideas lie in the background in Plato's exceptional foray into medical theory. When it comes to who can speak with authority about those problems to do with the origins of diseases (of which such play is made when he talks about trusting political and moral experts) it is not Hippocrates whom he chooses to cite, nor Philistion nor Philolaus nor any other of the writers cited in *Anonymus Londinensis* nor any of the nameless authors of the treatises that came to be associated with Hippocrates. No. The authority on the origins of diseases—'clear', as we are told, 'to everyone'—is Timaeus, spokesman, as we said, for Plato's own views.

CHAPTER 6 TEXTS

6.1 Plato, *Gorgias* 477e7–478c7 (Socrates and Polus)

ΣΩ. Τίς οὖν τέχνη πενίας ἀπαλλάττει; οὐ χρηματιστική;
ΠΩΛ. Ναί.
ΣΩ. Τίς δὲ νόσου; οὐκ ἰατρική;
ΠΩΛ. Ἀνάγκη.
ΣΩ. Τίς δὲ πονηρίας καὶ ἀδικίας; εἰ μὴ οὕτως εὐπορεῖς, ὧδε σκόπει· ποῖ ἄγομεν καὶ παρὰ τίνας τοὺς κάμνοντας τὰ σώματα;
ΠΩΛ. Παρὰ τοὺς ἰατρούς, ὦ Σώκρατες.
ΣΩ. Ποῖ δὲ τοὺς ἀδικοῦντας καὶ τοὺς ἀκολασταίνοντας;
ΠΩΛ. Παρὰ τοὺς δικαστὰς λέγεις;
ΣΩ. Οὐκοῦν δίκην δώσοντας;
ΠΩΛ. Φημί.
ΣΩ. Ἆρ' οὖν οὐ δικαιοσύνῃ τινὶ χρώμενοι κολάζουσιν οἱ ὀρθῶς κολάζοντες;
ΠΩΛ. Δῆλον δή.
ΣΩ. Χρηματιστικὴ μὲν ἄρα πενίας ἀπαλλάττει, ἰατρικὴ δὲ νόσου, δίκη δὲ ἀκολασίας καὶ ἀδικίας.
ΠΩΛ. Φαίνεται.
ΣΩ. Τί οὖν τούτων κάλλιστόν ἐστιν [ὧν λέγεις];
ΠΩΛ. Τίνων λέγεις;
ΣΩ. Χρηματιστικῆς, ἰατρικῆς, δίκης.
ΠΩΛ. Πολὺ διαφέρει, ὦ Σώκρατες, ἡ δίκη.
ΣΩ. Οὐκοῦν αὖ ἤτοι ἡδονὴν πλείστην ποιεῖ ἢ ὠφελίαν ἢ ἀμφότερα, εἴπερ κάλλιστόν ἐστιν;
ΠΩΛ. Ναί.
ΣΩ. Ἆρ' οὖν τὸ ἰατρεύεσθαι ἡδύ ἐστιν, καὶ χαίρουσιν οἱ ἰατρευόμενοι;
ΠΩΛ. Οὐκ ἔμοιγε δοκεῖ.
ΣΩ. Ἀλλ' ὠφέλιμόν γε. ἦ γάρ;
ΠΩΛ. Ναί.
ΣΩ. Μεγάλου γὰρ κακοῦ ἀπαλλάττεται, ὥστε λυσιτελεῖ ὑπομεῖναι τὴν ἀλγηδόνα καὶ ὑγιῆ εἶναι.
ΠΩΛ. Πῶς γὰρ οὔ;
ΣΩ. Ἆρ' οὖν οὕτως ἂν περὶ σῶμα εὐδαιμονέστατος ἄνθρωπος εἴη, ἰατρευόμενος, ἢ μηδὲ κάμνων ἀρχήν;

CHAPTER 6 TEXTS

6.1 Plato, *Gorgias* 477e7–478c7 (Socrates and Polus)

SOC. Now what is the art that relieves from poverty? Is it not money-making?
POL. Yes.
SOC. And what from disease? Is it not medicine?
POL. It must be.
SOC. And what from wickedness and injustice? If you are not ready for that offhand, consider it thus: whither and to whom do we take whose who are in bodily sickness?
POL. To the doctor, Socrates.
SOC. And whither the wrongdoers and libertines?
POL. To the law-court, do you mean?
SOC. Yes, and to pay the penalty?
POL. I agree.
SOC. Then is it not by employing a kind of justice that those punish who punish aright?
POL. Clearly so.
SOC. Then money-making relieves us from poverty, medicine from disease, and justice from licentiousness and injustice.
POL. Apparently.
SOC. Which then is the fairest of these things?
POL. Of what things, pray?
SOC. Money-making, medicine, justice.
POL. Justice, Socrates, is far above the others.
SOC. Now again, if it is fairest, it causes either most pleasure or benefit or both.
POL. Yes.
SOC. Well then, is it pleasant to be medically treated, and do those who undergo such treatment enjoy it?
POL. I do not think so.
SOC. But it is beneficial, is it not?
POL. Yes.
SOC. Because one is relieved of a great evil, and hence it is worth while to endure the pain and be well.
POL. Of course.
SOC. Is this then the happiest state of body for a man to be in—that of being medically treated— or that of never being ill at all?

ΠΩΛ. Δῆλον ὅτι μηδὲ κάμνων.
ΣΩ. Οὐ γὰρ τοῦτ' ἦν εὐδαιμονία, ὡς ἔοικε, κακοῦ ἀπαλλαγή, ἀλλὰ τὴν ἀρχὴν μηδὲ κτῆσις.
ΠΩΛ. Ἔστι ταῦτα.

6.2 Plato, *Gorgias* 505a6–b12 (Socrates and Callicles)

505   ΣΩ. Οὐκοῦν καὶ τὰς ἐπιθυμίας ἀποπιμπλάναι, οἷον πεινῶντα φαγεῖν ὅσον βούλεται ἢ διψῶντα πιεῖν, ὑγιαίνοντα μὲν ἐῶσιν οἱ ἰατροὶ ὡς τὰ πολλά, κάμνοντα δὲ ὡς ἔπος εἰπεῖν οὐδέποτ' ἐῶσιν ἐμπίμπλασθαι ὧν ἐπιθυμεῖ; συγχωρεῖς τοῦτό γε καὶ σύ;
KAΛ. Ἔγωγε.
b   ΣΩ. Περὶ δὲ ψυχήν, ὦ ἄριστε, οὐχ ὁ αὐτὸς τρόπος; ἕως μὲν ἂν πονηρὰ ᾖ, ἀνόητός τε οὖσα καὶ ἀκόλαστος καὶ ἄδικος καὶ ἀνόσιος, εἴργειν αὐτὴν δεῖ τῶν ἐπιθυμιῶν καὶ μὴ ἐπιτρέπειν ἄλλ' ἄττα ποιεῖν ἢ ἀφ' ὧν βελτίων ἔσται· φῂς ἢ οὔ;
KAΛ. Φημί.
ΣΩ. Οὕτω γάρ που αὐτῇ ἄμεινον τῇ ψυχῇ;
KAΛ. Πάνυ γε.
ΣΩ. Οὐκοῦν τὸ εἴργειν ἐστὶν ἀφ' ὧν ἐπιθυμεῖ κολάζειν;
KAΛ. Ναί.
ΣΩ. Τὸ κολάζεσθαι ἄρα τῇ ψυχῇ ἄμεινόν ἐστιν ἢ ἡ ἀκολασία, ὥσπερ σὺ νυνδὴ ᾤου.

6.3 Plato, *The Republic* 2. 372c2–e8

372c   Καὶ ὁ Γλαύκων ὑπολαβών, Ἄνευ ὄψου, ἔφη, ὡς ἔοικας, ποιεῖς τοὺς ἄνδρας ἑστιωμένους.
Ἀληθῆ, ἦν δ' ἐγώ, λέγεις. ἐπελαθόμην ὅτι καὶ ὄψον ἕξουσιν, ἅλας τε δῆλον ὅτι καὶ ἐλάας καὶ τυρόν, καὶ βολβοὺς καὶ λάχανά γε, οἷα δὴ ἐν ἀγροῖς ἑψήματα, ἑψήσονται. καὶ τραγήματά που παραθήσομεν αὐτοῖς τῶν τε σύκων καὶ ἐρεβίνθων καὶ κυάμων, καὶ μύρτα καὶ φηγοὺς σποδιοῦσιν πρὸς
d   τὸ πῦρ, μετρίως ὑποπίνοντες· καὶ οὕτω διάγοντες τὸν βίον ἐν εἰρήνῃ μετὰ ὑγιείας, ὡς εἰκός, γηραιοὶ τελευτῶντες ἄλλον τοιοῦτον βίον τοῖς ἐκγόνοις παραδώσουσιν.
Καὶ ὅς, Εἰ δὲ ὑῶν πόλιν, ὦ Σώκρατες, ἔφη, κατεσκεύαζες, τί ἂν αὐτὰς ἄλλο ἢ ταῦτα ἐχόρταζες;
Ἀλλὰ πῶς χρή, ἦν δ' ἐγώ, ὦ Γλαύκων;

POL. Clearly, never being ill.

SOC. Yes, for what we regarded as happiness, it seems, was not this relief from evil, but its non-acquisition at any time.

6.2 Plato, *Gorgias* 505a6–b12 (Socrates and Callicles)

SOC. And so the satisfaction of one's desires—if one is hungry, eating as much as one likes, or if thirsty, drinking—is generally allowed by doctors when one is in health; but they practically never allow one in sickness to take one's fill of things that one desires: do you agree with me in this?

CALL. I do.

SOC. And does not the same rule, my excellent friend, apply to the soul? So long as it is in a bad state—thoughtless, licentious, unjust and unholy—we must restrain its desires and not permit it to do anything except what will help it to be better: do you grant this, or not?

CALL. I do.

SOC. For thus, I take it, the soul itself is better off?

CALL. To be sure.

SOC. And is restraining a person from what he desires correcting him?

CALL. Yes.

SOC. Then correction is better for the soul than uncorrected licence, as you were thinking just now.

6.3 Plato, *The Republic* 2. 372c2–e8

Here Glaucon broke in: 'No relishes apparently,' he said, 'for the men you describe as feasting.' 'True,' said I; 'I forgot that they will also have relishes—salt, of course, and olives and cheese; and onions and greens, the sort of things they boil in the country, they will boil up together. But for dessert we will serve them figs and chickpeas and beans, and they will toast myrtle-berries and acorns before the fire, washing them down with moderate potations; and so, living in peace and health, they will probably die in old age and hand on a like life to their offspring.' And he said, 'If you were founding a city of pigs, Socrates, what other fodder than this would you provide?' 'Why, what would you have, Glaucon?' said I. 'What is customary,' he replied; 'they must recline on

Ἅπερ νομίζεται, ἔφη· ἐπί τε κλινῶν κατακεῖσθαι οἶμαι τοὺς μέλλοντας
e μὴ ταλαιπωρεῖσθαι, καὶ ἀπὸ τραπεζῶν δειπνεῖν, καὶ ὄψα ἅπερ καὶ οἱ νῦν
ἔχουσι καὶ τραγήματα.
Εἶεν, ἦν δ' ἐγώ· μανθάνω. οὐ πόλιν, ὡς ἔοικε, σκοποῦμεν μόνον ὅπως
γίγνεται, ἀλλὰ καὶ τρυφῶσαν πόλιν. ἴσως οὖν οὐδὲ κακῶς ἔχει· σκοποῦντες
γὰρ καὶ τοιαύτην τάχ' ἂν κατίδοιμεν τήν τε δικαιοσύνην καὶ ἀδικίαν ὅπῃ
ποτὲ ταῖς πόλεσιν ἐμφύονται. ἡ μὲν οὖν ἀληθινὴ πόλις δοκεῖ μοι εἶναι ἣν
διεληλύθαμεν, ὥσπερ ὑγιής τις· εἰ δ' αὖ βούλεσθε, καὶ φλεγμαίνουσαν
πόλιν θεωρήσωμεν· οὐδὲν ἀποκωλύει.

6.4 Plato, *The Republic* 4. 444c8–e2

444c Τὰ μέν που ὑγιεινὰ ὑγίειαν ἐμποιεῖ, τὰ δὲ νοσώδη νόσον.
Ναί.
d Οὐκοῦν καὶ τὸ μὲν δίκαια πράττειν δικαιοσύνην ἐμποιεῖ, τὸ δ' ἄδικα
ἀδικίαν;
Ἀνάγκη.
Ἔστι δὲ τὸ μὲν ὑγίειαν ποιεῖν τὰ ἐν τῷ σώματι κατὰ φύσιν καθιστάναι
κρατεῖν τε καὶ κρατεῖσθαι ὑπ' ἀλλήλων, τὸ δὲ νόσον παρὰ φύσιν ἄρχειν τε
καὶ ἄρχεσθαι ἄλλο ὑπ' ἄλλου.
Ἔστι γάρ.
Οὐκοῦν αὖ, ἔφην, τὸ δικαιοσύνην ἐμποιεῖν τὰ ἐν τῇ ψυχῇ κατὰ φύσιν
καθιστάναι κρατεῖν τε καὶ κρατεῖσθαι ὑπ' ἀλλήλων, τὸ δὲ ἀδικίαν παρὰ
φύσιν ἄρχειν τε καὶ ἄρχεσθαι ἄλλο ὑπ' ἄλλου;
Κομιδῇ, ἔφη.
e Ἀρετὴ μὲν ἄρα, ὡς ἔοικεν, ὑγίειά τέ τις ἂν εἴη καὶ κάλλος καὶ εὐεξία
ψυχῆς, κακία δὲ νόσος τε καὶ αἶσχος καὶ ἀσθένεια.

6.5 Plato, *The Republic* 5. 459c2–e3

459c Ὅτι ἀνάγκη αὐτοῖς, ἦν δ' ἐγώ, φαρμάκοις πολλοῖς χρῆσθαι. ἰατρὸν
δέ που μὴ δεομένοις μὲν σώμασι φαρμάκων, ἀλλὰ διαίτῃ ἐθελόντων
ὑπακούειν, καὶ φαυλότερον ἐξαρκεῖν ἡγούμεθα εἶναι· ὅταν δὲ δὴ καὶ
φαρμακεύειν δέῃ, ἴσμεν ὅτι ἀνδρειοτέρου δεῖ τοῦ ἰατροῦ.
Ἀληθῆ· ἀλλὰ πρὸς τί λέγεις;
Πρὸς τόδε, ἦν δ' ἐγώ· συχνῷ τῷ ψεύδει καὶ τῇ ἀπάτῃ κινδυνεύει ἡμῖν
d δεήσειν χρῆσθαι τοὺς ἄρχοντας ἐπ' ὠφελίᾳ τῶν ἀρχομένων. ἔφαμεν δέ που

couches, I presume, if they are not to be uncomfortable, and dine from tables and have made dishes and sweetmeats such as are now in use.' 'Good,' said I, 'I understand. It is not merely the origin of a city, it seems, that we are considering but the origin of a luxurious city. Perhaps that isn't such a bad suggestion, either. For by observation of such a city it may be we could discern the origin of justice and injustice in states. The true state I believe to be the one we have described—the healthy state, as it were. But if it is your pleasure that we contemplate also a fevered state, there is nothing to hinder.'

6.4 Plato, *The Republic* 4. 444c8–e2

'Healthful things, surely engender health and diseaseful disease.

'Yes.'

'Then does not doing just acts engender justice and unjust injustice?'

'Of necessity.'

'But to produce health is to establish the elements in a body in the natural relation of dominating and being dominated by one another, while to cause disease is to bring it about that one rules or is ruled by the other contrary to nature.'

'Yes, that is so.'

'And is it not likewise the production of justice in the soul to establish its principles in the natural relation of controlling and being controlled by one another, while injustice is to cause the one to rule or be ruled by the other contrary to nature?'

'Exactly, so,' he said.

'Virtue, then, as it seems, would be a kind of health and beauty and good condition of the soul, and vice would be disease, ugliness, and weakness.'

6.5 Plato, *The Republic* 5. 459c2–e3

'This,' said I, 'that they will have to employ many of those drugs of which we were speaking. We thought that an inferior physician sufficed for bodies that do not need drugs but yield to diet and regimen. But when it is necessary to prescribe drugs we know that a more enterprising and venturesome physician is required.'

'True; but what is the pertinency?'

'This,' said I: 'it seems likely that our rulers will have to make considerable use of falsehood and deception for the benefit of their

ἐν φαρμάκου εἴδει πάντα τὰ τοιαῦτα χρήσιμα εἶναι.

Καὶ ὀρθῶς γε, ἔφη.

Ἐν τοῖς γάμοις τοίνυν καὶ παιδοποιίαις ἔοικε τὸ ὀρθὸν τοῦτο γίγνεσθαι οὐκ ἐλάχιστον.

Πῶς δή;

Δεῖ μέν, εἶπον, ἐκ τῶν ὡμολογημένων τοὺς ἀρίστους ταῖς ἀρίσταις συγγίγνεσθαι ὡς πλειστάκις, τοὺς δὲ φαυλοτάτους ταῖς φαυλοτάταις
e τοὐναντίον, καὶ τῶν μὲν τὰ ἔκγονα τρέφειν, τῶν δὲ μή, εἰ μέλλει τὸ ποίμνιον ὅτι ἀκρότατον εἶναι, καὶ ταῦτα πάντα γιγνόμενα λανθάνειν πλὴν αὐτοὺς τοὺς ἄρχοντας, εἰ αὖ ἡ ἀγέλη τῶν φυλάκων ὅτι μάλιστα ἀστασίαστος ἔσται.

6.6 Plato, *The Republic* 8. 563e6–564b2

563e Ταὐτόν, ἦν δ' ἐγώ, ὅπερ ἐν τῇ ὀλιγαρχίᾳ νόσημα ἐγγενόμενον ἀπώλεσεν αὐτήν, τοῦτο καὶ ἐν ταύτῃ πλέον τε καὶ ἰσχυρότερον ἐκ τῆς ἐξουσίας ἐγγενόμενον καταδουλοῦται δημοκρατίαν. καὶ τῷ ὄντι τὸ ἄγαν τι ποιεῖν μεγάλην φιλεῖ εἰς τοὐναντίον μεταβολὴν ἀνταποδιδόναι, ἐν ὥραις τε
564 καὶ ἐν φυτοῖς καὶ ἐν σώμασιν, καὶ δὴ καὶ ἐν πολιτείαις οὐχ ἥκιστα.

Εἰκός, ἔφη.

Ἡ γὰρ ἄγαν ἐλευθερία ἔοικεν οὐκ εἰς ἄλλο τι ἢ εἰς ἄγαν δουλείαν μεταβάλλειν καὶ ἰδιώτῃ καὶ πόλει.

Εἰκός, γάρ.

Εἰκότως τοίνυν, εἶπον, οὐκ ἐξ ἄλλης πολιτείας τυραννὶς καθίσταται ἢ ἐκ δημοκρατίας, ἐξ οἶμαι τῆς ἀκροτάτης ἐλευθερίας δουλεία πλείστη τε καὶ ἀγριωτάτη.

Ἔχει γάρ, ἔφη, λόγον.

b Ἀλλ' οὐ τοῦτ' οἶμαι, ἦν δ' ἐγώ, ἠρώτας, ἀλλὰ ποῖον νόσημα ἐν ὀλιγαρχίᾳ τε φυόμενον ταὐτὸν καὶ ἐν δημοκρατίᾳ δουλοῦται αὐτήν.

6.7 Plato, *Sophist* 227c7–228b10 (Theaetetus and Visitor)

227c ΘΕΑΙ. Ἀλλὰ μεμάθηκα, καὶ συγχωρῶ δύο μὲν εἴδη καθάρσεως, ἓν δὲ τὸ περὶ τὴν ψυχὴν εἶδος εἶναι, τοῦ περὶ τὸ σῶμα χωρὶς ὄν.

ΞΕ. Πάντων κάλλιστα. καί μοι τὸ μετὰ τοῦτο ἐπάκουε πειρώμενος αὖ
d τὸ λεχθὲν διχῇ τέμνειν.

ΘΕΑΙ. Καθ' ὁποῖ' ἂν ὑφηγῇ πειράσομαί σοι συντέμνειν.

subjects. We said, I believe, that the use of that sort of thing was in the category of medicine.'

'And that was right,' he said.

'In our marriages, then, and the procreation of children, it seems there will be no slight need of this kind of "right."'

'How so?'

'It follows from our former admissions,' I said, 'that the best men must cohabit with the best women in as many cases as possible and the worst with the worst in the fewest, and that the offspring of the one must be reared and that of the other not, if the flock is to be as perfect as possible. And the way in which all this is brought to pass must be unknown to any but the rulers, if, again, the herd of guardians is to be as free as possible from dissension.'

6.6 Plato, *The Republic* 8. 563e6–564b2

'The same malady,' I said, 'that, arising in oligarchy, destroyed it, this more widely diffused and more violent as a result of this licence, enslaves democracy. And in truth, any excess is wont to bring about a corresponding reaction to the opposite in the seasons, in plants, in animal bodies, and most especially in political societies.'

'Probably,' he said.

'And so the probable outcome of too much freedom is only too much slavery in the individual and the state.'

'Yes, that is probable.'

'Probably, then, tyranny develops out of no other constitution than democracy—from the height of liberty, I take it, the fiercest extreme of servitude.'

'That is reasonable,' he said.

'That, however, I believe, was not your question, but what identical malady arising in democracy as well as in oligarchy enslaves it?'

6.7 Plato, *Sophist* 227c7–228b10 (Theaetetus and Visitor)

THT. I do understand, and I agree that there are two types of cleansing, one dealing with the soul and a separate one dealing with the body.

VIS. Fine. Next listen and try to cut the one we've mentioned in two.

ΞΕ. Πονηρίαν ἕτερον ἀρετῆς ἐν ψυχῇ λέγομέν τι;
ΘΕΑΙ. Πῶς γὰρ οὔ;
ΞΕ. Καὶ μὴν καθαρμός γ' ἦν τὸ λείπειν μὲν θάτερον, ἐκβάλλειν δὲ ὅσον ἂν ᾖ πού τι φλαῦρον.
ΘΕΑΙ. Ἦν γὰρ οὖν.
ΞΕ. Καὶ ψυχῆς ἄρα, καθ' ὅσον ἂν εὑρίσκωμεν κακίας ἀφαίρεσίν τινα, καθαρμὸν αὐτὸν λέγοντες ἐν μέλει φθεγξόμεθα.
ΘΕΑΙ. Καὶ μάλα γε.
ΞΕ. Δύο μὲν εἴδη κακίας περὶ ψυχὴν ῥητέον.
ΘΕΑΙ. Ποῖα;
228 ΞΕ. Τὸ μὲν οἷον νόσον ἐν σώματι, τὸ δ' οἷον αἶσχος ἐγγιγνόμενον.
ΘΕΑΙ. Οὐκ ἔμαθον.
ΞΕ. Νόσον ἴσως καὶ στάσιν οὐ ταὐτὸν νενόμικας;
ΘΕΑΙ. Οὐδ' αὖ πρὸς τοῦτο ἔχω τί χρή με ἀπικρίνασθαι.
ΞΕ. Πότερον ἄλλο τι στάσιν ἡγούμενος ἢ τὴν τοῦ φύσει συγγενοῦς ἔκ τινος διαφθορᾶς διαφοράν;
ΘΕΑΙ. Οὐδέν.
ΞΕ. Ἀλλ' αἶσχος ἄλλο τι πλὴν τὸ τῆς ἀμετρίας πανταχοῦ δυσειδὲς ἐνὸν γένος;
b ΘΕΑΙ. Οὐδαμῶς ἄλλο.
ΞΕ. Τί δέ; ἐν ψυχῇ δόξας ἐπιθυμίαις καὶ θυμὸν ἡδοναῖς καὶ λόγον λύπαις καὶ πάντα ἀλλήλοις ταῦτα τῶν φλαύρως ἐχόντων οὐκ ᾐσθήμεθα διαφερόμενα;
ΘΕΑΙ. Καὶ σφόδρα γε.
ΞΕ. Συγγενῆ γε μὴν ἐξ ἀνάγκης σύμπαντα γέγονεν.
ΘΕΑΙ. Πῶς γὰρ οὔ;
ΞΕ. Στάσιν ἄρα καὶ νόσον τῆς ψυχῆς πονηρίαν λέγοντες ὀρθῶς ἐροῦμεν.
ΘΕΑΙ. Ὀρθότατα μὲν οὖν.

6.8 Plato, *Laws* 5. 735b1–736a3

735b πᾶσαν ἀγέλην ποιμὴν καὶ βουκόλος τροφεύς τε ἵππων καὶ ὅσα ἄλλα τοιαῦτα παραλαβών, οὐκ ἄλλως μή ποτε ἐπιχειρήσει θεραπεύειν ἢ πρῶτον μὲν τὸν ἑκάστῃ προσήκοντα καθαρμὸν καθαρεῖ τῇ συνοικήσει, διαλέξας δὲ τά τε ὑγιῆ καὶ τὰ μὴ καὶ τὰ γενναῖα καὶ ἀγεννῆ, τὰ μὲν ἀποπέμψει πρὸς

THT. I'll try to follow your lead and cut it however you say.
VIS. Do we say that wickedness in the soul is something different from virtue?
THT. Of course.
VIS. And to cleanse something was to leave what's good and throw out whatever's inferior.
THT. Yes
VIS. So insofar as we can find some way to remove what's bad in the soul, it will be suitable to call it cleansing.
THT. Of course.
VIS. We have to say that there are two kinds of badness that affect the soul.
THT. What are they?
VIS. One is like bodily sickness, and the other is like ugliness.
THT. I don't understand.
VIS. Presumably you regard sickness and discord as the same thing, don't you?
THT. I don't know what I should say to that.
VIS. Do you think that discord is just dissension among things that are naturally of the same kind, and arises out of some kind of corruption?
THT. Yes
VIS. And ugliness is precisely a consistently unattractive sort of disproportion?
THT. Yes
VIS. Well then, don't we see that there's dissension in the souls of people in poor condition, between beliefs and desires, anger and pleasures, reason and pains, and all of those things with each other?
THT. Absolutely.
VIS. But all of them do have to be akin to each other.
THT. Of course.
VIS. So we'd be right if we said that wickedness is discord and sickness of the soul.
THT. Absolutely right.

6.8 Plato, *Laws* 5. 735b1–736a3

In dealing with a flock of any kind, the shepherd or cowherd, or the keeper of horses or any such animals, will never attempt to look after it until he has first applied to each group of animals the appropriate purge—which is to separate the sound from the unsound, and the

ἄλλας τινὰς ἀγέλας, τὰ δὲ θεραπεύσει, διανοούμενος ὡς μάταιος ἂν ὁ πόνος
c εἴη καὶ ἀνήνυτος περί τε σῶμα καὶ ψυχάς, ἃς φύσις καὶ πονηρὰ τροφὴ
διεφθαρκυῖα προσαπόλλυσιν τὸ τῶν ὑγιῶν καὶ ἀκηράτων ἠθῶν τε καὶ
σωμάτων γένος ἐν ἑκάστοις τῶν κτημάτων, ἄν τις τὰ ὑπάρχοντα μὴ
διακαθαίρηται. τὰ μὲν δὴ τῶν ἄλλων ζῴων ἐλάττων τε σπουδὴ καὶ
παραδείγματος ἕνεκα μόνον ἄξια παραθέσθαι τῷ λόγῳ, τὰ δὲ τῶν
ἀνθρώπων σπουδῆς τῆς μεγίστης τῷ τε νομοθέτῃ διερευνᾶσθαι καὶ
d φράζειν τὸ προσῆκον ἑκάστοις καθαρμοῦ τε πέρι καὶ συμπασῶν τῶν ἄλλων
πράξεων. αὐτίκα γὰρ τὸ περὶ καθαρμοὺς πόλεως ὧδ' ἔχον ἂν εἴη· πολλῶν
οὐσῶν τῶν διακαθάρσεων αἱ μὲν ῥᾴους εἰσίν, αἱ δὲ χαλεπώτεραι, καὶ τὰς
μὲν τύραννος μὲν ὢν καὶ νομοθέτης ὁ αὐτός, ὅσαι χαλεπαί τ' εἰσὶν καὶ
ἄρισται, δύναιτ' ἂν καθῆραι, νομοθέτης δὲ ἄνευ τυραννίδος καθιστὰς
πολιτείαν καινὴν καὶ νόμους, εἰ καὶ τὸν πρᾳότατον τῶν καθαρμῶν
καθήρειεν, ἀγαπώντως ἂν καὶ τὸ τοιοῦτον δράσειεν. ἔστι δ' ὁ μὲν ἄριστος
e ἀλγεινός, καθάπερ ὅσα τῶν φαρμάκων τοιουτότροπα, ὁ τῇ δίκῃ μετὰ
τιμωρίας εἰς τὸ κολάζειν ἄγων, θάνατον ἢ φυγὴν τῇ τιμωρίᾳ τὸ τέλος
ἐπιτιθείς· τοὺς γὰρ μέγιστα ἐξημαρτηκότας, ἀνιάτους δὲ ὄντας, μεγίστην
δὲ οὖσαν βλάβην πόλεως, ἀπαλλάττειν εἴωθεν. ὁ δὲ πρᾳότερός ἐστι τῶν
καθαρμῶν ὁ τοιόσδε ἡμῖν· ὅσοι διὰ τὴν τῆς τροφῆς ἀπορίαν τοῖς ἡγεμόσιν
ἐπὶ τὰ τῶν ἐχόντων μὴ ἔχοντες ἑτοίμους αὑτοὺς ἐνδείκνυνται
736 παρεσκευακότες ἕπεσθαι, τούτοις ὡς νοσήματι πόλεως ἐμπεφυκότι, δι'
εὐφημίας ἀπαλλαγήν, ὄνομα ἀποικίαν τεθέμενος, εὐμενῶς ὅτι μάλιστα
ἐξεπέμψατο.

6.9 Plato, *Phaedrus* 244a5–b3, 244d5–245a8

244a εἰ μὲν γὰρ ἦν ἁπλοῦν τὸ μανίαν κακὸν εἶναι, καλῶς ἂν ἐλέγετο· νῦν δὲ τὰ
μέγιστα τῶν ἀγαθῶν ἡμῖν γίγνεται διὰ μανίας, θείᾳ μέντοι δόσει
b διδομένης. ἥ τε γὰρ δὴ ἐν Δελφοῖς προφῆτις αἵ τ' ἐν Δωδώνῃ ἱέρειαι
μανεῖσαι μὲν πολλὰ δὴ καὶ καλὰ ἰδίᾳ τε καὶ δημοσίᾳ τὴν Ἑλλάδα
ἠργάσαντο, σωφρονοῦσαι δὲ βραχέα ἢ οὐδέν·

244d ἀλλὰ μὴν νόσων γε καὶ πόνων τῶν μεγίστων, ἃ δὴ παλαιῶν ἐκ μηνιμάτων
ποθὲν ἔν τισι τῶν γενῶν ἡ μανία ἐγγενομένη καὶ προφητεύσασα, οἷς ἔδει
e ἀπαλλαγὴν ηὕρετο, καταφυγοῦσα πρὸς θεῶν εὐχάς τε καὶ λατρείας, ὅθεν

well-bred from the ill-bred, and to send off the latter to other herds, while keeping the former under his own care; for he reckons that his labour would be fruitless and unending if it were spent on bodies and souls which nature and ill-nurture have combined to ruin, and which themselves bring ruin on a stock that is sound and clean both in habit and in body,—whatever the class of beast,—unless a thorough purge be made in the existing herd. This is a matter of minor importance in the case of other animals, and deserves mention only by way of illustration; but in the case of man it is of the highest importance for the lawgiver to search out and to declare what is proper for each class both as regards purging out and all other modes of treatment. For instance, in respect of civic purgings, this would be the way of it. Of the many possible modes of purging, some are milder, some more severe; those that are severest and best a lawgiver who was also a despot might be able to effect, but a lawgiver without despotic power might be well content if, in establishing a new polity and laws, he could effect even the mildest of purgations. The best purge is painful, like all medicines of a drastic nature,—the purge which hales to punishments by means of justice linked with vengeance, crowning the vengeance with exile or death: it, as a rule, clears out the greatest criminals when they are incurable and cause serious damage to the State. A milder form of purge is one of the following kind:—when, owing to scarcity of food, people are in want, and display a readiness to follow their leaders in an attack on the property of the wealthy,—then the lawgiver, regarding all such as a plague inherent in the body politic, ships them abroad as gently as possible, giving the euphemistic title of 'emigration' to their evacuation.

6.9 Plato, *Phaedrus* 244a5–b3, 244d5–245a8

That would be right if it were an invariable truth that madness is an evil: but in reality, the greatest blessings come by way of madness, indeed of madness that is heaven-sent. It was when they were mad that the prophetess at Delphi and the priestesses at Dodona achieved so much for which both states and individuals in Greece are thankful: when sane they did little or nothing.

And in the second place, when grievous maladies and afflictions have beset certain families by reason of some ancient sin, madness has appeared amongst them, and breaking out into prophecy has

δὴ καθαρμῶν τε καὶ τελετῶν τυχοῦσα ἐξάντη ἐποίησε τὸν [ἑαυτῆς] ἔχοντα πρός τε τὸν παρόντα καὶ τὸν ἔπειτα χρόνον, λύσιν τῷ ὀρθῶς μανέντι τε καὶ
245 κατασχομένῳ τῶν παρόντων κακῶν εὑρομένη. τρίτη δὲ ἀπὸ Μουσῶν κατοκωχή τε καὶ μανία, λαβοῦσα ἁπαλὴν καὶ ἄβατον ψυχήν, ἐγείρουσα καὶ ἐκβακχεύουσα κατά τε ᾠδὰς καὶ κατὰ τὴν ἄλλην ποίησιν, μυρία τῶν παλαιῶν ἔργα κοσμοῦσα τοὺς ἐπιγιγνομένους παιδεύει· ὃς δ' ἂν ἄνευ μανίας Μουσῶν ἐπὶ ποιητικὰς θύρας ἀφίκηται, πεισθεὶς ὡς ἄρα ἐκ τέχνης ἱκανὸς ποιητὴς ἐσόμενος, ἀτελὴς αὐτός τε καὶ ἡ ποίησις ὑπὸ τῆς τῶν μαινομένων ἡ τοῦ σωφρονοῦντος ἠφανίσθη.

6.10 Plato, *Phaedrus* 253e5–254e5

253e ὅταν δ' οὖν ὁ ἡνίοχος ἰδὼν τὸ ἐρωτικὸν ὄμμα, πᾶσαν αἰσθήσει διαθερμήνας
254 τὴν ψυχήν, γαργαλισμοῦ τε καὶ πόθου κέντρων ὑποπλησθῇ, ὁ μὲν εὐπειθὴς τῷ ἡνιόχῳ τῶν ἵππων, ἀεί τε καὶ τότε αἰδοῖ βιαζόμενος, ἑαυτὸν κατέχει μὴ ἐπιπηδᾶν τῷ ἐρωμένῳ. ὁ δὲ οὔτε κέντρων ἡνιοχικῶν οὔτε μάστιγος ἔτι ἐντρέπεται, σκιρτῶν δὲ βίᾳ φέρεται, καὶ πάντα πράγματα παρέχων τῷ σύζυγί τε καὶ ἡνιόχῳ ἀναγκάζει ἰέναι τε πρὸς τὰ παιδικὰ καὶ μνείαν ποιεῖσθαι τῆς τῶν ἀφροδισίων χάριτος. τὼ δὲ κατ' ἀρχὰς μὲν ἀντιτείνετον
b ἀγανακτοῦντε, ὡς δεινὰ καὶ παράνομα ἀναγκαζομένω· τελευτῶντε δέ, ὅταν μηδὲν ᾖ πέρας κακοῦ, πορεύεσθον ἀγομένω, εἴξαντε καὶ ὁμολογήσαντε ποιήσειν τὸ κελευόμενον. καὶ πρὸς αὐτῷ τ' ἐγένοντο καὶ εἶδον τὴν ὄψιν τὴν τῶν παιδικῶν ἀστράπτουσαν. ἰδόντος δὲ τοῦ ἡνιόχου ἡ μνήμη πρὸς τὴν τοῦ κάλλους φύσιν ἠνέχθη, καὶ πάλιν εἶδεν αὐτὴν μετὰ σωφροσύνης ἐν ἁγνῷ βάθρῳ βεβῶσαν· ἰδοῦσα δὲ ἔδεισέ τε καὶ σεφθεῖσα
c ἀνέπεσεν ὑπτία, καὶ ἅμα ἠναγκάσθη εἰς τοὐπίσω ἑλκύσαι τὰς ἡνίας οὕτω σφόδρα, ὥστ' ἐπὶ τὰ ἰσχία ἄμφω καθίσαι τὼ ἵππω, τὸν μὲν ἑκόντα διὰ τὸ μὴ ἀντιτείνειν, τὸν δὲ ὑβριστὴν μάλ' ἄκοντα. ἀπελθόντε δὲ ἀπωτέρω, ὁ μὲν ὑπ' αἰσχύνης τε καὶ θάμβους ἱδρῶτι πᾶσαν ἔβρεξε τὴν ψυχήν, ὁ δὲ λήξας τῆς ὀδύνης, ἣν ὑπὸ τοῦ χαλινοῦ τε ἔσχεν καὶ τοῦ πτώματος, μόγις ἐξαναπνεύσας ἐλοιδόρησεν ὀργῇ, πολλὰ κακίζων τόν τε ἡνίοχον καὶ τὸν ὁμόζυγα
d ὡς δειλίᾳ τε καὶ ἀνανδρίᾳ λιπόντε τὴν τάξιν καὶ ὁμολογίαν· καὶ πάλιν οὐκ ἐθέλοντας προσιέναι ἀναγκάζων μόγις συνεχώρησεν δεομένων εἰς αὖθις

secured relief by finding the means thereto, namely by recourse to prayer and worship; and in consequence thereof rites and means of purification were established, and the sufferer was brought out of danger, alike for the present and for the future. Thus did madness secure, for him that was maddened aright and possessed, deliverance from his troubles.

There is a third form of possession or madness, of which the Muses are the source. This seizes a tender, virgin soul and stimulates it to rapt passionate expresssion, especially in lyric poetry, glorifying the countless mighty deeds of ancient times for the instruction of posterity. But if any man come to the gates of poetry without the madness of the Muses, persuaded that skill alone will make him a good poet, then shall he and his works of sanity with him be brought to naught by the poetry of madness, and behold, their place is nowhere to be found.

6.10 Plato, *Phaedrus* 253e5–254e5

Now when the driver beholds the person of the beloved, and causes a sensation of warmth to suffuse the whole soul, he begins to experience a tickling or pricking of desire; and the obedient steed, constrained now as always by modesty, refrains from leaping upon the beloved; but his fellow, heeding no more the driver's goad or whip, leaps and dashes on, sorely troubling his companion and his driver, and forcing them to approach the loved one and remind him of the delights of love's commerce. For a while they struggle, indignant that he should force them to a monstrous and forbidden act; but at last, finding no end to their evil plight, they yield and agree to do his bidding. And so he draws them on, and now they are quite close and behold the spectacle of the beloved flashing upon them. At that sight the driver's memory goes back to that form of Beauty, and he sees her once again enthroned by the side of Temperance upon her holy seat; then in awe and reverence he falls upon his back, and therewith is compelled to pull the reins so violently that he brings both steeds down on their haunches, the good one willing and unresistant, but the wanton sore against his will. Now that they are a little way off, the good horse in shame and horror drenches the whole soul with sweat, while the other, contriving to recover his wind after the pain of the bit and his fall, bursts into angry abuse, railing at the charioteer and his yoke-fellow as cowardly treacherous deserters. Once again he tries to force them to advance, and when

ὑπερβαλέσθαι. ἐλθόντος δὲ τοῦ συντεθέντος χρόνου [οὗ] ἀμνημονεῖν προσποιουμένῳ ἀναμιμνήσκων, βιαζόμενος, χρεμετίζων, ἕλκων ἠνάγκασεν αὖ προσελθεῖν τοῖς παιδικοῖς ἐπὶ τοὺς αὐτοὺς λόγους, καὶ ἐπειδὴ ἐγγὺς ἦσαν, ἐγκύψας καὶ ἐκτείνας τὴν κέρκον, ἐνδακὼν τὸν χαλινόν, μετ' ἀναιδείας
e ἕλκει· ὁ δ' ἡνίοχος ἔτι μᾶλλον ταὐτὸν πάθος παθών, ὥσπερ ἀπὸ ὕσπληγος ἀναπεσών, ἔτι μᾶλλον τοῦ ὑβριστοῦ ἵππου ἐκ τῶν ὀδόντων βίᾳ ὀπίσω σπάσας τὸν χαλινόν, τήν τε κακηγόρον γλῶτταν καὶ τὰς γνάθους καθῄμαξεν καὶ τὰ σκέλη τε καὶ τὰ ἰσχία πρὸς τὴν γῆν ἐρείσας ὀδύναις ἔδωκεν.

6.11 Plato, *Timaeus* 81e6–82a7

82 Τὸ δὲ τῶν νόσων ὅθεν συνίσταται, δῆλόν που καὶ παντί. τεττάρων γὰρ ὄντων γενῶν ἐξ ὧν συμπέπηγεν τὸ σῶμα, γῆς πυρὸς ὕδατός τε καὶ ἀέρος, τούτων ἡ παρὰ φύσιν πλεονεξία καὶ ἔνδεια καὶ τῆς χώρας μετάστασις ἐξ οἰκείας ἐπ' ἀλλοτρίαν γιγνομένη, πυρός τε αὖ καὶ τῶν ἑτέρων ἐπειδὴ γένη πλείονα ἑνὸς ὄντα τυγχάνει, τὸ μὴ προσῆκον ἕκαστον ἑαυτῷ προσλαμβάνειν, καὶ πάνθ' ὅσα τοιαῦτα, στάσεις καὶ νόσους παρέχει·

6.12 Plato, *Timaeus* 82e7–83a5

παλιναίρετα γὰρ πάντα γεγονότα καὶ διεφθαρμένα τό τε αἷμα αὐτὸ πρῶτον
83 διόλλυσι, καὶ αὐτὰ οὐδεμίαν τροφὴν ἔτι τῷ σώματι παρέχοντα φέρεται πάντῃ διὰ τῶν φλεβῶν, τάξιν τῶν κατὰ φύσιν οὐκέτ' ἴσχοντα περιόδων, ἐχθρὰ μὲν αὐτὰ αὑτοῖς διὰ τὸ μηδεμίαν ἀπόλαυσιν ἑαυτῶν ἔχειν, τῷ συνεστῶτι δὲ τοῦ σώματος καὶ μένοντι κατὰ χώραν πολέμια, διολλύντα καὶ τήκοντα.

6.13 Plato, *Timaeus* 85e2–86a2

85e πλείων δ' ἐπιρρέουσα, τῇ παρ' αὑτῆς θερμότητι κρατήσασα τὰς ἶνας εἰς ἀταξίαν ζέσασα διέσεισεν· καὶ ἐὰν μὲν ἱκανὴ διὰ τέλους κρατῆσαι γένηται, πρὸς τὸ τοῦ μυελοῦ διαπεράσασα γένος κάουσα ἔλυσεν τὰ τῆς ψυχῆς αὐτόθεν οἷον νεὼς πείσματα μεθῆκέν τε ἐλευθέραν, ὅταν δ' ἐλάττων ᾖ τό τε σῶμα ἀντίσχῃ τηκόμενον, αὐτὴ κρατηθεῖσα ἢ κατὰ πᾶν τὸ σῶμα ἐξέπεσεν, ἢ διὰ τῶν φλεβῶν εἰς τὴν κάτω συνωσθεῖσα ἢ τὴν ἄνω κοιλίαν,

Chapter 6 Texts   173

they beg him to delay awhile he grudgingly consents. But when the time appointed is come, and they feign to have forgotten, he reminds them of it, struggling and neighing and pulling until he compels them a second time to approach the beloved and renew their offer; and when they have come close, with head down and tail stretched out he takes the bit between his teeth and shamelessly plunges on. But the driver, with resentment even stronger than before, like a racer recoiling from the starting-rope, jerks back the bit in the mouth of the wanton horse with an even stronger pull, bespatters his railing tongue and his jaws with blood, and forcing him down on legs and haunches delivers him over to anguish.

6.11   Plato, *Timaeus* 81e6–82a7

As regards diseases, how they originate is clear in a way to everyone. Since there are four kinds from which the body is constituted—earth, fire, water and air—when there is, contrary to nature, an excess or deficiency in these, or a transfer from their proper region to an alien one, or again since fire or the others have more than one variety, when the body admits an inappropriate one, all such and similar occurrences bring about strifes and diseases.

6.12   Plato, *Timaeus* 82e7–83a5

For when all the substances become reversed and corrupted, first of all they destroy the blood, and then themselves no longer afford nourishment to the body and move through the veins in every kind of way: they no longer maintain the order of their natural movements, but being at enmity with themselves they have no enjoyment of themselves and being at war with the established and regular, stable, constitution of the body they destroy and dissolve it.

6.13   Plato, *Timaeus* 85e2–86a2

But when [the bile] flows in, in greater quantity, it overcomes the fibres by the heat it contains and shakes it into disorder by boiling up. And if it is enough to overcome completely, it penetrates to the nature of the marrow and loosens from there the mooring-ropes of the soul, as it were of a ship, by burning them, and lets it free. But when it is less and the body resists being dissolved, then the bile itself is overcome, and either it is ejected all over the body or else it

86 οἷον φυγὰς ἐκ πόλεως στασιασάσης ἐκ τοῦ σώματος ἐκπίπτουσα, διαρροίας καὶ δυσεντερίας καὶ τὰ τοιαῦτα νοσήματα πάντα παρέσχετο.

6.14, Plato *Timaeus* 86b1–7

86b Καὶ τὰ μὲν περὶ τὸ σῶμα νοσήματα ταύτῃ συμβαίνει γιγνόμενα, τὰ δὲ περὶ ψυχὴν διὰ σώματος ἕξιν τῇδε. νόσον μὲν δὴ ψυχῆς ἄνοιαν συγχωρητέον, δύο δ' ἀνοίας γένη, τὸ μὲν μανίαν, τὸ δὲ ἀμαθίαν. πᾶν οὖν ὅτι πάσχων τις πάθος ὁπότερον αὐτῶν ἴσχει, νόσον προσρητέον, ἡδονὰς δὲ καὶ λύπας ὑπερβαλλούσας τῶν νόσων μεγίστας θετέον τῇ ψυχῇ.

6.15, Plato *Timaeus* 87c4–d3

87c πᾶν δὴ τὸ ἀγαθὸν καλόν, τὸ δὲ καλὸν οὐκ ἄμετρον· καὶ ζῷον οὖν τὸ τοιοῦτον ἐσόμενον σύμμετρον θετέον. συμμετριῶν δὲ τὰ μὲν σμικρὰ **d** διαισθανόμενοι συλλογιζόμεθα, τὰ δὲ κυριώτατα καὶ μέγιστα ἀλογίστως ἔχομεν. πρὸς γὰρ ὑγιείας καὶ νόσους ἀρετάς τε καὶ κακίας οὐδεμία συμμετρία καὶ ἀμετρία μείζων ἢ ψυχῆς αὐτῆς πρὸς σῶμα αὐτό.

is forced through the veins into the lower or upper gut, and is ejected from the body like exiles from a city in a state of faction: and it produces diarrhoea and dysentery and suchlike diseases.

6.14 Plato, *Timaeus* 86b1–7

That is the way in which diseases of the body occur: and those of the soul that are due to the condition of the body happen in the following way. We must agree that folly is a disease of the soul, and of folly there are two kinds. one being madness, the other ignorance. Whenever anyone suffers either of these affections, we must call it a disease, and we must suppose that excessive pleasures and pains are the greatest of the soul's diseases.

6.15 Plato, *Timaeus* 87c4–d3

All that is good is fair and what is fair does not lack due measure. So the living creature that is to be fair must be symmetrical. Of symmetries, we perceive distinctly and reason about the minor ones, but of the most important and greatest ones we have no rational comprehension. For as regards health and disease, and virtues and vices, there is no symmetry or lack of symmetry that is greater than that between the soul itself and the body itself.

7
Aristotle

Aristotle was the son of a doctor and contemplated writing a treatise *On Health and Disease*, though if he did so, it is no longer extant. We can organize our discussion of what he has to say about disease that is germane to our study under five main heads.

1. The importance of medicine in natural philosophy, 'physics', *phusike*, in Aristotle's sense.
2. His development of the comparison between the state and the body and of the nature of the healthy organism as the model for well-being in both the individual and the state.
3. The support the ideas of health and disease lend to the theses of the objectivity of the good and the existence of experts who can speak with authority on the subject—topics that we have just been discussing in relation to Plato, although Aristotle's position diverges from his in fundamental respects.
4. Further conclusions concerning good and deviant political constitutions that again draw on notions that have resonance in the sphere of medicine.
5. Aristotle's famous, but famously obscure, notion that the function of tragedy is to produce a *katharsis,* a purification or purgation.

In many cases there are anticipations of Aristotle's ideas in earlier writers. But it is not my chief aim here to assess his originality, but rather to explore the ramifications of the idea of disease in different areas of his work—and of its grip on his imagination.

Aristotle

1. In two prominent texts in the *Parva Naturalia*, namely at *On the Senses* 436ª17 ff. [T 7.1] and *On Respiration* 480ᵇ22 ff. [T 7.2], Aristotle makes the claim that the investigation of the first principles and causes of diseases is the job not just of the doctor (*iatros*) but also of the natural philosopher (*phusikos*). We recall the importance of the concept of nature in the Hippocratic treatise *On the Sacred Disease* in its refutation of the idea that that disease is the result of divine intervention. It is precisely as a student of nature, *phusis*, that Aristotle engages in his extensive inquiries into animals and into the inanimate world. *Phusis* stakes out a territory over which the *phusikos* can claim expertise. But now we see a wedge driven between the *phusikos* and the doctor. It is the more philosophically inclined doctors, he says in *On the Senses* 436ª19 ff., that share the interest in primary causes that most of the students of nature engage in. The latter end their inquiries with medicine, the former start their investigations of medicine from the study of nature. Similarly at the end of *On Respiration*, 480ᵇ24 ff., Aristotle says that we should not fail to recognise how the two groups differ. It is the more subtle doctors who derive their principles from the study of nature, and the most polished (*chariestatoi*) of the students of nature who end up by considering medical principles.

This concern with boundaries, both between doctors and naturalists, and within each group, is what we have come to expect in areas of Greek intellectual life where rivalry is endemic and claims to superiority repeatedly challenged. But Aristotle's own understanding of those boundaries is distinctive. It is not that he identifies the study of medicine with that of nature as a whole. However much the author of *On the Sacred Disease* went into battle under the banner of 'nature', there are, in Aristotle's view, still clear differences between doctors (even the 'more subtle' ones) and students of nature. The most obvious, of course, would be that the aim of medicine is not just theoretical knowledge, but to heal the sick.[1]

---

[1] See below, p. 182, on *Nicomachean Ethics* 1097ª11 ff., and cf. 1137ª23 ff.

In practice, to be sure, many natural philosophers claimed expertise on the subject of the causes of health and disease, whether or not they were medical practitioners. Plato is the most striking of a number of examples, among whom we may include several of the theorists mentioned in *Anonymus Londinensis* such as Philolaus, as well as the authors of some of the *epideixeis* in the Hippocratic Corpus.

Furthermore if Aristotle himself wrote on health and disease, he would count as another case, and in any event we find him pronouncing in general terms on medical problems in his extant treatises. It is true that when in the *Topics*, $139^{b}20$f., $145^{b}7$ff., and *Physics*, $246^{b}4$f., he refers to health being a balance or proportion, *summetria*, between opposites such as hot and cold, he is repeating what may be taken as a commonplace of Greek thought. However in *On the Parts of Animals* 2 chs. 2–4, for instance, he goes into the question of the innate constitution of different types of animals with some care, suggesting that their character and intelligence depend (in part) on the quality of their blood. Again in the *Parva Naturalia* he discusses the causes of old age and death in animals (see King 2001). Although he does not, in the treatises that have come down to us, present a fully fledged theory of disease, in the manner of Plato's *Timaeus*, his natural philosophical interests extend to the study of what preserves the normal healthy state of the animal and of what threatens to undermine that.

So we can see that that convergence of the studies of the more philosophical doctors and those of the more polished of the natural philosophers enables Aristotle to claim the former as his allies while maintaining the right of the natural philosophers to pronounce on matters that others might consider belonged to the domain of medicine. At the same time he scores a point against both the less philosophical doctors and those natural philosophers who did not go into the problem of the first principles of diseases. The former lack the basic theory on which their practical skills depend. The latter ignore an important part of the domain of the study of nature. While Aristotle makes his own views clear, we should remember that there were Hippocratic authors who would strongly have resisted that convergence. The author of *On Ancient Medicine*, in particular, objected to what he considered the invasion of medicine by 'philosophy', represented, precisely, by those who sought to derive the whole of medicine from a limited number of 'hypotheses', postulates, or as Aristotle might have said 'first principles', concerning the causes of diseases. The objection to them, according to the Hippocratic author, is that they narrow down the principles of disease and introduce factors that are unverifiable, a fatal mistake in a branch of knowledge such as medicine that depends on experience. So not all the more subtle doctors in our sources would have agreed with that convergence that Aristotle wished for: they for their part would have insisted on the autonomy of medicine from the focus on the types of causal explanations in the study of nature as a whole that Aristotle advocated.

2. Our second topic is again one on which Aristotle draws on predecessors, Plato especially. The Aristotelian versions of the idea of the body as modelled on the state and that of the state as the body politic have precedents in, for example, the analogy between the individual and the state in the *Republic*. Yet the context in which Aristotle introduces the first image, in *On the Movement of Animals* 703^{a}29ff. [T 7.3], is very different, namely the investigation of how animals move. The leading idea here is that there is a controlling element in the soul that is responsible not just for movement, that is voluntary motions, but also for perception and indeed life itself. He believes that the heart, where this control centre is located, is the first part of the animal to be formed, and he claims direct evidence for this from his detailed investigation of the development of hen's eggs. In a famous experiment in the *History of Animals* 6 ch. 3, 561^{a}4ff., he describes the dissection of eggs at different stages of growth and reports that the first part to be formed (the first visible to the naked eye, that is) is what later came to be called the *punctum saliens*, corresponding to the heart.

In *On the Movement of Animals*, after a discussion of the modalities of movement in which he alludes (at 703ª14ff.) to the primacy of the heart, he proceeds: 'we must suppose that an animal is constituted like a well-governed city-state. For once order is established in the city, there is no need of a monarch to be present at every activity, but individuals each play their own part as they are ordered, and one thing follows another because of habituation. So in animals the same thing happens because of nature, each part naturally doing its own work as constituted by nature. So there is no need for soul in each part, but it resides in a kind of source of authority, *arche* [here ruling part, as much as principle] in the body, and the other parts live by being naturally connected to it, and they perform their own work because of nature' (703ª29–b2).

Here we see Aristotle making the most of the analogy between living organism and state for the sake of some 'biological' conclusions. But as we shall see in greater detail later in this chapter, the analogy works also in the reverse direction. The constitution (*politeia*) he says at *Politics*, 1295ª40f. [T 7.4], is a kind of life (*bios tis*) for the state. But by kind of life he means not just being alive, but more especially a manner of living. Although *phusis,* nature, as a whole, corresponds to what is good, often picking out the final causes of objects or events—and so in *On the Movement of Animals* a normal animal is compared with a *well-ordered* city—there are of course better and worse manners of life and better and worse political constitutions. In the *Politics* passage, Aristotle's concern is to suggest that the best constitution is one where the *mesoi*— 'middle class' in the sense of those who are neither very rich nor very poor—are the dominant group.

It is in fact the healthy organism that serves as the model for the well-run state, and the notion of disease is, as we shall see, in the background in his account of deviant constitutions. We said that it was the well-governed state that serves as the analogue for the way the control centre in the animal should and normally does operate, and what Aristotle called the *arche* in the triple sense of principle and starting-point and source of rule was later to enter into discussions of how the soul governs the body under the label of the *hegemonikon*. The modelling of the idea of psychic control on political rule (already present in Plato) thus became profoundly embedded in Greek thought, and as we shall see in the next chapter, was common ground to theorists who interpreted it in quite different ways to support divergent psychologies.

3. The normative function of health takes us to our next topics, the way in which the medical analogue underpins claims that in ethics values such as the good and the pleasant are objective, and the idea that there are experts who can pronounce on this with authority. Plato too, as we saw, used medicine to justify his ideas of the role of the philosopher-kings and to support the Socratic thesis that it is better to undergo punishment (the cure of the wrongdoings of your soul) than not to do so. But for Plato the ultimate source of the objectivity of ethical values is the corresponding Forms, of Justice, Courage, the Good itself. Aristotle uses the same analogy, and shares a belief in objectivity in the moral domain, but now gives a very different account of that from Plato's.

Moral virtue or excellence, *arete*, in the famous definition in the *Nicomachean Ethics*, 1106^{b}36ff., is a state that lies in a mean relative to us and as the person with practical wisdom would define it. This is not an arithmetic mean halfway between the excesses either side of it, of course, but virtue lies, nevertheless, between excess and defect, courage between foolhardiness and cowardice, generosity between profligacy and miserliness, and so on. Courage is not just a matter of doing a few courageous acts: it must reflect the disposition to behave in such a way. The deeds stem from the disposition, which they nevertheless help to build up. The actions must also reflect knowledge of all the relevant circumstances of the case. Obviously if the soldier is unaware of the danger he runs, he is not behaving courageously. So the appeals to the knowledge of the context of the action, and to how the person of practical wisdom, the *phronimos*, would decide, are essential.

It is the *phronimos* who can tell the right thing to do, at the right time and for the right motives.

But what that right solution will be will vary from one individual to another, for one aspect of the knowledge required relates to the agent's own circumstances. It is easiest to illustrate this in the case of generosity. Clearly what would be a generous donation to a charitable cause on the part of a poor person would not count as generosity in a multi-millionaire.

But if what will count as a virtuous act and a virtuous disposition varies from one person to another, that does not mean that Aristotle has abandoned the claim to objectivity in ethics. Certainly not. There *is* a right solution in each case for each individual, even though we have to take those differences into account.

The analogy with health and disease is repeatedly invoked to support different aspects of Aristotle's position. He uses it first in relation to the basic point that ethics is a practical, not a theoretical, branch of knowledge. The doctor, he says at *Nicomachean Ethics* $1097^{a}11$ ff. [T 7.5] in an argument objecting to Plato's conception of the form of the Good, focuses not on health in general, but on that of a human being, or rather on that of this human being. For it is the individual whom he cures. Both general, that is abstract, knowledge on the one hand, and knowledge of the particular circumstances of the case, have their distinct roles to play. In medicine, he says at $1137^{a}13$ ff. [T 7.6], optimistically, in all conscience, it is easy to know what honey, wine, hellebore, cautery, and surgery are: but to know how and when to apply them so as to bring about a cure is no less a task than that of being a doctor. To be a physician and cure patients is not a matter of employing or not employing surgery or drugs, but of doing so in a certain manner.

Then three other contexts in which the health analogy is put to work are in relation to the basic idea of the moral disposition as a mean, with regard to his views on how moral dispositions are formed, and to his conception of the good person as the judge or criterion of right and wrong.

Thus at 1104ª11ff. [T 7.7] in first introducing the mean Aristotle remarks that moral qualities are destroyed by excesses and deficiencies and he cites the analogies with strength and health to support this. Both those two are ruined by too much, or too little, exercise, or food and drink, while the right amount preserves and increases them. He continues with the food analogy at 1106ª29 ff. [T 7.8] when pointing out that the mean varies from one individual to another. The correct amount for an athlete such as Milo would not be right for ordinary people.

Then at 1114ª11 ff.[T 7.9] and 1115ª1–3, when discussing how moral dispositions are formed, his key point is that we are directly responsible for our individual actions and so indirectly for our dispositions or characters. The latter, once formed, are hard to change. The case is argued by reference to a sick person. He or she may have become ill because of intemperate living or ignoring the doctor's orders. But once sick, it may not be possible voluntarily to become well again. While it was once open to the patient not to become sick, that may eventually not be an option. So once we have become unjust or self-indulgent, for example, it may no longer be possible not to be so.[2]

Some had claimed that views on the subject of pleasure, for instance, are subjective. But Aristotle counters this and argues that the good person is the true judge of what is really pleasant. The case is analogous to health, where it is the person of sound constitution who can be used as a standard. Aristotle is aware that sick people have a different view of what is sweet or bitter, for example, from healthy individuals. But that does not lead him to qualify the claim that we can talk about what is really sweet and bitter for he believes we can use the healthy person as the judge of this (1113ª25 ff., 1173ᵇ22 ff. [T 7.10], 1176ª12 ff. [T 7.11]). It is the morally sound person who must be taken to be the one who can determine what is

---

[2] Aristotle also uses a comparison with throwing a stone to make the same point: once you have let it go, it is too late to recover it, *Nicomachean Ethics* 1114ª16–19 [T 7.9].

truly pleasant or painful not just in the physical domain but right across the board.

There are, of course, difficulties in Aristotle's position here, because even the question of who *is* healthy can be problematic, and a fortiori who is morally sound is likely to be. Here there is a difference between the medical and the moral situations that Aristotle leaves implicit. We may distinguish between the question of whether we can believe there are morally sound individuals, and the further issue of how we would recognise them, if they exist. Doctors are those who, in principle at least, are supposed to be able to tell the healthy from the sick, though the appearances may well be deceptive and the ordinary lay person may well get it wrong. Of course in the medical domain being healthy is quite distinct from being able to say who or what is healthy. In the sphere of morality, however, soundness of moral judgement, in Aristotle's judgement at least, does double service. Knowledge here is indissociable from morality itself (1144^a1 ff.). A person who is just intellectually knowledgeable is not a man of practical wisdom, but just someone who is clever (*deinos*, 1144^a23 ff.). Conversely, without knowledge of the appropriate kind the person who has a good disposition possesses not moral, but merely natural excellence (1144^b4 ff.). But that means that the person who does fulfil both criteria, having both moral excellence and practical wisdom, is the analogue both of the doctor (who can reason correctly about health) and of the person who is truly healthy.

The differences between Aristotle's and Plato's use of the medical analogy in ethics are worth spelling out as a conclusion to this section. For Plato the good is absolute, difficult as it is to describe the Form of the Good, let alone to attain it. But that and the other Forms correspond to what is in no sense relativised, whether to persons or respects or times or places. What is beautiful in itself is contrasted with what is beautiful in some respects but not others in such a text as *Symposium* 210e f. It is because they have apprehended the Forms and can give an account of them that the philosopher-kings are true statesmen. Even though Plato does not expect *doctors* to proceed by way of understanding the Forms, and their knowledge is accordingly inferior to that of the philosopher, they too are expected to be able to give the reasons for why the healthy are healthy, the sick sick, and for the remedies and treatments for the situations they encounter.

But Aristotle, without absolutes as moral standards, can and still does appeal to the medical analogy, to justify his different claims to objectivity. Indeed he can be said to use more of the medical situation to illustrate the moral one. In contrast, rather, to Plato, Aristotle uses the doctor as the analogue for the morally sound person in respect of the detailed appreciation of all the circumstances of the particular case that both will need to have. The doctor's decisions will depend on a grasp not just of the general principles of medicine, but of how to bring about a cure in the individual patient with whom he is faced. Just as in Plato, the doctor is the person in authority, but the way he exercises that authority is different, for it involves his practical understanding of all the relevant circumstances of the case. As in Plato, ordinary folk should agree with what the experts prescribe, and as in Plato, the desirability of being good is supported by the far less controversial desirability of being healthy. Yet given Aristotle's views on the difficulty of altering a disposition, once it has become ingrained, it is not that he sends an optimistic message about how the morally unsound may be 'cured'.

4. The political applications of the health analogy had, as we saw, supported Plato's view that the true statesman will be able to diagnose the diseases in the body politic and will move swiftly and surely from diagnosis to treatment, not shrinking from the most painful measures if they are necessary to purge the state of pathogens. Aristotle too has his accounts of the best, and of normal or natural, constitutions to propose, though these are far less idealistic than those Plato suggested in the *Republic* or even in the *Laws*. First Aristotle's view of the knowledge the statesman needs to possess incorporates

the same conception of *phronesis* or practical wisdom that we discussed in the last section. The *phronimoi* will be able to arrive at correct judgements about what to do, though they will certainly not do so by reference to absolutes. Rather, the skills they need to display are (as we have seen) like those of the doctor who has to take into account all the circumstances of a case in reaching a diagnosis and recommendations for therapy.

Here then is one context in which the medical analogy is relevant. Another relates to Aristotle's classification of political constitutions. Different suggestions are made at different places in the *Politics* on this issue, but in the most complex of his analyses, at 1279^{a}22 ff. [T 7.12] he contrasts three true constitutions with what he calls their deviations (*parekbaseis*). The three correct constitutions are the rule of one (monarchy), that of the few (aristocracy) and that of a greater number, which here goes by the general label 'constitution' (*politeia*)—the same term being used both generically of constitutions as a whole, and normatively of the *best* one. Those three are contrasted with three others on the criterion of *whose* interests are served. In each case the correct constitutions aim not just at the good of those who rule but of the whole state. The three corresponding deviant constitutions, tyranny, oligarchy, and democracy, have just the interests of the rulers at heart.

The term I have translated 'deviation', namely *parekbasis* (e.g. at 1279^{b}4 [T 7.13]) does not directly conjure up ideas of sickness. But the true constitutions are the natural ones, and in that sense these deviations are abnormal or unnatural. The 'soundness' of a state is compared with health and with seaworthy ships in such a context as 1320^{b}33 ff., to make the point that a weak state needs most safeguarding, just as a sickly body and unseaworthy ships are especially vulnerable. 'Nature' applies, we must remember, even in the political domain: for all humans are *by* nature political animals, more strictly ones that live in city-states (1253^{a}2 f.). Even though Aristotle is fully aware of important differences between the inquiry into nature (*phusike*) and moral and political philosophy, both deal with regularities and cause–effect relationships, to describe which the same term 'nature' can be used, on occasion, in both contexts. The person who knows—Aristotle himself in the first instance—can contrast the natural with unnatural social arrangements, where the former correspond to the natures of human beings as the social animals they are.

5. Aristotle's famous essay on literary criticism has more in common (I shall claim) with the other aspects of his thought that we have been discussing than one might at first expect. His account of poetry can be seen as restoring it to the place of importance and prestige that it normally occupied in Greek perceptions, but which had been challenged by Plato's attacks in the *Republic*. Plato had banned most Greek poetry, epic and tragedy included, first for purveying false tales about the gods and false morality in general, and then for promoting dangerous psychological tendencies—encouraging people to live with images or representations rather than training their souls to study reality. For Aristotle poetry in general and tragedy in particular had positive value, but quite what he wishes to claim for them is much disputed. Tragedy, in his well-known but elliptical phrase (*Poetics* 1449^{b}24ff. [T 7.14]) procures, through pity and fear, a *katharsis* of such affections.

What kind of *katharsis* is this? Three main lines of interpretation have been put forward, that it is or is like a medical purge, that it is basically a ritual or religious one, and that it is no purification or purgation at all, but rather a clarification (Nussbaum 1986, 388–90). That last, cognitive, view does not sufficiently explain the reciprocity involved in the *katharsis of* certain emotions *through* them. On that view Aristotle would seem to owe us an account of why in certain circumstances (but not in others) such a 'clarification' of emotions should occur by their very experience.

We have to concede, to be sure, that the *Poetics* itself gives us very little to go on. Ritual purifications can indeed be exemplified in extant tragedy: the end of Aeschylus' *Oresteia* is one notable instance. Yet the claim Aristotle makes is a quite general one about tragedy as a whole, and too specific an application to what happens only in particular plays can be faulted on those grounds.

Our main clue to understanding must come from the account of the aims and effects of different kinds of music in *Politics* 8, where Aristotle deals with education in relation to his ideal state. This text has, of course, often been brought to bear, but some have been reluctant to allow the medical ideas it introduces to be the key to the statement about tragedy in the *Poetics*.

At 1341^{b}32 ff. [T 7.15] he distinguishes three types of melodies, 'ethical' ones, melodies relating to actions, and 'enthusiastic' ones. Music should be used not just for one kind of benefit but for many, for it serves the purposes both of education and of *katharsis* (^{b}38). He says he will use the term *katharsis* for the present without qualification or explanation, *haplos*, though 'we will speak more clearly about it again in the *Poetics*'. Unfortunately that does not happen in what we have of that work, and if Aristotle's promise was fulfilled, that must have been in the parts that we know were written but are not extant. Then thirdly, the third purpose it serves is for *diagoge*, amusement, helping to relax us and affording relief from tension.

Using this threefold analysis of aims and of benefits, he says that all should be used, and attempts some correlations between his earlier account of melodies and the corresponding benefits. Thus the ethical melodies should be used for education. The two others (active and enthusiastic) are to be employed on other occasions, in listening to others' performances. He then opens a convoluted digression in an already complicated analysis. Any *pathos*, feeling, affection, or emotion (but the term is of course also used of disease) that occurs violently in some souls is found in all, some to a greater, some to a less, extent. That includes pity and fear and again 'enthusiasm'. Some people are liable to this change and possessed by it. 'We see them, under the influence of sacred melodies, when they use melodies that excite the soul to frenzy, being restored as if they had received a cure (*iatreia*) and a *katharsis*.'

The same experience must also come to the compassionate and the fearful and those who are generally given to feeling (*pathetikoi*) to the degree that it affects each type: all must undergo a certain *katharsis* and a feeling of relief accompanied by pleasure. And similarly also the purgative (*kathartika*) melodies offer harmless delight to people.

This text is, as remarked, highly convoluted, and yet it provides us with important insights. First the correlations between melodies and purposes are not straightforward. While educational aims are served by 'ethical' melodies, the other two purposes are divided between the other two types of melody. The juxtaposition with cure at 1342ª10ff. suggests that the *katharsis* in question there is thought of partly as a medical purge. Yet this clear reference to a medical purgation relates to the experience of those who suffer from religious fervour or possession (*enthousiasmos*) who listen to sacred melodies. Aristotle evidently moves without strain from the religious to the medical context—and this is in line with what we have already found in Chapter 3, for instance, namely that, just as *pharmaka* may be spells or drugs, so 'purifications' span both rituals and physical purges. Moreover in the *Politics* the cures in question are pleasurable. This is implicit perhaps at 1342a10f. where the *katharsis* involves a restoration (*kathistamenous*) to a normal state. But it is explicit in the second reference at a14f. which speaks of the pleasant feeling of relief that accompanies *katharsis* there, and the point is repeated in the mention of the 'harmless delight' that purgative melodies offer.

The central question must now be faced. How far is the *Politics* passage relevant to the claims in the *Poetics* about tragedy? Evidently the discussion in the *Politics* concerns music of different kinds, while the *Poetics* offers an account of the experience of tragedy in particular. Yet two lines of argument strongly suggest that we can and should relate the two texts. First there is the explicit cross-reference to the *Poetics* in the *Politics*. Even though that appears to be to a part of the *Poetics* we no longer have, it would be surprising if that part conflicted in what it had to say on *katharsis* with the mention of that term in the definition of tragedy. Secondly, both texts refer to the same emotions or affections, pity and fear, and their removal.

Yet the stumbling block to using the *Politics*, and to the whole medical line of interpretation of *katharsis*, has been thought to be that medical purgations deal with the sick, while tragedy can be appreciated by the healthy and there is no suggestion that Aristotle thought anything different. Why should *we* need this kind of medical treatment? Why should the citizens of Greek city-states do so especially, or, to turn the question round, if, as this interpretation suggests, there is need for a cure for certain feelings, how do those who have not got the chance to go to tragedies (or to listen to the appropriate music), how do they manage to stay healthy?

These questions are understandable, but they arise from mistaken assumptions. What Aristotle appears to believe— indeed what he states in so many words—is that any ordinary person can suffer from some emotional excess or disturbance. The affections that occur in violent form in some souls come to all to a greater or less degree (*Politics* 1342^{a}4 ff.). Even under the best political constitution, then, the citizens may well come to be disturbed. This is not the same problem we had in Plato, where spirit and appetite have to be controlled by the reasoning faculty, even (in the *Phaedrus* image of the chariot-team) with some violence. Aristotle thinks here not so much of a struggle in the soul, as of the feelings by which it may be swayed. At one extreme these include religious possession or Bacchic frenzy (where we might compare the *Bacchae*): but at the milder end of the spectrum, there are still disturbing emotions that may affect anyone—which it may be the function of tragedy to alleviate.

If so, what is claimed is not that tragedy is a cure for the abnormal, but rather of the emotions that fall within the range of anyone's experience. No one can be said to be free of those affections of pity and fear and the like: indeed they contribute to education, in this sense that growing up involves learning to cope with them. The experience of watching a tragedy enables the audience to find the necessary release from them. Even the good person is not immune. To say that we need a purification is not to equate those emotions with disease, nor with religious frenzy, but to allow that common human experience may include powerful affections from which we need relief. And if tragedy is therapeutic in that sense, it is also pleasurable. But these aesthetic pleasures are no more than an extrapolation from Aristotle's general view of pleasure as the accompaniment of natural activity, for in this case the pleasure arises from the return to the norm.

When we say that health is natural, nature is both descriptive and normative. In the descriptive sense, disease and old age are *also* natural, in that they occur as a matter of course. Strong feelings are also natural, in the sense of regular, for everyone is liable to them. But we need relief, to return to a state of full well-being, and can obtain that through tragedy and music of certain types. This is true even if we live as citizens in the best type of political constitution. Even in ideal conditions, the good life is not easy. The *Politics* identifies the different roles that music can play, educational, cathartic, entertaining, each useful and in their different ways pleasurable. Our own understanding of strong feelings, if we follow Aristotle, has been taken further. We have learnt that we may all be subject to them: we need relief from them and we see how that is forthcoming in aesthetic experience.

The concept of *phusis* will enable me to draw some of the threads of our discussion together, for it provides an important connecting link between Aristotle's views on such disparate subjects as medicine itself, the study of nature, ethics and politics, and poetry. While that was the concept that some of the medical writers used to distance themselves from the 'purifiers' and others who believed in divine intervention in diseases, Aristotle drives a wedge within the doctors, and recovers a positive sense for purification. First he distinguishes between those doctors that do and those that do not seek basic medical principles and the causes of health and disease. Those who do, converge in their interests with natural philosophy as he, Aristotle, defines it. Natural philosophy, we are to understand, will encompass the theoretical basis for medicine.

A second fundamental distinction is drawn between 'physics' on the one hand, and 'ethics' and 'politics' on the other. The former deals with the physical world, the latter with the realm of moral choice, political constitutions and the like, a domain where (as in physics) the exactness of mathematical disciplines cannot be expected. Yet the human body is like a well-run state, and the city like a living organism: and different political constitutions can be classified into true and deviant kinds, where the true picks out the normal and the natural.[3] That there is an objective good, and that there is what is objectively pleasant, as determined by the person of sound judgement, is argued in part on the analogy of health—a good that we all want. That there are experts in that domain, doctors, supports the conclusion that persons with objectively good judgement in ethics also exist (even if they do not play the authoritarian role they do in Plato).

Phusis finally underpins the account of the pleasure and relief obtained from watching tragedy, on the interpretation I have offered. Even ordinary people have feelings, of pity and

[3] In a remarkable passage in *Politics* 4 ch. 4, 1290^{b}21 ff., Aristotle suggests a further analogy between political constitutions and animals. To define the different types of constitution, one should proceed by first identifying the necessary parts in the state and then working out their theoretical combinations. Similarly one can classify all the different kinds of animals by identifying the necessary animal parts (sense-organs, organs of locomotion, those involved in nutrition and so on) and seeing how they combine. The interpretation of this passage is disputed, and it has to be said that in his zoological works Aristotle never attempts to classify animals according to the method here envisaged. The text is, however, one further indication of the ease with which Aristotle passes from the domain of (in his terms) physics to that of morality and politics.

fear, that some experience in a violent form. Tragedy fulfils the function of providing an agreeable release from such affections, to return to the norm, in the sense of the ideal condition. Even in the best city-states this will be needed—just as there will inevitably be old age and disease in such cities. Even though *phusis* is not directly invoked in our key texts in the *Poetics* and *Politics,* the latter passage allows us to infer that all human nature is liable to some emotional disturbance and needs such a release. 'Purifications', we have been learning throughout this study, are not limited to strictly medical ones, nor just to religious or ritual ones: where the 'purification' of pity and fear in tragedy is concerned, we can see that Aristotle exploits the full range of possibilities that his term *katharsis* offers.

CHAPTER 7 TEXTS

7.1 Aristotle, *On the Senses* 436ª17–ᵇ1

436a Φυσικοῦ δὲ καὶ περὶ ὑγιείας καὶ νόσου τὰς πρώτας ἰδεῖν ἀρχάς· οὔτε γὰρ ὑγίειαν οὔτε νόσον οἷόν τε γίνεσθαι τοῖς ἐστερημένοις ζωῆς. διὸ σχεδὸν τῶν τε περὶ φύσεως οἱ πλεῖστοι καὶ τῶν ἰατρῶν οἱ φιλοσοφωτέρως τὴν
b τέχνην μετιόντες, οἱ μὲν τελευτῶσιν εἰς τὰ περὶ ἰατρικῆς, οἱ δ' ἐκ τῶν περὶ φύσεως ἄρχονται περὶ τῆς ἰατρικῆς.

7.2 Aristotle, *On Respiration* 480ᵇ21–30

480ob Περὶ μὲν οὖν ζωῆς καὶ θανάτου καὶ τῶν συγγενῶν ταύτης τῆς σκέψεως, σχεδὸν εἴρηται περὶ πάντων. περὶ δὲ ὑγιείας καὶ νόσου οὐ μόνον ἐστὶν ἰατροῦ ἀλλὰ καὶ τοῦ φυσικοῦ μέχρι του τὰς αἰτίας εἰπεῖν. ᾗ δὲ διαφέρουσι καὶ ᾗ διαφέροντα θεωροῦσιν, οὐ δεῖ λανθάνειν, ἐπεὶ ὅτι γε σύνορος ἡ πραγματεία μέχρι τινός ἐστι, μαρτυρεῖ τὸ γινόμενον· τῶν τε γὰρ ἰατρῶν ὅσοι κομψοὶ ἢ περίεργοι, λέγουσί τι περὶ φύσεως καὶ τὰς ἀρχὰς ἐκεῖθεν ἀξιοῦσι λαμβάνειν, καὶ τῶν περὶ φύσεως πραγματευθέντων οἱ χαριέστατοι σχεδὸν τελευτῶσιν εἰς τὰς ἀρχὰς τὰς ἰατρικάς.

7.3 Aristotle, *Movement of Animals* 703ª28–ᵇ2

703a Ὅτι μὲν οὖν κινεῖ κινουμένῳ μορίῳ ἡ ψυχή, εἴρηται, καὶ δι' ἣν αἰτίαν· ὑποληπτέον δὲ συνεστάναι τὸ ζῷον ὥσπερ πόλιν εὐνομουμένην. ἔν τε γὰρ τῇ πόλει ὅταν ἅπαξ συστῇ ἡ τάξις, οὐδὲν δεῖ κεχωρισμένου μονάρχου, ὃν δεῖ παρεῖναι παρ' ἕκαστον τῶν γινομένων, ἀλλ' αὐτὸς ἕκαστος ποιεῖ τὰ αὑτοῦ ὡς τέτακται, καὶ γίνεται τόδε μετὰ τόδε διὰ τὸ ἔθος· ἔν τε τοῖς ζῴοις τὸ αὐτὸ τοῦτο διὰ τὴν φύσιν γίνεται καὶ τῷ πεφυκέναι ἕκαστον οὕτω συστάντων ποιεῖν τὸ αὑτοῦ ἔργον, ὥστε μηδὲν δεῖν ἐν ἑκάστῳ εἶναι ψυχήν,
b ἀλλ' ἔν τινι ἀρχῇ τοῦ σώματος οὔσης τἆλλα ζῆν μὲν τῷ προσπεφυκέναι, ποιεῖν δὲ τὸ ἔργον τὸ αὑτῶν διὰ τὴν φύσιν.

7.4 Aristotle, *Politics* 1295ª40–ᵇ1

1295a τοὺς δὲ αὐτοὺς τούτους ὅρους ἀναγκαῖον εἶναι καὶ πόλεως ἀρετῆς καὶ
b κακίας καὶ πολιτείας, ἡ γὰρ πολιτεία βίος τίς ἐστι πόλεως.

CHAPTER 7 TEXTS

7.1 Aristotle, *On the Senses* 436^{a}17–^{b}1

It is the business of the student of nature to inquire into the first principles of health and disease. For neither health nor disease can come to be in things deprived of life. So generally speaking, most of those who study nature end by dealing with medicine, while those of the doctors who practise their art in a more philosophical manner take their medical principles from nature.

7.2 Aristotle, *On Respiration* 480^{b}21–30

Our inquiry into life and death and related matters is now practically complete. As for health and disease it is not just the business of the doctor, but also of the student of nature, to discuss their causes up to a point. But we should not fail to recognize the way in which they differ and consider different issues, since the facts show that up to a point these inquiries border one another. For those doctors who are more subtle and inquisitive have something to say about the study of nature and claim to derive their principles from it, while the most polished of those who study nature generally end up by considering medical principles.

7.3 Aristotle, *Movement of Animals* 703^{a}28–^{b}2

We have now said what the part is which is moved when the soul initiates movement and what the reason for this is. We must suppose that the animal is constituted like a well-governed city-state. For once order is established in the city, there is no need of a monarch to be present at every activity, but individuals each play their own part as they are ordered, and one thing follows another because of habituation. So in animals the same thing happens because of nature, each part naturally doing its own work as constituted by nature. So there is no need for soul in each part, but it resides in a kind of source of authority in the body, and the other parts live by being naturally connected to it and they perform their own work because of nature.

7.4 Aristotle, *Politics* 1295^{a}40–^{b}1

The same criteria necessarily apply also to the goodness and badness of a city-state, and of a constitution: for the constitution is a kind of life for the state.

7.5 Aristotle, *Nicomachean Ethics* 1097ᵃ11–13

1097a φαίνεται μὲν γὰρ οὐδὲ τὴν ὑγίειαν οὕτως ἐπισκοπεῖν ὁ ἰατρός, ἀλλὰ τὴν ἀνθρώπου, μᾶλλον δ' ἴσως τὴν τοῦδε· καθ' ἕκαστον γὰρ ἰατρεύει.

7.6 Aristotle, *Nicomachean Ethics* 1137ᵃ11–17

1137a ἀλλ' οὐ ταῦτ' ἐστὶ τὰ δίκαια ἀλλ' ἢ κατὰ συμβεβηκός· ἀλλὰ πῶς πραττόμενα καὶ πῶς νεμόμενα δίκαια; τοῦτο δὴ πλέον ἔργον ἢ τὰ ὑγιεινὰ εἰδέναι· ἐπεὶ κἀκεῖ μέλι καὶ οἶνον καὶ ἐλλέβορον καὶ καῦσιν καὶ τομὴν εἰδέναι ῥᾴδιον, ἀλλὰ πῶς δεῖ νεῖμαι πρὸς ὑγίειαν καὶ τίνι καὶ πότε, τοσοῦτον ἔργον ὅσον ἰατρὸν εἶναι.

7.7 Aristotle, *Nicomachean Ethics* 1104ᵃ11–19

1104a Πρῶτον οὖν τοῦτο θεωρητέον, ὅτι τὰ τοιαῦτα πέφυκεν ὑπὸ ἐνδείας καὶ ὑπερβολῆς φθείρεσθαι, (δεῖ γὰρ ὑπὲρ τῶν ἀφανῶν τοῖς φανεροῖς μαρτυρίοις χρῆσθαι) ὥσπερ ἐπὶ τῆς ἰσχύος καὶ τῆς ὑγιείας ὁρῶμεν· τά τε γὰρ ὑπερβάλλοντα γυμνάσια καὶ τὰ ἐλλείποντα φθείρει τὴν ἰσχύν, ὁμοίως δὲ καὶ τὰ ποτὰ καὶ τὰ σιτία πλείω καὶ ἐλάττω γινόμενα φθείρει τὴν ὑγίειαν, τὰ δὲ σύμμετρα καὶ ποιεῖ καὶ αὔξει καὶ σώζει. οὕτως οὖν καὶ ἐπὶ σωφροσύνης καὶ ἀνδρείας ἔχει καὶ τῶν ἄλλων ἀρετῶν.

7.8 Aristotle, *Nicomachean Ethics* 1106ᵃ29–ᵇ7

1106a λέγω δὲ τοῦ μὲν πράγματος μέσον τὸ ἴσον ἀπέχον ἀφ' ἑκατέρου τῶν ἄκρων, ὅπερ ἐστὶν ἓν καὶ ταὐτὸν πᾶσιν, πρὸς ἡμᾶς δὲ ὃ μήτε πλεονάζει μήτε ἐλλείπει· τοῦτο δ' οὐχ ἕν, οὐδὲ ταὐτὸν πᾶσιν. οἷον εἰ τὰ δέκα πολλὰ τὰ δὲ δύο ὀλίγα, τὰ ἓξ μέσα λαμβάνουσι κατὰ τὸ πρᾶγμα· ἴσῳ γὰρ ὑπερέχει τε καὶ ὑπερέχεται, τοῦτο δὲ μέσον ἐστὶ κατὰ τὴν ἀριθμητικὴν ἀνα-
1106b λογίαν. τὸ δὲ πρὸς ἡμᾶς οὐχ οὕτω ληπτέον· οὐ γὰρ εἴ τῳ δέκα μναῖ φαγεῖν πολὺ δύο δὲ ὀλίγον, ὁ ἀλείπτης ἓξ μνᾶς προστάξει· ἔστι γὰρ ἴσως καὶ τοῦτο πολὺ τῷ ληψομένῳ ἢ ὀλίγον· Μίλωνι μὲν γὰρ ὀλίγον, τῷ δὲ ἀρχομένῳ τῶν γυμνασίων πολύ· ὁμοίως ⟨δ'⟩ ἐπὶ δρόμου καὶ πάλης. οὕτω δὴ πᾶς ἐπιστήμων τὴν ὑπερβολὴν μὲν καὶ τὴν ἔλλειψιν φεύγει, τὸ δὲ μέσον ζητεῖ καὶ τοῦθ' αἱρεῖται, μέσον δὲ οὐ τὸ τοῦ πράγματος ἀλλὰ τὸ πρὸς ἡμᾶς.

Chapter 7 Texts

7.5 Aristotle, *Nicomachean Ethics* 1097ª11–13

For a doctor does not seem to study health in such a way [viz in general], but rather the health of a human being, or rather perhaps the health of a particular human. For it is the individual whom he cures.

7.6 Aristotle, *Nicomachean Ethics* 1137ª11–17

But the actions prescribed by law are only accidentally just actions. But to know how actions should be performed, and how distributions should be made, in order to be just, is harder than to know what is good for health. And even there, while it is easy to know what honey, wine, hellebore, cautery and surgery are, to know how and to whom and when they should be applied in order to produce health is no less a task than that of being a doctor.

7.7 Aristotle, *Nicomachean Ethics* 1104ª11–19

First then we should observe this, that it is the nature of such things [viz moral qualities] to be destroyed by deficiency and excess, as we see in the case of strength and of health (for we must use clear cases as evidence concerning unclear ones). Both excessive and deficient exercises destroy strength, and similarly too much or too little drink and food destroys health, while what is proportionate produces and increases and preserves it. The same holds also of temperance and courage and the other virtues.

7.8 Aristotle, *Nicomachean Ethics* 1106ª29–ᵇ7

By the mean of the thing I mean that which is equidistant from each of the extremes, which is one and the same for everybody. By the mean relative to us, that which is neither too much nor too little, and this is not one, nor the same for everybody. For example, if ten be many and two is few, then six is the mean with respect to the thing: for it exceeds and is exceeded by an equal amount, and this is the mean according to arithmetical proportion. But the mean relative to us is not to be grasped in the same way. Suppose that ten pounds is too much for a particular person to eat and two too little: it does not follow that the trainer will prescribe six pounds. For this is perhaps too much for the person who is to consume it, or too little. For Milo it is too little, but for the person who is beginning to engage in athletics too much. Similarly with the amount of running and wrestling. In the same way every expert avoids excess, and deficien-

7.9 Aristotle, *Nicomachean Ethics* 1114ᵃ11–19

1114a ἔτι δ' ἄλογον τὸν ἀδικοῦντα μὴ βούλεσθαι ἄδικον εἶναι ἢ τὸν ἀκολασταίνοντα ἀκόλαστον· οὐ μὴν ἐάν γε βούληται, ἄδικος ὢν παύσεται καὶ ἔσται δίκαιος· οὐδὲ γὰρ ὁ νοσῶν ὑγιής, καί⟨τοι⟩, εἰ οὕτως ἔτυχεν, ἑκὼν νοσεῖ, ἀκρατῶς βιοτεύων καὶ ἀπειθῶν τοῖς ἰατροῖς. τότε μὲν οὖν ἐξῆν αὐτῷ μὴ νοσεῖν, προεμένῳ δ' οὐκέτι, ὥσπερ οὐδ' ἀφέντι λίθον ἔτ' αὐτὸν δυνατὸν ἀναλαβεῖν· ἀλλ' ὅμως ἐπ' αὐτῷ τὸ λαβεῖν καὶ ῥῖψαι· ἡ γὰρ ἀρχὴ ἐν αὐτῷ.

7.10 Aristotle, *Nicomachean Ethics* 1173ᵇ22–25

1173b οὐ γὰρ εἰ τοῖς κακῶς διακειμένοις ἡδέα ἐστίν, οἰητέον αὐτὰ καὶ ἡδέα εἶναι πλὴν τούτοις, καθάπερ οὐδὲ τὰ τοῖς κάμνουσιν ὑγιεινὰ ἢ γλυκέα ἢ πικρά, οὐδ' αὖ λευκὰ τὰ φαινόμενα τοῖς ὀφθαλμιῶσιν.

7.11 Aristotle, *Nicomachean Ethics* 1176ᵃ12–16

1176a καὶ ἐπὶ γλυκέων δὲ τοῦτο συμβαίνει· οὐ γὰρ τὰ αὐτὰ δοκεῖ τῷ πυρέττοντι καὶ τῷ ὑγιαίνοντι, οὐδὲ θερμὸν εἶναι τῷ ἀσθενεῖ καὶ τῷ εὐεκτικῷ. ὁμοίως δὲ τοῦτο καὶ ἐφ' ἑτέρων συμβαίνει. δοκεῖ δ' ἐν ἅπασι τοῖς τοιούτοις εἶναι τὸ φαινόμενον τῷ σπουδαίῳ.

7.12 Aristotle, *Politics* 1279ᵃ22–31

1279a Διωρισμένων δὲ τούτων ἐχόμενόν ἐστι τὰς πολιτείας ἐπισκέψασθαι, πόσαι τὸν ἀριθμὸν καὶ τίνες εἰσί, καὶ πρῶτον τὰς ὀρθὰς αὐτῶν· καὶ γὰρ αἱ παρεκβάσεις ἔσονται φανεραὶ τούτων διορισθεισῶν. ἐπεὶ δὲ πολιτεία μὲν καὶ πολίτευμα σημαίνει ταὐτόν, πολίτευμα δ' ἐστὶ τὸ κύριον τῶν πόλεων, ἀνάγκη δ' εἶναι κύριον ἢ ἕνα ἢ ὀλίγους ἢ τοὺς πολλούς, ὅταν μὲν ὁ εἷς ἢ οἱ ὀλίγοι ἢ οἱ πολλοὶ πρὸς τὸ κοινὸν συμφέρον ἄρχωσι, ταύτας μὲν ὀρθὰς ἀναγκαῖον εἶναι τὰς πολιτείας, τὰς δὲ πρὸς τὸ ἴδιον ἢ τοῦ ἑνὸς ἢ τῶν ὀλίγων ἢ τοῦ πλήθους παρεκβάσεις.

cy, and seeks and chooses the mean, but not the mean of the thing, but rather the mean relative to us.

7.9 Aristotle, *Nicomachean Ethics* 1114ª11–19

Again it is irrational to suppose that a person who acts unjustly or self-indulgently does not wish to be unjust or self-indulgent. Yet it does not follow that, if he wishes, he can stop being unjust and be just. For neither can a sick person become healthy [by wishing], although possibly he became ill voluntarily, by living intemperately and disobeying the doctors. At that point, then, it was possible for him not to be ill, but that is no longer the case, once he has let go the chance—just as once you have thrown a stone, it is no longer possible to recall it. But still it was in your power to pick up the stone and throw it, for the origin of the act was in you.

7.10 Aristotle, *Nicomachean Ethics* 1173ᵇ22–25

If things are pleasant to people of bad character, one must not suppose that they are also pleasant to others besides them—any more than what is healthy or sweet or bitter to those who are sick [is really so] or again what seems white to those suffering from disease of the eyes [is really so].

7.11 Aristotle, *Nicomachean Ethics* 1176ª12–16

This happens too in the case of sweet things: the same things do not seem sweet to a person with a fever and to a healthy person—nor hot to a sickly person and to one in good condition. The same happens in other cases as well. But it is agreed that in all such matters what appears to the good person is really so.

7.12 Aristotle, *Politics* 1279ª22–31

Having determined these points, we have next to consider how many constitutions there are and what they are, and first study the true ones: for once these are determined, the deviations will become clear. But since constitution and government have the same meaning, and the government has the supreme authority in the state, and this must be in the hands of one person, or few, or the many, then whenever the one or the few or the many govern with a view to the common interest, these are necessarily the true constitutions. But those governed with a view to the private interest of the one or the few or the many are deviations.

7.13 Aristotle, *Politics* 1279ᵇ4–10

παρεκβάσεις δὲ τῶν εἰρημένων τυραννὶς μὲν βασιλείας ὀλιγαρχία δὲ ἀριστοκρατίας δημοκρατία δὲ πολιτείας· ἡ μὲν γὰρ τυραννίς ἐστι μοναρχία πρὸς τὸ συμφέρον τὸ τοῦ μοναρχοῦντος, ἡ δ' ὀλιγαρχία πρὸς τὸ τῶν εὐπόρων, ἡ δὲ δημοκρατία πρὸς τὸ συμφέρον τὸ τῶν ἀπόρων. πρὸς δὲ τὸ τῷ κοινῷ λυσιτελοῦν οὐδεμία αὐτῶν.

7.14 Aristotle, *Poetics* 1449ᵇ24–8

ἔστιν οὖν τραγῳδία μίμησις πράξεως σπουδαίας καὶ τελείας μέγεθος ἐχούσης, ἡδυσμένῳ λόγῳ χωρὶς ἑκάστῳ τῶν εἰδῶν ἐν τοῖς μορίοις, δρώντων καὶ οὐ δι' ἀπαγγελίας, δι' ἐλέου καὶ φόβου περαίνουσα τὴν τῶν τοιούτων παθημάτων κάθαρσιν.

7.15 Aristotle, *Politics* 1341ᵇ32–1342ᵃ16

ἐπεὶ δὲ τὴν διαίρεσιν ἀποδεχόμεθα τῶν μελῶν ὡς διαιροῦσί τινες τῶν ἐν φιλοσοφίᾳ, τὰ μὲν ἠθικὰ τὰ δὲ πρακτικὰ τὰ δ' ἐνθουσιαστικὰ τιθέντες, καὶ τῶν ἁρμονιῶν τὴν φύσιν πρὸς ἕκαστα τούτων οἰκείαν ἄλλην πρὸς ἄλλο μέρος τιθέασι, φαμὲν δ' οὐ μιᾶς ἕνεκεν ὠφελείας τῇ μουσικῇ χρῆσθαι δεῖν ἀλλὰ καὶ πλειόνων χάριν (καὶ γὰρ παιδείας ἕνεκεν καὶ καθάρσεως—τί δὲ λέγομεν τὴν κάθαρσιν, νῦν μὲν ἁπλῶς, πάλιν δ' ἐν τοῖς περὶ ποιητικῆς ἐροῦμεν σαφέστερον,—τρίτον δὲ πρὸς διαγωγήν, πρὸς ἄνεσίν τε καὶ πρὸς τὴν τῆς συντονίας ἀνάπαυσιν), φανερὸν ὅτι χρηστέον μὲν πάσαις ταῖς ἁρμονίαις, οὐ τὸν αὐτὸν δὲ τρόπον πάσαις χρηστέον, ἀλλὰ πρὸς μὲν τὴν παιδείαν ταῖς ἠθικωτάταις, πρὸς δὲ ἀκρόασιν ἑτέρων χειρουργούντων καὶ ταῖς πρακτικαῖς καὶ ταῖς ἐνθουσιαστικαῖς (ὃ γὰρ περὶ ἐνίας συμβαίνει πάθος ψυχὰς ἰσχυρῶς, τοῦτο ἐν πάσαις ὑπάρχει, τῷ δὲ ἧττον διαφέρει καὶ τῷ μᾶλλον—οἷον ἔλεος καὶ φόβος, ἔτι δ' ἐνθουσιασμός, καὶ γὰρ ὑπὸ ταύτης τῆς κινήσεως κατακώχιμοί τινές εἰσιν, ἐκ δὲ τῶν ἱερῶν μελῶν ὁρῶμεν τούτους ὅταν χρήσωνται τοῖς ἐξοργιάζουσι τὴν ψυχὴν μέλεσι καθισταμένους ὥσπερ ἰατρείας τυχόντας καὶ καθάρσεως· ταὐτὸ δὴ τοῦτο ἀναγκαῖον πάσχειν καὶ τοὺς ἐλεήμονας καὶ τοὺς φοβητικοὺς καὶ τοὺς ὅλως παθητικοὺς τοὺς ἄλλους καθ' ὅσον ἐπιβάλλει τῶν τοιούτων ἑκάστῳ, καὶ πᾶσι γίγνεσθαί τινα κάθαρσιν καὶ κουφίζεσθαι μεθ' ἡδονῆς· ὁμοίως δὲ καὶ τὰ μέλη τὰ καθαρτικὰ παρέχει χαρὰν ἀβλαβῆ τοῖς ἀνθρώποις).

7.13 Aristotle, *Politics* 1279^b4–10

Deviations to the constitutions mentioned are tyranny corresponding to kingship, oligarchy corresponding to aristocracy, democracy corresponding to constitutional government. For tyranny is monarchy in the interest of the monarch, oligarchy in the interest of the wealthy, democracy in that of the poor, and none of these is for the benefit of the community as a whole.

7.14 Aristotle, *Poetics* 1449^b24–8

Tragedy is a representation of an action that is serious, complete and of a certain magnitude, by means of language embellished with ornament of different kinds for each part, in a dramatic and not in a narrative form, procuring through pity and fear a purgation of suchlike affections.

7.15 Aristotle, *Politics* 1341^b32–1342^a16

We accept the division of melodies made by some philosophers, as ethical ones, melodies relating to actions, and enthusiastic ones, and we distribute the various harmonies among them as being in nature akin to one or to another. And we say that music ought to be used not just for one kind of benefit but for many, for it serves both for education and for purgation (we talk of purgation for the present without qualification, but we shall speak more clearly about it again in the *Poetics*). Thirdly it serves for amusement, for relaxation and to afford relief from tension. It is clear, therefore, that we should use all the harmonies, yet not all in the same way, but the most ethical ones for education, and the active and enthusiastic ones for listening to when others are performing: for the affections that occur violently in some souls, happen to all, though with different degrees of intensity, for example pity and fear, and again enthusiasm. For some people are possessed by such a change, and we see them, under the influence of sacred melodies, when they use melodies that excite the soul to frenzy, being restored as if they had received a cure and a purgation. The same experience must also come to the compassionate and the fearful and other emotional people, to the degree that it affects each type, and all must undergo a certain purgation and a feeling of relief accompanied by pleasure. And similarly the purgative melodies offer harmless delight to people.

8

After Aristotle: Or Did Anything Change?

Real and imaginary plagues continued to haunt the Greek—and the Roman—imagination long after Aristotle. Galen the famous medical theorist from the second century CE, whose account of the passions we shall be considering later in this chapter, lived through a particularly nasty plague, that struck Rome in 166—or rather it would be more accurate to say, not that he lived through it, but left Rome to escape it. As for the continued reflections on previous plagues, we shall be discussing Lucretius' account of the Athenian plague, the actual historical one described by Thucydides, but now overlaid with new imaginings. Why should this staunch advocate of the Epicurean philosophy have ended his poem with a detailed and graphic—and intensely gloomy—account of that plague? I shall try to answer that question at the end of the chapter.

The principal question I now want to raise is whether, as I put it, anything changed from the classical period to late antiquity on the issues that we are concerned with, the attitudes to, preoccupation with, and understanding of, disease. In certain respects or in some senses the answer can be a straightforward yes. But those respects turn out to be peripheral and unimportant compared with those in which the similarities between earlier and later periods are more striking than the contrasts.

Aristotle himself had already recommended, and practised, the dissection of animals in pursuit of his inquiry into their

After Aristotle: Or Did Anything Change?

forms and functions. *On the Parts of Animals* 1 ch. 5 is eloquent advocacy of the method, though it also reveals that he had to overcome considerable inhibitions on the subject among his contemporaries. The practice of dissection—and of vivisection—was extended to humans for a brief period in Alexandria with the anatomists Herophilus and Erasistratus. The knowledge that thereby became available was impressive (von Staden 1989). Herophilus distinguished the nerves from the other structures (tendons, ligaments) that had regularly been confused with them, and among the nerves he distinguished between the sensory and the motor. He was aware of the ventricles of the brain. He gave some detailed descriptions of the reproductive organs, undertook a comparative anatomy of the liver, and many other examples can be cited. There is conflicting evidence as to whether he knew of the valves of the heart, but Erasistratus certainly did, and this turned out to be a particularly important discovery, not least for the further problems it posed for investigation. If there are one-way valves controlling entry into, and exit, from the two sides of the heart, what is the connection between them? Are their contents identical? How does blood get into the left side? It was often thought to originate in the liver, but if from there it entered and then exited from the right side, how did it get into the arterial system? Some thought that the arteries naturally contained air, not blood at all, and the questions of the contents of the two systems, and the transport of blood and air into and out of the two sides of the heart, continued to reverberate down to Harvey.

Human dissection practically ceased after the generation of Herophilus and Erasistratus, and dissection as a whole remained controversial, since some argued that the knowledge it provided was relevant only to dead bodies (Lloyd 1987, 160ff.). Yet Galen, for one, continued Herophilus' explorations of the nervous system, and of the processes of digestion, for instance, even though his work was no longer on human, but on animal, subjects, the pig, the Barbary ape, even on one famous occasion, an elephant.

But while knowledge of anatomy and physiology (as we like to call them) increased, that does not answer the question of whether there were any advances in pathology. We should not underestimate the improvements in surgical practices that could result from increased understanding of, for example, the nervous system. But my chief question relates to diseases as such. Medical theories based on humours, the elements, other kinds of opposites (like repletion and depletion, cf. above Ch. 6 n. 2) and so on, continued to proliferate. Yet there was no resolution of the disputes and controversies these generated, no intellectual resolution at least. Eventually the theory based on four humours (blood, phlegm, yellow and black bile) correlated with the four simple bodies and the four primary opposites came to predominate over all others. But that was because it was the theory that Galen maintained. It was the prestige he attained some 200 years after his death that led to this becoming something of an orthodoxy. But in the centuries that preceded Galen there was no agreement either about which the important humours were, or on whether they were the causes, or the products, of diseases.

Galen, it is true, saw his own theory as being based on, indeed as merely repeating, the one he ascribed to Hippocrates, for which he used the treatise *On the Nature of Man* as his chief evidence (Lloyd 1991, ch. 17). Yet that was Galen's reconstruction, on the basis of his particular interpretation not just of that treatise but also of what Plato said about Hippocrates in the *Phaedrus*. Few scholars would now go along with Galen's views on the latter, and as to the former, Galen himself ascribed parts of *On the Nature of Man* not to Hippocrates himself but to his son-in-law Polybus. Yet it was Galen's adoption of that theory that ensured its prominence in later medical teaching—thanks to the authority that Galen himself acquired as the most learned, most articulate, and in certain respects, such as in anatomy, undoubtedly the most knowledgeable theorist of his day. I shall be returning to this in the Epilogue.

Yet the reaction of some doctors to the ongoing theoretical

After Aristotle: Or Did Anything Change? 205

disputes that were such a feature of the classical and Hellenistic periods was to reject theory in favour of practice. Some argued that it was less important to know why any particular treatment worked, than *that* it worked. In the Proem to book 1 of his *On Medicine* (39) [T 8.1] Celsus reports the Empiricists as arguing: 'nor do we have any need to inquire into how we breathe, but what relieves difficult and laboured breathing: nor what may move the blood-vessels, but what the various types of movement signify . . . A man of few words who learns by practice to discern well would make an altogether better doctor than one who, unpractised, cultivates his tongue excessively.' Such knowledge was to be built up from experience (from which the Empiricist doctors got their name) and theory was pointless.

The so-called Methodists went a good deal further and rejected the entire gamut of traditional Greek medical ideas about disease entities as such (Lloyd 1983, Part III chs. 5–6; Frede 1987, ch. 14). Instead of focusing on 'pleuritis', 'pneumonia', 'peripneumonia', and the like, they argued that what counted was the overall state of the patient, his or her 'common conditions', where they distinguished the constricted, the lax, and the mixed—to be countered, in each case, by attempting to restore a balanced, healthy state. For them too the emphasis was on therapy, on what worked, or at least what helped to alleviate the patients' conditions. But while this practical turn was sensible, it also reflected a widespread disillusion with theory.

After these preliminaries we may now concentrate on the two main topics for discussion, first the ongoing debate as to what disease consists in and how the 'affections' are to be interpreted, and secondly the continued controversy between those who adopted an entirely naturalistic approach to medicine and those who still believed that the gods are at work.

Many of the philosophers in the period after Aristotle remained aloof from, some were quite ignorant of, the advances that came from the anatomical studies I have described. Their chief interest was in ethics, to which indeed the study of nature was subordinated. The main function of philosophy was to provide the wherewithal to achieve happiness, and that—everyone agreed—depended on peace of mind, freedom from disturbance, *ataraxia*. The study of nature was only relevant—so many philosophers argued—insofar as you could not achieve peace of mind without some understanding of the basic constitution of the universe and of the causes of phenomena. Unfortunately the philosophers were as divided on the former question as the medical theorists were on the causes of disease.

For ethics you certainly needed an account of the soul or mind, *psuche*. Ever since Plato had distinguished three functions of the soul, reason, spirit, and appetite, the question of what was needed, in addition to the reasoning faculty, to account for human cognitive, conative, or affective abilities was controversial. Aristotle had distinguished the rational faculty from such others as nutrition and reproduction, perception, locomotion, desire, and the imagination. He used that account of the faculties of the soul in part to organize his ideas of the hierarchy of nature and of the place of humans and other animals in it. For him 'reason' covers both practical and more especially theoretical reason, but he does not have a separate faculty corresponding to the spirited part, and his 'desire' (*orektikon*) cuts across all three of the Platonic parts. While his fully worked out theory in *On the Soul* has these faculties, for the purposes of his ethical discussions he often uses a simpler contrast between the rational and irrational parts of the soul. We saw in the last chapter how he argues that practical wisdom and moral character are interdependent. The latter is built up through training in the right reactions to pleasures and pains. His total picture of the harmonious and wise individual is rather different, therefore, from Plato's, where everything depends on the rational part doing the governing, while the other parts should obey orders and be under its control.

The major positive post-Aristotelian philosophical systems, Stoic and Epicurean, were as split on the analysis of the soul as Plato and Aristotle had been. The Stoic position is particularly interesting since they adopted a quite radical solution to the problems, denying that there are distinct parts of the soul and claiming that its sole constituent is reason.

On that view the *pathe* (feelings or passions, though, as we shall see, the word retains its association with diseases) do not belong to a separate part of the soul, but to the rational part itself. Just as reason rules in the universe, so too in the microcosm of the individual person the rational element should be in control. Of course it sometimes fails, but on the Stoic view this is not because it is overcome by some other part of the soul: there is no other part. Rather, the feelings are excessive impulses (*hormai*). While the Stoics allow joy, watchfulness, and wishing (which are called well-reasoned impulses, *eupatheiai*, in our sources[1]) the *pathe* in general are disturbances of the rational faculty. The comparison that is attributed to Chrysippus is that of the difference between someone walking—where his movements are under control—and someone running—where they are not.[2] All impulses imply assent. The affections do not just incorporate judgements (*kriseis*): they *are* judgements, even though the kind of mistake that may be made can be distinguished from a mere error of fact: it is rather a matter of an excessive conation, contrary to reason in the sense that the excess goes beyond what reason, if in full control, would determine.[3]

This looks like an extreme instance of the intellectualizing tendencies that have often been found in Greek philosophy, especially in the Platonic representation of Socrates, for whom 'virtue' is 'knowledge'.[4] Yet caution is necessary on two

[1] Diogenes Laertius 7. 116. But whether the Stoics themselves used the term is disputed, Long and Sedley 1987, ii. 407.
[2] Galen, *On the Opinions of Hippocrates and Plato* 240. 35 ff. [T 8.2]
[3] Galen, *On the Opinions of Hippocrates and Plato* 242. 32 ff.
[4] We should bear in mind, however, that many Greek cognitive terms incorporate also a dispositional element. This applies particularly to *phronesis* and its cognates. *Phronein turannika*, for instance (as in Aristophanes *Wasps* 507) is not so much to think tyrannical thoughts as to have a tyrannical disposition, to be intent on tyranny.

counts. First to intellectualize the affections is at the same time to extend the notion of reason to cover many other phenomena besides those we would normally associate with the intellect. By the time we get to talk of the diseases of the soul, we see that the converse of the intellectualizing of the feelings is the pathologizing of the intellect.

But then the second methodological reason for caution is that our sources for Stoic views are not complete works of the leading members of the school (Zeno, Cleanthes, Chrysippus) but reports in generally hostile witnesses, Galen especially. Galen himself accepted the Platonic doctrine of the three main faculties of the soul. Against the monistic views of the Stoics he brings a series of objections. He is intent, first, on showing that their monism is internally inconsistent. He attacks Chrysippus on that score repeatedly.[5] Affection is an irrational and unnatural movement of the soul and an excessive impulse that Galen glosses as 'irrational' or 'without reason (*logos*) and judgement': but with that gloss Galen can accuse Chrysippus of having contradicted himself, both asserting and denying that affection is a judgement. Whether or not Galen has cited Chrysippus correctly, it is clear that he has distorted his views, for what Chrysippus more probably meant was that affections lack right judgement, not that they were not judgements at all. Furthermore Galen seeks to drive a wedge, within Stoic theorists, between Chrysippus and Zeno and more especially between Chrysippus and the later Stoic Posidonius, whom Galen represents as returning more or less to tripartition.[6]

It is striking that both the monistic and the tripartite views of the soul make use of the model or analogy or image of disease to account for evil. In the tripartite view evil is an imbalance between the parts, just as disease itself can be, and frequently was, explained in terms of a similar imbalance between opposite elements within the body. But on the monistic view too evil is seen as an excess, an affection that

[5] *On the Opinions of Hippocrates and Plato* 234. 22 ff., 238.4–240. 29.
[6] *On the Opinions of Hippocrates and Plato* 246. 38 ff., 248. 3 ff.

afflicts the rational faculty itself, as if that faculty were diseased. Whatever psychological theory was upheld, so it seems, evil could be construed in terms of illness. Yet unlike in some modern views (cf. below, Ch. 9) that did not go with a sense of diminished personal responsibility for wrongdoing. Rather, the argument was that the individual can be held responsible for the state their soul was in.

Indeed in *On the Opinions of Hippocrates and Plato* (294. 33 ff.) Galen represents Chrysippus as making much of the analogy between the diseases of the soul and those of the body. The *pathe* do not arise in the souls of good persons at all: but the souls of inferior people are like the bodies of people prone to fall into fever on a small triggering cause (*prophasis*). Posidonius, Galen goes on, criticized Chrysippus at this point on the grounds that while there are some souls that are immune to the *pathe*, there are no bodies that are totally immune to disease. But rather than accept Posidonius' modification of Chrysippus' view (that the souls of inferior people are either like vulnerable physical constitutions or actually diseased) we find Galen offering the Stoics a five-level analogy setting out at each stage the comparison between physical and bodily ailments (296. 18 ff.) [T 8.3]. The souls of the good are like bodies that are invulnerable to disease (whether or not such bodies exist). Those who are progressing towards sagehood are like those with a strong or robust constitution, *euexia*. Moderately good people are like those who are healthy but lack that *euexia*. The many inferior people are like those who are diseased from a small cause (*prophasis*), while fifthly and finally those who are repeatedly angry or enraged are like those who are already ill.

One of the great strengths of the Stoic position is the clear, if uncompromising, emphasis on reasoning and responsibility. While in the Stoic universe everything is determined in the sense of there being an inexorable chain of cause and effect, the individual person is responsible for his or her reason and so also for his or her feelings. When things go wrong, this is like the disease of the rational part. All the more need, then, for a physician of the soul. All the more need for philosophy as a remedy for suffering. If you believe the Stoics, the soul is, *in principle*, invulnerable to evil, in the sense that the only source of that is judgement, and you can (if you are a Stoic sage at least) be in total control of your judgements. The ultimate goal was such an immunity to evil or to distress. Nevertheless they recognized that the sage is an ideal rarely if ever encountered in real life. Heracles was one example, but he was legendary. Socrates may be another, but he was safely dead.

Galen's criticism of the Stoic, especially the Chrysippean, view starts from his assumption that of course there must be different sources of psychic activities. Plato was right to insist that psychic struggles occur between the rational faculty and the spirited and appetitive parts. That struggle too, as explained, could be imagined as a disease needing remedies that only the doctor of the soul can provide. Galen's position on the affections is that they do not belong to the reasoning faculty, but to the other parts, but that does not stop him, too, treating imbalance within the soul on the model of sickness in the body.

Those ideas appear in his treatise *On the Opinions of Hippocrates and Plato* especially. But in another work he makes even stronger claims. In the short treatise entitled *That the Faculties of the Soul Follow the Mixtures of the Body* (hereafter *QAM*) he embarks on an ambitious project proposing a picture of the doctor as able to cure not just the body, but also the soul. In the view that he there develops, character is made to depend on the physiological constitution or state of the body.

It had, of course, always been part of traditional medical theory that there were important differences between different physical constitutions. The Hippocratic work *On Airs Waters Places* associates these physical differences with corresponding climatic and ecological conditions (while allowing a place also for social and political factors in influencing character-formation). But the extra point in Galen's *QAM* is that he urges that you can—on the advice of the doctor—modify your physical constitution by diet and regimen and consequently also your character. Insofar as character depends on physiology (and the claim is that it does), this means that the doctor will be in a position to help those whom he advises to modify their characters, indeed to improve them.

If so, the doctor can make you a better person. In the course of the argument Galen engages in some—highly selective—citations from Plato and others (ignoring, for example, what Plato has to say in the *Timaeus* on the role of education in training people to be good, cf. Lloyd 1988). But if we believe Galen, then putting ourselves in the hands of doctors and following their advice on food, drink, and exercise, can turn us into upright and honourable people. 'So it would be wise of my opponents,' he says at *QAM* ch. 9 [T 8.4], with no apparent sign of his tongue being in his cheek, 'to come to me even now and receive instruction on their diet. They would derive enormous benefit from this in their command of ethics; and the improvement in their intellectual faculties, too, would have an effect on their virtue, as they acquired greater powers of understanding and memory.' Here was a medical writer infiltrating the domain of philosophy and taking over the traditional role of the philosopher as the source of moral advice and guidance for your improvement.

Both the Stoics and Galen, in their different ways, thus extend the domain of therapeutics. In that regard, both do introduce and develop new ideas and in that sense too we can say that something changed after Aristotle. For the Stoics psychotherapeutics has as its aim the removal of all those excessive impulses that constitute the *pathe*. As disturbances, they are like diseases: but unlike the diseases that affect the body they are ones for which the remedy is at hand—in principle at least—when the rational faculty takes full control, even though they recognised how difficult it was to attain sagehood.

But if psychotherapeutics is a Stoic speciality, Galen's emphasis, in *QAM*, on modifying your character via modifying your physical constitution reflects a determined claim to extend the role of the doctor into that of a source of moral improvement in his patients. Adopting and adapting Plato's tripartite psychology, he sees evil as an imbalance between the faculties. The extremely wide definition of 'disease' which we saw Plato offer in the *Sophist* (above Ch. 6, p. 146) is taken up with approval by Galen in *On the Opinions of Hippocrates and Plato* (302. 17ff.) [T 8.5]. Plato had said that disease is the destruction of what is by nature congenial as a result of some difference.[7] What Galen finds attractive in this, among other things, is that it covers far more than just the diseases of the body. 'It is not difficult to ascertain,' Galen writes, 'that this formulation is at a higher level and accurately covers all particular diseases, those of our soul, those of our body, those found in other animals and plants, even those of whole cities. Thus we say, I believe, that cities divided by civil war (*stasiazousais*) are internally diseased, as though their components, congenial by nature, had come to blows.' It is clear that this talk of *diseases* in the state is no mere figure of speech, transferred from the body to those other contexts. The sphere of disease is a generic one that includes every kind of disorder. We could hardly have a more vivid illustration and proof of the wide extensions of which the terms *nosema* and *pathos* are capable.

But if both the Stoics and Galen do thereby represent certain new trends in the period after Aristotle, our final two sources show first that traditional views continued to be vigorously maintained and secondly that there was still nothing like unanimity on diseases and their cures. We may consider first the evidence in Aelius Aristides that demonstrates the continued belief in the role of the gods. Then we shall backtrack to discuss what a representative of the other major Hellenistic philosophical school besides the Stoics has to say on the problems. This is the Epicurean poet Lucretius.

Galen himself from time to time suggests that he was in some sense divinely inspired. He became a doctor because his

[7] To judge from *On the Opinions of Hippocrates and Plato* 302. 18f., cf 310. 26, Galen may have read a slightly different text of Plato's *Sophist* 228a8.

After Aristotle: Or Did Anything Change? 213

father had a dream that that was what he was to do. He says that some of the treatments he used came to him in dreams. But of course the whole tenor of his work is naturalistic. He explicitly disclaims any suggestion that his ability was in any way 'magical', though one feels he was flattered by the suggestion that his diagnostic insights were so extraordinary that they defied ordinary explanation.[8] He just puts it down to his particular skill in the interpretation of the pulse and so on.

But we can use the *Sacred Tales* of his contemporary Aelius Aristides to illustrate how not just ordinary folk, but some of the most distinguished members of the literate elite, continued to be devoted to the cult of Asclepius. Aelius Aristides was a famous orator, widely acclaimed as such by his fellow-citizens and indeed across the Greek-speaking provinces of the Roman world. He was also a confirmed hypochondriac, constantly afflicted, on his own account, by terrible complaints. But for these the ordinary doctors he consulted were usually no good. In any case they often disagreed among themselves (e.g. *Sacred Tales* 47. 62) [T 8.6] and were often quite at a loss as to how to treat him (48. 39 [T 8.7], cf. 63). The god, on the other hand, was his salvation. He often contradicted the advice that ordinary mortal doctors had given (47. 62f.). Their remedies failed, but his were really effective, and the more enlightened doctors, according to Aelius Aristides, came to appreciate that this was so. 'From here on, the doctors stopped their criticisms,' and 'expressed extraordinary admiration for the providence of the god in each particular' (47. 67).

The god works through dreams and visions, and in the text it is sometimes hard to know what register we are in: is it

---

[8] Galen tells us that his use of the pulse in diagnosis was considered to be mere divination by his critics, *On Prognosis, CMG* V 8 1, 94. 18f. cf. 84. 5ff., 106. 21 ff. He was evidently suspected of magic and charlatanry, even while he himself accused others in similar vein. It is clear, too, that he sometimes deliberately sought to amaze his audience, especially in the context of spectacular exhibition dissections, while he criticizes others for doing the same (see Kollesch 1965, Vegetti 1981, Lloyd 1987, 42f.).

Aelius Aristides speaking, or the god speaking to him in his dreams? As was the case with the much earlier Epidaurus inscriptions that we discussed in Chapter 2, the god uses many standard therapies, though sometimes in a less than standard way. At one point (48. 47) he orders venesection at the elbow, drawing off 120 *litrai* of blood indeed—which would come to an unbelievable 25 to 30 litres. That evokes the response from the temple assistants that they had never known anyone who had been venesected so much.[9]

Just as the severity of his complaints is exceptional, so too is the rigour of what the god tells him to do to remedy them. He is commanded to run barefoot in winter (47. 65) [T 8.6], indeed to do the rounds of all the temples at Pergamum (48. 75), and other drastic treatments include horseback riding and taking to sea in a storm. He himself becomes, naturally enough, something of an expert in both diagnosis and treatment. After one vision of the goddess Athena (48. 41 ff.) [T 8.7] he says: 'it immediately occurred to me to have an enema of Attic honey.' However in places his account is indeterminate. Zosimus and he have a dream at 47. 66 [T 8.6] about a certain drug—but Aelius Aristides cannot remember what it contained, except salt. On other occasions he is hesitant about precisely what remedies were used when he was under the god's care. 48. 43 [T 8.7] is one instance of this: 'First, I think, goose-liver after much refusal of all food. Then a sausage ...'

The amazement with which he says both his terrible ailments and his miraculous cures were greeted indicates an element of what we may call competitive hypochondria. He never comments on why it is that he gets all these diseases. No sooner does the god achieve one astonishing cure, than Aelius Aristides falls sick again: he certainly keeps the god busy. While his confidence in ordinary doctors is minimal, his expression of faith in Asclepius is unqualified. The god may act like a human from time to time, but his cures are unfailing.

---

[9] Aelius Aristides adds 'with the exception of Ischuron': but his was a strange case, and even so his own case surpassed it.

After Aristotle: Or Did Anything Change? 215

His appearance in visions and dreams is marvellously reassuring. He is the healer par excellence, the source of indescribable solace, hailed as the Saviour (*soter*).

Aelius Aristides is, to be sure, an exceptional case. The detail he provides of his dreams—as he reports them—has provoked attempts at retrospective psychoanalysis. That is not my purpose here. Rather we may use the evidence he provides to illuminate the dilemma that many must have faced, in choosing what mode of therapy to employ for the complaints from which they suffered. How effective were naturalistic treatments? Of course the question cannot be answered. Some of the drugs we know to have been used certainly contained some powerful ingredients: some indeed were highly toxic.[10] Some of the surgical interventions too were drastic, cutting for the stone, trepanning, cautery, the reduction of fractures by stretching on the so-called Hippocratic bench, the use of a ladder on which the patient was strapped upside down, and then bounced on the floor or earth, employed again in reduction or even for cases of difficult childbirth.[11] Already in the classical period some doctors warned against the remedies their own colleagues were using, and as I noted already in Chapter 3 (n. 7) some even confess that their own treatments did more harm than good.[12]

---

[10] This applies particularly to those that incorporated minerals, not least the various arsenical compounds that were employed. See Caley and Richards 1956, 171f., on *sandarache* (realgar) and *arrenikon* (orpiment), used at *On Diseases of Women* II ch. 203 (L VIII 388. 11ff.), *On Superfetation* chs. 32 and 33 (*CMG* I 2 2, 90. 26, 94. 14), *On Wounds* chs. 16 and 17 (L VI 418. 22ff., 420. 6ff.). There are further references to primary and secondary literature in Lloyd 1987, 19 and n. 58.

[11] See e.g. *On Diseases of Women* I ch. 68 (L VIII 142. 20ff.) and *On the Excision of the Foetus* ch. 4 (L VIII 514. 14ff.). At *Epidemics* V 103 (L V 258. 9ff.) one case of a woman who had been succussed in childbirth is reported that ends fatally, though success in the use of succussion in a case where a patient suffers from a liver complaint is claimed at *Epidemics* VI 8. 28 (L V 354. 4f.).

[12] The various contexts in which medical writers warn against the dangers of commonly employed remedies include surgical procedures (e.g. *On Joints* chs. 42 and 44, L IV 182. 13ff., 188. 1ff. as well as those noted in

Whatever the physical results of therapies may have been, often the psychological effects and preconceptions were as important or more important. The extra dimension provided by the fact that temple medicine came under the aegis of Asclepius and Apollo certainly weighed with many. Aelius Aristides himself evidently enjoyed an iron constitution—to judge from the way he survived even the most rigorous therapies that he undertook on the god's orders. But it was his unshakeable belief that he was special, and specially favoured by the gods, that bolsters him in the darkest moments of his illnesses.

This is not to ignore the differences that existed between healing in different modes. If recourse to diet and drugs was common to most traditions, the Hippocratic surgical treatises show that specialists developed a variety of techniques for dealing with fractures and dislocations, not all of which were as drastic as the use of the Hippocratic bench could be, and several stand comparison with modern orthopaedic procedures. But if we try to understand the continuing pluralism of medicine in the Graeco-Roman world, it is as well to appreciate that the competition in persuasion was for their patients' minds and related as much to what they could be got to believe as to obviously verifiable results. The effects of a given treatment were always a matter of interpretation, where there would be plenty of room for disagreement among different practitioners as to why the patient died or recovered.

Although a fundamental gap opened up between those who thought the divine was involved directly in diseases and their

Ch. 3 n. 7, and cf. above n. 11), drugs (e.g. Dioscorides 5. 104–5), excessive and inappropriate exercise (*Epidemics* VI 3. 18, L V 302. 1 ff., cf. Plato, *Republic* 406a–c on Herodicus), and the use of what was called a 'starvation diet', *limoktonia* (*On Regimen* III 71, *CMG* I 2 4, 204. 10, criticized, for instance, in *On Regimen in Acute Diseases*, ch. 11 Littré II 310. 1 ff., 316. 9 ff., chs. 39–44 Jones). Even the Methodists, who avoided drastic remedies in principle, and criticized some of those used in mental cases in particular, give a limited endorsement to some harsh measures to 'cure' madness (Caelius Aurelianus *On Chronic Diseases* I 144 ff., 155 ff., 171 ff.). See Lloyd 1987, 19 ff., 25 ff., 68 ff.

After Aristotle: Or Did Anything Change? 217

cures, and those who denied that, we have seen that there was, in practice, considerable overlap both in the remedies used and in the discourse employed to justify them. Temple medicine adopted many of the therapies lay doctors used. Both traditions aimed to foretell the courses of diseases, and both used dreams as diagnostic tools, even though differences remained as to whether they were sent from the gods, or merely indicators of physical disturbances in the body.

On the patients' side of the equation, there were no doubt those who were convinced by the naturalists' arguments, just as there were many who doubted divination. Some may well have been relieved that those arguments implied the denial of the view that diseases were punishments sent by the gods for some offence that you yourself, or your ancestors, had committed. But just as many, if not more, were led to seek the protection of the gods—in disease as in other matters—putting their trust in their own piety and their use of traditional rituals to placate the gods or otherwise to negotiate a deal with them. The naturalists could point to the increased knowledge of anatomy that came from the use of the methods that some of them, at least, favoured. Some might further argue that their own research extended knowledge in such matters as the properties and effects of drugs. The supernaturalists were not short of apparent successes that they could chalk up to the efficacy of prayer. At least there is no reason to believe that every patient in the temples succumbed to their diseases, any more than there is to credit the 100 per cent success rate claimed in the inscriptions the priests set up to advertise the power of the god. And who was to say that those who survived and were cured owed that to the gods or to nature?

The struggle was for the beliefs of patients, then, and in the wider battle, the arguments between belief and agnosticism, and between different modes of belief, were complex and more evenly balanced than we might suppose, at least until the third century. Then, however, the institutionalization of Christianity, when it was adopted as the official religion of the Roman emperor, added a new and eventually in many respects decisive factor. I shall have more to say on this in the Epilogue.

The question of the relevance of the gods takes me to my final source, for whom we need to go back in time, to the first century BCE. Lucretius is in many respects an exceptional writer, an Epicurean who chose to advocate that philosophy in poetry. On two separate occasions in his poem, 1. 936ff. [T 8.8] and 4. 11ff., he represents the poetry as like the honey on a cup of bitter medicine that will persuade children to drink it down. That immediately suggests—what will be our main theme—the therapeutic function of his philosophy.

The poem, *On the Nature of Things*, ends with some 200 lines devoted to disease, first Lucretius' explanation of its origins and causes and then his account of the plague that struck Athens in the Peloponnesian War. From one point of view this is just what we should expect, in that Epicureanism was all about providing people with the knowledge that would free them from fear, particularly of fear that the gods are at work in the world. So naturally an explanation of diseases, how they vary from one climate to another, how the 'seeds of disease' as Lucretius calls them, may be transported from place to place in the air or in the water, affecting animals as well as humans, all that is understandable in terms of Lucretius' programme.

Yet the graphic detail of the plague at Athens, where Lucretius goes over and elaborates the material in Thucydides (and it may well be other sources) provides an unexpected culmination of the poem. Nor can we dismiss the problem on the grounds that the poem was left unfinished at his death. When we think that Lucretius' message is supposed to be one of consolation, it is striking that he should have ended his poem with the story of the total despair to which the plague reduced the Athenians, their despondency (6. 1156ff. [T 8.9], 1230ff.), the failure of ordinary doctors (1179ff.), the filling of the temples and the sanctuaries with the bodies of the dead (1272). Why should he have left his readers, at the end, with this bleak, sustained, description of human miseries?

Yet on reflection we can see that this is the perfect, or at

After Aristotle: Or Did Anything Change? 219

least the most powerful, conclusion that there could be. Although the message is left implicit, it is clear. Despair at disease is precisely what ordinary mortals suffer, *if* they have not learned the lessons of Epicurus (as the Athenians when that plague struck—before Epicurus himself lived—were certainly in no position to do). What seems like misery, pain, unbearable suffering, is not. Epicurus tells us that death itself is 'nothing to us', and that the Epicurean sage is happy even on the rack, under torture that is. In a letter that Epicurus is purported to have written on the final day of his life, he refers to his suffering from strangury and dysentery, and yet describes the day as blissful and talks of the joy that his memories of his conversations with his friends give him.[13] The message is like that of the Stoics, though with a very different doctrinal underpinning, namely that philosophy is the key to happiness. With philosophy you are safe, immune to the apparent ills that surround and afflict you. Philosophy, in other words, is the supreme therapy.[14]

Once again we see the power of the discourse of health and disease. If philosophy is the true therapy, what it cures you of is disturbance in your soul. But disturbances in the soul, those that affect your body, even those that the state may suffer from, are all ills from which you need release. Lucretius joins the long list of writers for whom disease is not limited to what affects your body, except that now he finesses the idea that either disease or death is truly evil. Philosophy is the sovereign remedy, one that can make you immune to every kind of ill, both real and imaginary. Or so the claim was.

---

[13] Diogenes Laertius 10. 22, Long and Sedley 1987, 24D.
[14] Porphyry, *To Marcella* 31, Long and Sedley 1987, 25C, cites Epicurus: 'Empty are the words of that philosopher who offers therapy for no human suffering. For just as there is no use in medical expertise if it does not give therapy for bodily diseases, so too there is no use in philosophy if it does not expel the suffering of the soul.'

CHAPTER 8 TEXTS

8.1 Celsus, *On Medicine* I Prooemium 39

Neque quaerendum esse quomodo spiremus, sed quid gravem et tardum spiritum expediat; neque quid venas moveat, sed quid quaeque motus genera significent. Haec autem cognosci experimentis. Et in omnibus eiusmodi cogitationibus in utramque partem disseri posse; itaque ingenium et facundiam vincere, morbos autem non eloquentia sed remediis curari. Quae si quis elinguis usu discreta bene norit, hunc aliquanto maiorem medicum futurum, quam si sine usu linguam suam excoluerit.

8.2 Galen, *On The Opinions of Hippocrates and Plato* IV, 240.11–242.11

Καὶ γὰρ οὐ κατὰ ταῦτα μόνον αὐτὸς ἑαυτῷ διαφέρεται φανερῶς, ἀλλὰ κἀπειδὰν ὑπὲρ τῶν κατὰ τὸ πάθος ὁρισμῶν γράφων ἄλογόν τε καὶ παρὰ φύσιν κίνησιν ψυχῆς αὐτὸ φάσκῃ καὶ πλεονάζουσαν ὁρμήν, εἶτα τὸ μὲν ἄλογον ἐξηγούμενος τὸ χωρὶς λόγου τε καὶ κρίσεως εἰρῆσθαι φάσκῃ, τῆς δὲ πλεοναζούσης ὁρμῆς παράδειγμα τοὺς τρέχοντας σφοδρῶς παραλαμβάνῃ· ταυτὶ γὰρ ἀμφότερα μάχεται τῷ κρίσεις εἶναι τὰ πάθη. εἰσόμεθα δ᾽ ἐναργέστερον αὐτὰς τὰς ῥήσεις αὐτοῦ παραγράψαντες· ἔχει δ᾽ ἡ μὲν ἑτέρα τόνδε τὸν τρόπον· "δεῖ δὲ πρῶτον ἐντεθυμῆσθαι ὅτι τὸ λογικὸν ζῷον ἀκολουθητικὸν φύσει ἐστὶ τῷ λόγῳ καὶ κατὰ τὸν λόγον ὡς ἂν ἡγεμόνα πρακτικόν. πολλάκις μέντοι καὶ ἄλλως φέρεται ἐπί τινα καὶ ἀπό τινων ἀπειθῶς τῷ λόγῳ ὠθούμενον ἐπὶ πλεῖον, καθ᾽ ἣν φορὰν ἀμφότεροι ἔχουσιν οἱ ὅροι, τῆς παρὰ φύσιν κινήσεως ἀλόγως οὕτως γινομένης καὶ τοῦ ἐν ταῖς ὁρμαῖς πλεονασμοῦ. τὸ γὰρ ἄλογον τουτὶ ληπτέον ἀπειθὲς λόγῳ καὶ ἀπεστραμμένον τὸν λόγον, καθ᾽ ἣν φορὰν καὶ ἐν τῷ ἔθει τινάς φαμεν ὠθεῖσθαι καὶ ἀλόγως φέρεσθαι ἄνευ λόγου ⟨καὶ⟩ κρίσεως· ⟨οὐ γὰρ⟩ ὡς εἰ διημαρτημένως φέρεται καὶ παριδών τι κατὰ τὸν λόγον, ταῦτ᾽ ἐπισημαινόμεθα, ἀλλὰ μάλιστα καθ᾽ ἣν ὑπογράφει φοράν, οὐ πεφυκότος τοῦ λογικοῦ ζῴου κινεῖσθαι οὕτως κατὰ τὴν ψυχήν, ἀλλὰ κατὰ τὸν λόγον."

Ἡ μὲν οὖν ἑτέρα τῶν τοῦ Χρυσίππου ῥήσεων ἐξηγουμένη τὸν πρότερον τῶν ὅρων τοῦ πάθους ἐνταυθοῖ τελευτᾷ. τὴν δ᾽ ὑπόλοιπον ἐν ᾗ τὸν ἕτερον ὅρον ἐξηγεῖται γεγραμμένην ἐφεξῆς τῇδε κατὰ τὸ πρῶτον σύγγραμμα Περὶ παθῶν ἤδη σοι παραθήσομαι· "κατὰ τοῦτο δὲ καὶ ὁ πλεονασμὸς τῆς

CHAPTER 8 TEXTS

8.1 Celsus, *On Medicine* I Prooemium 39

Nor do we have any need to inquire into how we breathe, but what relieves difficult and laboured breathing: nor what may move the blood-vessels, but what the various types of movement signify. This is to be learnt through experiences. And in all theorising of such a kind it is possible to argue on either side, and so cleverness and fluency may win the victory. But it is not by eloquence but by remedies that diseases are cured. A man of few words who learns by practice to discern well would make an altogether better doctor than one who, unpractised, cultivates his tongue excessively.

8.2 Galen, *On The Opinions of Hippocrates and Plato* IV, 240.11–242.11

These are not the only definitions in which he clearly contradicts himself. He does so also in his accoount of the definitions of affection, when he says that affection is an irrational and unnatural movement of the soul and an excessive conation, then says, in explaining 'irrational', that it means 'without reason and judgment' and takes as a model of excessive conation persons who are running hard. These are both in conflict with the statement that affections are judgments. We shall see this more clearly when we have quoted his own words. The first passage is as follows: 'First one must keep in mind that the rational animal is by nature such as to follow reason and to act with reason as his guide. But often he moves in another way toward some things and away from some things in disobedience to reason when he is pushed too much. Both definitions refer to this movement; the unnatural motion arises irrationally in this way, and also the excess in the conations. For this irrationality must be understood as disobedient to reason and rejecting it; and with reference to this motion we say in ordinary usage that some persons are pushed and moved irrationally, without reason and judgment. For when we use these expressions it is not as if a person is carried away by error and from a misapprehension of something that is in accord with reason; we use them most of all with reference to the movement that he describes, since it is not the nature of a rational animal to move thus in his soul, but in accordance with reason.'

The first passage from Chrysippus, expounding the first of the

ὁρμῆς εἴρηται, διὰ τὸ τὴν καθ' αὑτοὺς καὶ φυσικὴν τῶν ὁρμῶν συμμετρίαν ὑπερβαίνειν. γένοιτο δ' ἂν τὸ λεγόμενον διὰ τούτων γνωριμώτερον, οἷον ἐπὶ τοῦ πορεύεσθαι καθ' ὁρμὴν οὐ πλεονάζει ἡ τῶν σκελῶν κίνησις ἀλλὰ συναπαρτίζει τι τῇ ὁρμῇ ὥστε καὶ στῆναι, ὅταν ἐθέλῃ, καὶ μεταβάλλειν. ἐπὶ δὲ τῶν τρεχόντων καθ' ὁρμὴν οὐκέτι τοιοῦτον γίνεται, ἀλλὰ πλεονάζει παρὰ τὴν ὁρμὴν ἡ τῶν σκελῶν κίνησις ὥστε ἐκφέρεσθαι καὶ μὴ μεταβάλλειν εὐπειθῶς οὕτως εὐθὺς ἐναρξαμένων. αἷς οἶμαί τι παραπλήσιον καὶ ἐπὶ τῶν ὁρμῶν γίνεσθαι διὰ τὸ τὴν κατὰ λόγον ὑπερβαίνειν συμμετρίαν, ὥσθ' ὅταν ὁρμᾷ μὴ εὐπειθῶς ἔχειν πρὸς αὐτόν, ἐπὶ μὲν τοῦ δρόμου τοῦ πλεονασμοῦ λεγομένου παρὰ τὴν ὁρμήν, ἐπὶ δὲ τῆς ὁρμῆς παρὰ τὸν λόγον. συμμετρία γάρ ἐστι φυσικῆς ὁρμῆς ἡ κατὰ τὸν λόγον καὶ ἕως τοσούτου, [καὶ] ἕως αὐτὸς ἀξιοῖ. διὸ δὴ καὶ τῆς ὑπερβάσεως κατὰ τοῦτο καὶ οὕτως γινομένης πλεονάζουσά τε ὁρμὴ λέγεται εἶναι καὶ παρὰ φύσιν καὶ ἄλογος κίνησις ψυχῆς."

8.3 Galen, *On The Opinions of Hippocrates and Plato*
V, 296.18–27

Ἐν τούτοις τὸν Ποσειδώνιον ἐπαινῶ μὲν ὅτι τοῖς ὑγιαίνουσι σώμασιν ὁμοίως ἔχειν φησὶ τὰς τῶν φαύλων ψυχὰς ὅταν ἔξω παθῶν καθεστήκωσιν, οὐκ ἐπαινῶ δὲ νόσον ὀνομάζοντα τὴν τοιαύτην κατάστασιν. ἐχρῆν γάρ, εἴπερ ὀρθῶς εἴκαζε, τὰς μὲν τῶν σπουδαίων ψυχὰς ὁμοίως ἔχειν φάναι τοῖς ἀπαθέσι σώμασιν, εἴτ' οὖν ἐστιν εἴτ' οὐκ ἔστιν τινὰ τοιαῦτα, περιττὸν γὰρ ὡς πρὸς τὴν προκειμένην εἰκόνα διασκέπτεσθαι τοῦτο, τὰ⟨ς⟩ δὲ τῶν προκοπτόντων τοῖς εὐεκτικοῖς, τὰς δὲ τῶν μετρίων ἀνδρῶν τοῖς ὑγιαίνουσι χωρὶς εὐεξίας, τὰς δὲ τῶν πολλῶν τε καὶ φαύλων τοῖς ἐπὶ σμικρᾷ προφάσει νοσοῦσι, τὰς δὲ τῶν ὀργιζομένων ἢ θυμουμένων ἢ ὅλως ἐν πάθει τινὶ καθεστώτων τοῖς ἤδη νοσοῦσιν.

definitions of affection, ends here. The remaining passage, in which he expounds the second definition, comes next after this in the first book *On the Affections*; I shall now place it before you. 'In this context we have spoken also of excess of conation, because their conations exceed the measure that accords with themselves and with nature. My meaning would be made clearer by the following examples. When a man walks in accordance with a conation, the motion of his legs is not excessive but is in some way commensurate with the conation, so that he may stop when he wishes, or change his pace. But when persons run in accordance with a conation, this sort of thing no longer happens. The movement of the legs exceeds the conation, so that they are carried away and do not obediently change their pace (as they did before) the moment they set out to do so. I think that something similar to these [movements of the legs] happens also in conations because of an excess beyond the rational measure, so that when a man exercises the conation he is not obedient to reason; and whereas the excess in running is termed contrary to the conation, the excess in conation is termed contrary to reason. For the proper measure of natural conation is that which is conformable to reason and which goes only so far as reason thinks right. Therefore when excess arises in this respect and under these conditions, it is said to be an excessive conation and an unnatural and irrational movement of the soul.'

8.3 Galen, *On The Opinions of Hippocrates and Plato* V, 296.18–27

In this passage I commend Posidonius for stating that the souls of inferior persons, when free from affections, are like healthy bodies; but I do not approve his calling such a state a disease. If the comparison were properly made, the souls of virtuous men ought to be compared to bodies immune to disease, whether any such bodies exist or not—for that inquiry is not germane to the analogy now before us—;the souls of those progressing in virtue should be compared to bodies of robust constitution, souls of intermediate persons to bodies that are healthy without being robust, souls of the multitude of ordinary men to bodies that become ill at a slight cause, and souls of men who are angry or enraged or in any affected state whatever to bodies that are actually diseased.

8.4 Galen, *That the Faculties of the Soul Follow the Mixtures of the Body* ch. 9

ὥστε σωφρονήσαντες [καὶ] νῦν γοῦν οἱ δυσχεραίνοντες, ⟨ὅτι⟩ τροφὴ δύναται τοὺς μὲν ⟨σωφρονεστέρους, τοὺς δ' ἀκολαστοτέρους ἐργάζεσθαι καὶ τοὺς μὲν⟩ ἐγκρατεστέρους, τοὺς δ' ἀκρατεστέρους καὶ θαρσαλέους καὶ δειλοὺς ἡμέρους τε καὶ πράους ἐριστικούς τε καὶ φιλονείκους, ἡκέτωσαν πρός με μαθησόμενοι, τίνα μὲν ἐσθίειν αὐτοὺς χρή, τίνα δὲ πίνειν. εἴς τε γὰρ τὴν ἠθικὴν φιλοσοφίαν ὀνήσονται μέγιστα καὶ πρὸς ταύτῃ κατὰ τὰς τοῦ λογιστικοῦ δυνάμεις ἐπιδώσουσιν εἰς ἀρετὴν συνετώτεροι καὶ μνημονικώτεροι γενόμενοι.

8.5 Galen, *On The Opinions of Hippocrates and Plato* V, 302. 17–30

Ἔστι γὰρ ἡ νόσος ἀνωτέρω καὶ καθόλου μᾶλλον ἢ ὡς μικρὸν ἔμπροσθεν εἴρηται. περιλάβωμεν οὖν αὐτῆς τὴν ἔννοιαν· ἡ τοῦ φύσει συγγενοῦς ἔκ τινος ⟨διαφορᾶς⟩ διαφ⟨θ⟩ορά· οὕτως γὰρ ἐν Σοφιστῇ Πλάτων ὡρίσατο. ὅτι δ' ἀνωτάτω τ' ἐστὶν ἡ ἀπόδειξις ἥδε καὶ πάσας τὰς κατὰ μέρος νόσους ἀκριβῶς ἐπιλαμβάνει, τάς τε τῆς ψυχῆς ἡμῶν καὶ τὰς τοῦ σώματος καὶ τὰς ἐν τοῖς ἄλλοις ζῴοις τε καὶ φυτοῖς, ἤδη δὲ κἂν ταῖς πόλεσιν ὅλαις, οὐ χαλεπὸν καταμαθεῖν. οὕτω γὰρ οἶμαι καὶ τὰς στασιαζούσας πόλεις ἐμφυλίῳ πολέμῳ νοσεῖν ἐν ἑαυταῖς λέγομεν, ὡς ἂν εἰς μάχην ἀφιγμένων τῶν ἐν αὐταῖς φύσει συγγενῶν. αὕτη μὲν ἡ γενικωτάτη νόσου πάσης ἔννοια. τῶν δ' ἁπλουστάτων μορίων ἡ πρὸς ἄλληλα στάσις ἧττον ταύτης ἐστὶ γενική, καὶ ταύτης ἔθ' ἧττον ἐπειδὰν θερμῶν καὶ ψυχρῶν καὶ ξηρῶν καὶ ὑγρῶν ἀμετρία τις εἶναι λέγηται. σώματος γὰρ αὕτη γε μόνου καὶ οὐδενὸς τῶν ἄλλων ἐστὶ νόσος, ὥσπερ γε καὶ ἡ τοῦ λογιστικοῦ στάσις οὐδενὸς τῶν ἄλλων ἐστὶ πλὴν ψυχῆς νόσος.

8.6 Aelius Aristides, *Sacred Tales* 47. 62–3, 65–7

62 καὶ γίγνεται φῦμα ἀπ' ἀρχῆς οὐδεμιᾶς φανερᾶς τὸ μὲν πρῶτον οἷον ἄν τῳ καὶ ἄλλῳ γένοιτο, ἔπειτα προῆλθεν εἰς ὄγκον ἐξαίσιον, καὶ ὅ τε βουβὼν μεστὸς ἦν καὶ πάντα ἐξῴδει, καὶ ὀδύναι παρηκολούθουν δειναὶ καὶ πυρετὸς ἔστιν ἃς ἡμέρας. ἐνταῦθα οἱ μὲν ἰατροὶ πάσας φωνὰς ἠφίεσαν, οἱ μὲν τέμνειν, οἱ δὲ ἐπικάειν φαρμάκοις, ἢ πάντως δεῖν ὑπόπυον γενόμενον
63 διαφθαρῆναι. ὁ δὲ θεὸς τὴν ἐναντίαν ἐτίθετο, ἀντέχειν καὶ τρέφειν τὸν ὄγκον· καὶ δηλαδὴ οὐχ αἵρεσις ἦν ἢ τῶν ἰατρῶν ἀκούειν ἢ τοῦ θεοῦ. ὁ δὲ ὄγκος ἔτι ἐπὶ μᾶλλον ᾔρετο καὶ ἦν ἀπορία πολλή. τῶν δὲ φίλων οἱ μὲν

8.4 Galen, *That the Faculties of the Soul Follow the Mixtures of the Body* ch. 9

So it would be wise of my opponents—those men who are unhappy at the idea that nourishment has this power to make men more or less temperate, more or less continent, brave or cowardly, soft and gentle or violent and quarrelsome—to come to me even now and receive instruction on their diet. They would derive enormous benefit from this in their command of ethics; and the improvement in their intellectual faculties, too, would have an effect on their virtue, as they acquired greater powers of understanding and memory.

8.5 Galen, *On The Opinions of Hippocrates and Plato* V, 302. 17–30

Disease is a higher and more general term than was indicated by the statement I made a moment ago. Let us therefore give a comprehensive definition of the concept: it is 'the destruction of what is by nature congenial as a result of some dissension'. That was Plato's definition in the *Sophist*. It is not difficult to ascertain that this formulation is at a higher level and accurately covers all particular diseases, those of our soul, those of our body, those found in other animals and plants, and even those of whole cities. Thus we say, I believe, that cities divided by civil war are internally diseased, as though their components, congenial by nature, had come to blows. This is the most generic concept of all disease. The mutual conflict of the simplest parts is less generic than this, and still less generic is the statement that disease is a lack of proportion of things hot, cold, dry and wet. For this (last) is disease of the body only, and of nothing else, just as the conflict of the rational is disease of nothing but the soul.

8.6 Aelius Aristides, *Sacred Tales* 47. 62–3, 65–7

(62) And a tumor grew from no apparent cause, at first as it might be for anyone else, and next it increased to an extraordinary size, and my groin was distended, and everything was swollen and terrible pains ensued, and a fever for some days. At this point, the doctors cried out all sorts of things, some said surgery, some said cauterization by drug, or that an infection would arise and I must surely die. (63) But the god gave a contrary opinion and told me to endure and foster the growth. And clearly there was no choice between listening to the doctors or to the god. But the growth increased even more,

ἐθαύμαζον τὴν καρτερίαν, οἱ δὲ ἐνεκάλουν ὡς λίαν ἅπαντα ἐπὶ τοῖς ὀνείρασιν ποιουμένῳ, τινὲς δὲ καὶ ὡς ἄτολμον ἐπῃτιῶντο, ἐπειδὴ οὐ παρεῖχον τέμνειν οὐδ᾽ αὖ φαρμάκων ἠνειχόμην. ὁ δ᾽ αὖ θεὸς διὰ τέλους ἀντεῖχεν κελεύων φέρειν τὸ παρόν, πάντως γὰρ αὐτὸ ὑπὲρ σωτηρίας εἶναι· εἶναι γὰρ τοῦ ῥεύματος τούτου τὰς πηγὰς ἄνω, τοὺς δὲ κηπουροὺς τούτους οὐκ εἰδέναι τοὺς ὀχετοὺς ᾗ χρὴ τρέπειν.

65 Πολλὰ μὲν οὖν καὶ παράδοξα ἐπετάχθημεν· ὧν δὲ ἀπομνημονεύω, δρόμος τέ ἐστιν ὃν ἔδει δραμεῖν ἀνυπόδητον χειμῶνος ὥρᾳ, καὶ πάλιν ἱππασία, πραγμάτων ἀπορώτατον, καί τι καὶ τοιοῦτον μέμνημαι. τοῦ γὰρ λιμένος κυμαίνοντος ἐξ ἀνέμου λιβὸς καὶ τῶν πλοίων ταραττομένων ἔδει διαπλεύσαντα εἰς τὸ ἀντιπέρας μέλιτος καὶ δρυὸς βαλάνων φαγόντα ἐμέσαι, καὶ γίγνεται δὴ κάθαρσις ἐντελής. πάντα δὲ ταῦτα ἐν ἀκμῇ τῆς φλεγμονῆς οὔσης ἐπράττετο καὶ δὴ πρὸς αὐτὸν ἀναχωρούσης τὸν ὀμφαλόν.
66 τέλος δὲ ὁ Σωτήρ σημαίνει τῆς αὐτῆς νυκτὸς ταὐτὸν ἐμοί τε καὶ τῷ τροφεῖ—περιῆν γὰρ δὴ τότε ὁ Ζώσιμος—, ὥστε ἐγὼ μὲν ἔπεμπον ἐκείνῳ φράσων ἃ εἰρηκὼς εἴη ὁ θεός, ὁ δ᾽ ἀπῆντα φράσων αὐτός μοι ἃ ἠκηκόει τοῦ θεοῦ. ἦν δέ τι φάρμακον οὗ τὰ μὲν καθ᾽ ἕκαστα οὐ μέμνημαι, ἁλῶν δὲ ὅτι μετεῖχεν· ὡς δὲ ἐπεπάσαμεν, ἔρρει δὴ ταχὺ τοῦ ὄγκου τὸ πλεῖστον, καὶ ἅμα
67 ἕῳ παρῆσαν οἱ ἐπιτήδειοι χαίροντες μετὰ ἀπιστίας. ἐντεῦθεν δὲ ἤδη τῶν μὲν ἐγκλημάτων ἐπαύσαντο οἱ ἰατροὶ καὶ ἐθαύμαζον ὑπερφυῶς ἐφ᾽ ἑκάστῳ τοῦ θεοῦ τὴν πρόνοιαν, καὶ ὡς ἕτερόν τι ἄρα ἦν μεῖζον, ὃ λάθρᾳ ἰᾶτο, τὸ δὲ τοῦ κόλπου τίνα ἂν τρόπον κατασταίη διεσκοποῦντο·

8.7 Aelius Aristides, *Sacred Tales* 48. 39–43

39 τέως μὲν οὖν ἀντεῖχον οὐδὲν ἧττον τῆς τῶν ἄλλων σωτηρίας ἢ τῆς ἐμαυτοῦ προνοούμενος, ἔπειτα ἐπέτεινέν τε ἡ νόσος καὶ κατελήφθην ὑπὸ δεινοῦ πυρὸς χολῆς παντοίας, ἣ συνεχῶς νύκτα καὶ ἡμέραν ἠνώχλει, καὶ τῆς τροφῆς ἀπεκεκλείμην καὶ ἡ δύναμις κατελέλυτο. καὶ οἱ ἰατροὶ ἀφίσταντο καὶ τελευτῶντες ἀπέγνωσαν παντάπασιν, καὶ διηγγέλθη ὡς οἰχησομένου αὐτίκα. τὸ μέντοι τοῦ Ὁμήρου κἂν τούτοις εἶπες ἂν τὸ "νόος γε μὲν ἔμπεδος ἦεν"· οὕτω παρηκολούθουν ἐμαυτῷ, ὥσπερ ἂν ἄλλῳ τινί, καὶ ᾐσθανόμην ὑπολείποντος αἰεὶ τοῦ σώματος, ἕως εἰς τοὔσχατον ἦλθον.

and there was much dismay. Some of my friends marveled at my endurance, others criticized me because I acted too much on acount of dreams, and some even blamed me for being cowardly, since I neither permitted surgery nor again suffered any cauterizing drugs. But the god remained firm throughout and ordered me to bear up with the present circumstances. *He said that this was wholly for my safety, for the source of this discharge was located above, and these gardeners did not know where they ought to turn the channels.*

(65) We were ordered to do many strange things. Of what I remember, there was a race, which it was necessary to run unshod in winter time. And again horse back riding, a most difficult matter. And I also remember some such thing. When the harbor was stormy from a southwest wind and the boats were being tossed about, I had to sail across to the opposite side, and having eaten honey and acorns, to vomit, and so the purge was complete. All these things were done while the inflamed tumor was at its worst and was spreading right up to my navel. (66) Finally the Saviour indicated on the same night the same thing to me and to my foster father—for Zosimus was then alive—, so that I sent to him to tell him what the god had said, but he himself came to see me to tell me what he had heard from the god. There was a certain drug, whose particulars I do not remember, except that it contained salt. When we applied this, most of the growth quickly disappeared, and at dawn my friends were present, happy and incredulous. (67) From here on, the doctors stopped their criticisms, expressed extraordinary admiration for the providence of the god in each particular, and said that it was some other greater disease, which he secretly cured. But they considered how the loose skin might be restored to normal.

8.7 Aelius Aristides, *Sacred Tales* 48. 39–43

(39) Meanwhile I persisted in my concern for the safety of the others, no less than for my own. Then the disease increased and I was attacked by the terrible burning of a bilious mixture, which troubled me continuously day and night, and I was prevented from taking nourishment and my strength failed. And the doctors gave up and finally despaired entirely, and it was announced that I would die immediately. However even here you could use that Homeric phrase, 'Still his mind was firm'. Thus I was conscious of myself as if I were another person, and I perceived my body ever slipping

40 τοιούτων δὲ ὄντων ἔτυχον μὲν εἰς τὸ εἴσω τετραμμένος τῆς κλίνης, ἔδοξα δὲ ὡς ὄναρ· αὐτὸ δὲ ἦν ἄρα ἡ λύσις· ἔδοξα δὲ καὶ δὴ ἐπὶ τέλει τοῦ δράματος εἶναι καὶ τοὺς ἐμβάτας ἀποτίθεσθαι καὶ τὰς κρηπῖδας μεταλήψεσθαι τοῦ πατρός. κἂν τούτοις ὄντα στρέφει με ὁ Σωτὴρ Ἀσκληπιὸς τὴν εἰς τὸ ἔξω 41 στροφὴν ἐξαίφνης. ἔπειτα οὐ πολὺ ὕστερον ἡ Ἀθηνᾶ φαίνεται τήν τε αἰγίδα ἔχουσα καὶ τὸ κάλλος καὶ τὸ μέγεθος καὶ σύμπαν δὴ σχῆμα οἷάπερ ἡ Ἀθήνησιν ἡ Φειδίου. ἀπῶζεν δὲ καὶ τῆς αἰγίδος ὅτι ἥδιστον καὶ ἦν κηρῷ τινι προσφερής, θαυμαστὴ καὶ αὕτη τὸ κάλλος καὶ τὸ μέγεθος. ἐφαίνετο μὲν δὴ μόνῳ στᾶσα καταντικρὺ καὶ ὅθεν αὐτὴν ὡς κάλλιστα ἔμελλον ὄψεσθαι. ἐγὼ δὲ ἐπεδείκνυν καὶ τοῖς παροῦσιν—δύο δ' ἤστην τῶν φίλων καὶ τροφός—βοῶν καὶ ὀνομάζων τὴν Ἀθηνᾶν ὅτι ἑστήκοι τε αὐτὴ ἀπαντικρὺ καὶ διαλέγοιτο, καὶ τὴν αἰγίδα ἀπεδείκνυν· οἱ δ' οὐκ εἶχον ὅ τι χρήσοιντο, ἀλλ' ἠπόρουν τε καὶ ἐδεδοίκεσαν μὴ παραληρῶν ἄρα τυγχάνω, πρίν γε δὴ τήν τε δύναμιν συνεώρων ἀναφερομένην καὶ τῶν λόγων ἤκου-
42 σαν ὧν ἤκουσα παρὰ τῆς θεοῦ. καὶ ἔστιν ἃ μέμνημαι τοιάδε. ἀνεμίμνησκέ με τῆς Ὀδυσσείας καὶ ἔφασκεν οὐ μύθους εἶναι ταῦτα, τεκμαίρεσθαι δὲ χρῆναι καὶ τοῖς παροῦσιν. δεῖν οὖν καρτερεῖν, εἶναι δ' αὐτὸν πάντως καὶ τὸν Ὀδυσσέα καὶ τὸν Τηλέμαχον καὶ δεῖν αὐτῷ βοηθεῖν· καὶ ἄλλα τοιουτότροπα ἤκουσα. οὕτως ἐφάνη τε ἡ θεὸς καὶ παρεμυθήσατο καὶ ἀνέσωσεν καὶ
43 δὴ κείμενον καὶ τῶν εἰς τὴν τελευτὴν οὐδενὸς ἔτι ἐλλείποντα. καὶ δῆτα εὐθύς με εἰσῆλθεν κλύσματι χρήσασθαι μέλιτος Ἀττικοῦ, καὶ ἐγένετο κάθαρσις χολῆς. καὶ μετὰ ταῦτα ἧκεν ἰάματα καὶ τροφαί· πρῶτον μὲν ἧπαρ, οἶμαι, χηνὸς μετὰ τὴν πολλὴν ἀπόρρησιν πρὸς ἅπαντα τὰ σιτία, ἔπειτα ὑείου τι ὑπογαστρίου.

8.8 Lucretius, *De Rerum Natura* 1. 936–50

sed veluti pueris absinthia taetra medentes
cum dare conantur, prius oras pocula circum
contingunt mellis dulci flavoque liquore,
ut puerorum aetas inprovida ludificetur
labrorum tenus, interea perpotet amarum 940
absinthi laticem deceptaque non capiatur,
sed potius tali pacto recreata valescat,
sic ego nunc, quoniam haec ratio plerumque videtur
tristior esse quibus non est tractata, retroque
volgus abhorret ab hac, volui tibi suaviloquenti 945

away, until I was near death. (40) During these circumstances I happened to have turned to the inside of my bed. *I seemed, as it were in a dream*—it was then the end—*I seemed even to be at the conclusion of the play and to put aside my buskins, and to be going to take my father's shoes.* And while I was about this, Asclepius, the Saviour, turned me suddenly to the outside. (41) *Then not much later, Athena appeared with her aegis and the beauty and magnitude and the whole form of the Athena of Phidias in Athens. There was also a scent from the aegis as sweet as could be, and it was like wax, and it too was marvelous in beauty and magnitude. She appeared to me alone, standing before me, even from where I would behold her as well as possible.* I also pointed her out to those present—they were two of my friends and my foster sister—and I cried out and I named her Athena, saying that she stood before me and spoke to me, and I pointed out the aegis. They did not know what they should do, but were at a loss, and were afraid that I had become delirious, until they saw that my strength was being restored and heard the words which I had heard from the goddess. And I remember the following: (42) *She reminded me of* The Odyssey *and said that these were not idle tales, but that this could be judged even by the present circumstances. It was necessary to persevere. I myself was indeed both Odysseus and Telemachus, and she must help me. And I heard other things of this sort.* Thus the goddess appeared and consoled me, and saved me, while I was in my sick bed and nothing was wanting for my death. (43) And it immediately occurred to me to have an enema of Attic honey, and there was a purge of my bile. And after this came drugs and nourishment. First, I think, goose liver after much refusal of all food. Then some sausage.

8.8 Lucretius, *De Rerum Natura* 1. 936–50

[B]ut as with children, when physicians try to administer rank wormwood, they first touch the rims about the cups with the sweet yellow fluid of honey, that unthinking childhood be deluded as far as the lips, and meanwhile may drink up the bitter juice of wormwood, and though beguiled be not betrayed, but rather by such means be restored and regain health, so now do I: since this doctrine commonly seems somewhat harsh to those who have not used it, and the people shrink back from it, I have chosen to set forth my doctrine to you in sweet-speaking Pierian song, and as it were to touch it with the Muses' delicious honey, if by chance in such a way I might

carmine Pierio rationem exponere nostram
et quasi musaeo dulci contingere melle,
si tibi forte animum tali ratione tenere
versibus in nostris possem, dum perspicis omnem
naturam rerum qua constet compta figura. 950

8.9 Lucretius, *De Rerum Natura* 6. 1156–81

atque animi prorsum tum vires totius, omne
languebat corpus leti iam limine in ipso.
intolerabilibusque malis erat anxius angor
adsidue comes et gemitu commixta querella.
singultusque frequens noctem per saepe diemque 1160
corripere adsidue nervos et membra coactans
dissoluebat eos, defessos ante, fatigans.
   Nec nimio cuiquam posses ardore tueri
corporis in summo summam fervescere partem,
sed potius tepidum manibus proponere tactum 1165
et simul ulceribus quasi inustis omne rubere
corpus, ut est per membra sacer dum diditur ignis.
intima pars hominum vero flagrabat ad ossa,
flagrabat stomacho flamma ut fornacibus intus.
nil adeo posses cuiquam leve tenveque membris 1170
vertere in utilitatem, at ventum et frigora semper.
in fluvios partim gelidos ardentia morbo
membra dabant nudum iacientes corpus in undas.
multi praecipites lymphis putealibus alte
inciderunt, ipso venientes ore patente: 1175
insedabiliter sitis arida, corpora mersans,
aequabat multum parvis umoribus imbrem.
   Nec requies erat ulla mali: defessa iacebant
corpora. mussabat tacito medicina timore,
quippe patentia cum totiens ardentia morbis 1180
lumina versarent oculorum expertia somno.

engage your mind in my verses, while you are learning to see in what shape is framed the whole nature of things.

8.9 Lucretius, *De Rerum Natura* 6. 1156–81

And then all the powers of the mind, the whole body, grew faint, being now on the very threshold of death. These intolerable sufferings were ever attended by torments of anxiety and laments mingled with moans. Retching persisted often through night and day, constantly causing cramps in the muscles and limbs, which quite broke them up, wearying those who were already wearied out.

Yet you could not perceive the outermost part of the body of anyone to be burning with excessive heat on the surface, but rather to give forth a sensation of warmth to the hand, and at the same time to be red all over with ulcers as it were burnt into it, like when the accursed fire spreads abroad over the limbs. But the inward parts in men burnt to the bones; a flame burnt in the stomach as in a furnace. There was nothing so light or thin that you could turn it to use for their bodies; only wind and cold always. Some cast their frame burning with the plague into cool streams, throwing the body naked into the waters. Many fell headlong from a height into wells of water, which they struck first with gaping mouth as they came. Dry thirst beyond all quenching drenched their bodies, and made a flood of water no more than a drop.

Nor was there any rest from pain: outwearied the bodies lay. Medicine muttered below her breath, scared into silence, because no doubt they so often rolled their staring eyes, fiery with the plague and knowing no sleep.

9

Epilogue

The account of Graeco-Roman ideas and attitudes towards disease that I have presented in these studies is very different from those histories that are limited to medicine in the strict sense, let alone from those that put the emphasis, within that field, on the achievements and discoveries of the ancients. There were indeed, as I explained, advances in knowledge of the internal structure of the body and on other subjects. But there was certainly no triumphant victory of naturalistic medicine over those traditional varieties that invoked personal gods and healing heroes.

The popularity of the shrines of Asclepius was as great in the second century CE as it had been in the fourth century BCE. Pagan temple healing, it is true, eventually declined—only to be replaced by a belief in Christ the healer (Dinkler 1980 Kollmann 1996). The relationships between paganism and Christianity on this, as on so many other issues, were complex and ambivalent. On the one hand Asclepius could be seen as a precursor. But on the other, he might also be seen as a rival and a threat (Temkin 1991, 113). Some of his shrines became Christian sanctuaries. As Nutton (1988, ch. 10) for instance has documented, a Christian basilica was constructed at the Asclepieion at Epidaurus. At Rome the Asclepieion became the church of San Bartolomeo and the healing spring was used as its font. Nor did this just affect Asclepius. There are instances where churches dedicated to St Michael replace the healing shrines of Heracles. Other Christian saints, Cosmas and Damian, Cyrus and John, especially, came to occupy other niches that the major pagan healing heroes had filled.

Epilogue

The miraculous cures ascribed to the former pair included replacing the leg of a wounded man with one taken from a corpse (Deubner 1907, 207–8), and again, as in the original Epidaurus inscriptions, doubters were punished. One who said that the cures of Saints Cyrus and John were natural and not miraculous was punished by an untreatable disease that was only removed after he had confessed to his impiety.[1]

Yet elsewhere the Christians did not appropriate and transform, they sought rather to destroy, the shrines where Asclepius had been worshipped,—or his statues—as happened for example at Pergamum. Nor should we underestimate the changes in the sets of beliefs that underpinned attitudes towards health and disease and god's role in them. Pagans and Christians both shared a belief in the possibility of god sending diseases as well as curing them. But as Nutton (1988, 8) remarked, when Cyprian in his *On Mortality* ch. 9, in 252 advised his congregation to accept a plague joyfully as proof of god's love—for by it the wicked would be sent more swiftly to hell, while the just would also obtain everlasting life more quickly—that set of ideas is hard, or indeed impossible, to parallel in pagan antiquity.[2]

In the wider context the triumph of Christianity over paganism also brought profound changes. Although not all those who put their faith in the new religion were totally hostile to all pagan inquiries into nature, there were many who were. Not only had pagan investigators lamentably failed to reach any kind of agreement about what to believe on fundamental cosmological, physical, medical—or moral—questions. In the view of many Christian apologists, from Tertullian on, their whole endeavour was mistaken. What humans needed was not inquiry, not curiosity, but faith.

---

[1] This is Sophronius on Gesius, an iatrosophist in Alexandria in the 5th cent., *On the Miracles of St Cyrus and St John* 30, PG 87. 3: 3514–20, cf. Fernandez Marcos 1975, 302 ff.

[2] Compare also Tertullian's view of famine and plague as the rightful reaction of god to the excessive prosperity and overpopulation of the time, *On the Soul* 30.

'What then has Athens to do with Jerusalem', Tertullian wrote (*On Prescriptions against Heretics* ch. 7), 'the Academy with the Church, the heretic with the Christian? . . . We have no need for curiosity after Jesus Christ, nor of research after the gospel.'

Yet the learned tradition represented by Galen was not, of course, altogether superfluous to requirements. In the Greek East especially that tradition continued, even though new research declined and such techniques as dissection became rarer and rarer. The turning of Galen into the key medical authority begins already a couple of hundred years after his death. The first extensive extant source where we can see this development is the encyclopaedia of Oribasius. He was physician to the emperor Julian, the so-called apostate who attempted—in vain—to revive the old pagan religion in the century after Constantine had made the decisive move of converting to Christianity. Oribasius compiled a massive compendium of all useful medical knowledge, for which Galen was the chief source. But even though Galen's sponsor (in a sense) was a pagan, like Galen himself, Galen's own learning was too valuable to be ignored, even by Christians.

Those who sought to practise medicine in the elite literate tradition took Galen, and Galen's interpretation of Hippocrates, as their models. Aspiring doctors, in that tradition, began with the group of works that Galen had written 'for beginners', graduating from them to the more advanced treatises.

Galen thereby craftily anticipated occupying a key role in the training of subsequent generations of doctors, and he had already paved the way for the argument in favour of medical authority by his own adoption of Hippocrates as his 'guide in all that is good'. He was not to know just how successful he was to be. He was acceptable, at least up to a point, to Christians, since he believed in teleology, divine craftsmanship, even divine providence. His medicine was, supposedly, based on the best, certainly one of the most comprehensive, physical theories, with the backing, so he claimed, not just of

Hippocrates, but (in certain respects) of both Plato and Aristotle. He was the most accomplished anatomist of his day—not that later doctors tried to follow him there: they were just grateful that his books told them what they needed to know.

Finally he insisted that 'the best doctor is also a philosopher', dedicating a short treatise with that title to various aspects of that thesis. The doctor needed to have studied logic (as indeed Galen had) in order to deliver valid arguments and proofs. He needed 'physics' in the sense already explained: his theories should be based on a sound grasp of how material objects are constituted, their elements and their modes of combining and mixture. Most reassuring of all, the doctor needed ethics, not (just) as a theoretical study, but to be good. He should not practise medicine for mercenary reasons. He should be a lover of humankind, *philanthropos*, selflessly dedicated to his patients' well-being. The model that he thus represented—that elite doctors were only too glad to claim to follow—was at once intellectually, morally, and ideologically respectable.

The history of later medicine in Europe is first of all one of continuing pluralism. Most people most of the time treated themselves or followed local practices and customs. At the scholarly end of the spectrum, however, that history is one of the long years of Galen's dominance, even though in the process of assimilation many of his ideas were modified. Where his theory of the humours had primarily addressed physiological and pathological questions, it came to provide a framework for the organization of thoughts about the diversity of human characters and personality in general. Since medicine did not belong to the subjects included in either the trivium or the quadrivium, it did not receive the attention, in primary education, that, say, grammar did. Yet in the medieval universities the doctors were as keen as the lawyers and the theologians to control access to the profession through the award of degrees. More importantly from the perspective of my inquiry here, ideas about health and disease continued to have widespread repercussions on notions of good and evil even when those notions acquired new theological overtones with the advent of Christianity.

When the challenge to Galen came, that was fuelled by the anatomical researches of Vesalius, Fabricius, Harvey. Yet as is well known Harvey remained close to Aristotle—and to Galen—in his teleology and in many other aspects of his work. Moreover when Galen was no longer the supreme medical authority, Hippocrates remained an ideal. Although what he stood for underwent many changes, he was admired, at different times, both for the ethical standards he was assumed to have set—the doctor's devotion to and care for his patients —and for his detailed and meticulous clinical observations. For Sydenham in the third edition of the *Observationes Medicae* (1676) he was an 'unrivalled historian of disease', who had 'founded the art of medicine on a solid and unshakeable basis', namely on the principle that 'our natures are the physicians of diseases' and the method of 'the exact description of nature'.

This is not the place to pursue these further topics of the history of medicine in Europe. Let me now turn back, in conclusion, to reflect on my principal theme, that of the grip of disease on the Greek imagination. What are the chief lessons that can be learnt from our studies of so much disparate material from so many different types of source?

From time to time, from the earliest beginnings of their recorded history, the Greeks were struck with terrible plagues, disease, and famine. Everyone who read the *Iliad*— and anyone who read anything read the *Iliad*—had the story of the imaginary plague hitting the Achaeans etched on their minds. But who could tell the causes and identify who or what was responsible? We have found the themes of disease as retribution, disease as the result of offences against the gods, common in writers of many different kinds, both poets and historians. The obverse of that belief was the idea that the gods could not just bring diseases, they could cure them. In any event experts were needed to say what had gone wrong

Epilogue

and how to put it right, and so the major issue of who could speak with authority on those subjects emerges. Appearances, in this matter as so often elsewhere, could deceive: the signs were always difficult to interpret. At a second level, too, *apparent* priests or prophets or diviners were not necessarily to be trusted, as honest let alone as correct. They might always be suspected of corruption, or at least of having their own agenda.

By the classical period the range of those who *claimed* expertise of one type or another encompassed Hippocratic naturalists at one end of the spectrum, and the advocates of the new pan-Hellenic cult of Asclepius at the other—with many other categories in between. Some concepts and arguments are distinctive—the invocation of nature on the one hand, the need for prayer and piety on the other. But we found a large area of overlap, where representatives of rival traditions appropriated one another's ideas and sought to reinterpret them within the framework of their own discourse. Dreams are used in the healing shrines and by naturalistic doctors, though the latter saw them as indications of the physical state of the body not as messages from god. Prognosis is practised, but on the basis of physical signs on the one side, of divine indications on the other. Above all a common aim was identified as 'purification', though what was meant by that differed profoundly. The purification you might receive could be a matter of a ritual cleansing, or of a physical purgation by means of suppositories or emetics.

The struggle for authority both between rival medical traditions, and within each, is striking. The priests who worked at an established shrine such as that at Epidaurus had institutional backing that the itinerant purifiers mentioned by Plato and attacked in *On the Sacred Disease* certainly lacked. The quarrels among literate naturalistic doctors ranged over every aspect of medical theory and practice.

This is all the more surprising when we think of the use made of medical authority to advocate authority in other fields. Those such as Plato and Aristotle who argued for objectivity in ethics and politics used the knowledge that doctors were assumed to possess as support. That there was objective right and wrong, good and evil, in the moral domain was argued on the analogy of the objectivity of the causes of diseases. As the doctor was supposed to be able both to diagnose the complaint and bring about a cure, so the experts in the moral field—philosopher-kings or the person of practical wisdom, the *phronimos* or *spoudaios*—were in a position to identify the disturbance to the health of the body politic and follow diagnosis up with prescriptions for treatment. The implication was that the ordinary lay individual or idiot (*idiotes*) was in no position to challenge what the true statesman laid down.

That ideal, of doctors confident in their understanding of diseases and in their ability to treat them, does not correspond to the reality revealed by many a Hippocratic writer honestly stating his own bafflement and helplessness. Moreover the postulated distance between expert practitioners and mere lay people did not square with what some of the latter themselves claimed. Thucydides, as we saw, presents his account of the Athenian plague as if he were in just as good a position to talk about it (having suffered from it) as any doctor—and he has a further motive for doing so, insofar as the objectivity of cause and effect in diseases stands as an analogue for the objectivity that governs human behaviour generally. Plato, most remarkably, turns from his use of the distinction between doctor and lay person to offer his own theory of diseases (with its distinctive agenda) in the *Timaeus* for all the world as if he could speak with authority on the question (which in a sense he believed he could, since his ideas reflected a true appreciation of the notions of order and disorder in the cosmos as a whole).

The new developments of the Hellenistic age include both philosophers (such as Chrysippus) taking over the role of prime therapists of the soul, and doctors (such as Galen) assimilating the ideal doctor to the philosopher. Yet the actual authority with which doctors could pronounce on the causes and cures of acute diseases, and proceed from diagnoses to successful treatment, was not substantially greater in the second century CE than it had been in the fourth BCE. In real-life medical practice doctors were as helpless in the face of severe conditions as they had always been, and the best remedy was (one may presume) to get the patient to rest and to hope that nature itself would effect a cure. The naturalists claimed that diseases could be explained and treated, using their methods, but that was an expression of an ideal, when not mere wish-fulfilment. The supernaturalists similarly claimed that gods could cure: they appealed to those who they said had been helped by Asclepius. Yet that too depended on a—different—act of faith.

One dispute was on the issue of who could claim authority in matters of diagnosis and treatment. A second related to the concept of disease itself. What did that include? Was passion a disease—love, for example, so often described in terms of a burning, of fire, indeed of a fever? How did that relate to madness or mental illness? What about feelings or emotions in general? We saw that the Stoics considered the *pathe* to be judgements, connected with excessive impulses, a sign that the rational faculty was not in proper control and therefore in need of therapy. But even the anti-Stoic Galen accepted that, in the most general acceptance of the term, disease, *nosema*, is to be defined in terms of the destruction of what is congenial, a genus that has species whose subjects ranged from bodies to souls to cities.

Disease is part of the human condition, a normal in the sense of frequent occurrence. But it conflicts with the norm when that is identified with the ideal, well-being—as we too naturally think of the healthy state of the body as the natural one. In that way, or thanks to that ambivalence, the concept of disease enables one to normalize the paranormal, to treat as natural what nevertheless goes against the ideal.

As to its origins, those who saw them in other than purely physical terms continued to invoke the gods. But those possessed by the gods, and afflicted with physical or with mental sickness, were they cursed, or blessed, or both at once? Or should such possession be treated like any ordinary disease? As for therapy, that ranged all the way from prayer and supplicating the gods, to spells, to taking drugs that might be poisons, to curing your rational soul by philosophy. The cacophony of conflicting advice, from priests, doctors, and philosophers, all claiming in their different ways to dispense the appropriate therapy, continued from the archaic period to late antiquity—and beyond.

Fundamental questions of values were at stake. What was presumed to be good was the healthy state of the body (if only that could be agreed). That was then taken as the basis for representations of what is good ethically and in the political domain. The rhetoric of the diseased body politic was no mere rhetoric, even though it undoubtedly contained large elements of hand-waving, simply because what counted as a disease in a state was even less agreed than physical sickness was. Everyone could see that physical disease was painful and to be avoided—despite the celebrations of madness we encounter in tragedy and in Plato. If you could successfully attach the term *nosos* to other things you disapproved of, you were halfway to getting other people to agree to your disapproval of them. Yet that depended on a remarkable feat of conceptual boot-strapping. Doctors and health and disease were good to think with—they were the assumed knowns by means of which the unknowns could be apprehended, from political disruption, to madness, to the emotions themselves. Except that doctors and health and disease were *not* knowns, but themselves highly problematic and contested.

The Greek imagination had, then, much grist to its mill. The lead was sometimes taken by those who had some experience as practitioners of one type or another, but more often by those who spoke on this complex of conceptual issues from the point of view of poetry, or sagehood, or historiography, or philosophy. What conceptually begins, in a sense, as a problem of how to treat someone who says they are ill spreads into one domain of inquiry after another. Who is sound in body, who in mind, what of the body politic and the disorders of society, and the causes and effects of good and evil in human history? The supposed objectivity of disease provides the opening for claims as various as those of Thucydides—for whom human history is a matter of the impact of certain recurrent factors in human nature—or of Plato—for whom the ideal state is one run on the basis of ungainsayable authority—or of Chrysippus—whose message was that reason alone is or should be in control—or of Galen, whose claim is that the doctor can tell you how to become not just a healthier but a better person. And if these were among the chief theory-builders, there were others among the poets and historians who underlined not the supposed knowns but the large unknowns—the ambivalent messages of the sickness or pollution of Oedipus or the folly of Pentheus or the frenzy of the Bacchants, the unsure pronouncements in Herodotus on quite what caused the madness of Cambyses or Cleomenes (even though he makes his own preferred views clear). Meanwhile as a counterpoint to the belief in the total infallibility of divine healing we can set the expressions of doubt and difficulty in the Hippocratics, their admissions of defeat and honest confessions that the therapies not just that their colleagues, but they themselves, used, did more harm than good.

I asked whether anything changed in the ancient world. But we may now follow that up, in conclusion, by asking the same question of the modern. The salient points here relate to what we now believe we understand and the grounds for that. On the one hand there are the extraordinary advances in biomedicine, both a knowledge of the causes of diseases and in the development of effective therapies. True, there are some diseases that evade the one and elude the other, where precisely what we are dealing with still poses problems, or is too multiform to be readily encompassed by a single diagnosis, or where there is either no known cure or only one that has side-effects that are almost as bad as the disease itself.

Yet on the whole and in comparison with the ancient world, modern biomedicine exudes a well-grounded confidence concerning its control of many diseases. The obverse of that confidence is, however, that lay patients are not on anything like equal terms with their physicians, and in no position to challenge their advice. Indeed they are often given no intelligible explanation of the medical condition they suffer from or the rationale for the treatments prescribed—not unless they are rich or curious or stubborn enough to demand them. Gone are the dialogues between patients and doctors to which some Hippocratic writers refer and which even Plato expects the real doctor to undertake.

Yet when we consider how the ancients finessed the problems in their constructions of medical authority, on that score they manifest an apparent confidence that eludes us in the modern, indeed the post-modern, world. We no longer believe that there are experts who can pronounce with the authority of physicians on the cause–effect relations in human affairs, let alone on the values that should guide behaviour. Some would say that we are better off *not* having such authoritarian models of the objectively good, to be invoked to justify political regimes with doubtful aims and methods. Yet two points might be adduced to moderate any sense that we might have of our own superiority in this respect. First the absence of an agreed sense that there is an objective good in morality leads rather to a vacuum of values—other than the dubious one of materialism. Second even in the absence of the ancient belief in objectivity in the matter of political goods, the rhetoric of disease still infects our political and moral discourse to an alarming degree. Even though we may think we are no longer in thrall to the idea of the pathology of politics, the rhetoric of politicians is still full of that imagery.

If we probe deeper, however, we may see that in certain respects our own situation is not so totally different from that which the ancients faced, even though we may not face it by deploying the *same* resources of the complex of concepts surrounding disease. In three areas especially we should admit to being rather at a loss. Madness is one, criminality a second, the creative imagination a third.

The modern discourse of mental illness, largely a product of the last fifty years, is now, to be sure, relatively stable. The definition of schizophrenia is accepted more or less across the world. That is distinguished from other complaints, differentiated from it often by the degree of severity involved, such as manic depression, bipolar disorder, anxiety disorder, and so on. The trainee psychiatrist learns all about this and much else besides from Kaplan and Sadock's *Pocket Handbook of Clinical Psychiatry*.

Yet as a recent study by Tanya Luhrmann (2000) has shown, the ways in which in practice psychiatric patients are recognized as patients, diagnosed and treated, may vary as much with the institutions handling them as with any other factor. Luhrmann examined the tensions and accommodations between what theory taught and what practice necessitated in the experience of those training as psychiatrists in institutions in the USA, varying from busy public hospitals at one end of the spectrum to rich private clinics at the other. Responsibility for admissions, in the former, is often in the hands of relatively junior staff, who are faced with tricky decisions to distinguish those genuinely needing treatment from others referred to the hospitals, whether by the police, or by relatives or friends, for apparently uncontrollable behaviour. Some of the patients themselves become quite canny about what they need to say or do to ensure that they get admitted. Talk of suicide, for instance, cannot be ignored. Meanwhile the psychiatrist taking the patient's history often focuses more on the level of dosage of drugs to control the immediate situation than with any long-term therapy, the availability of which will, in any event, reflect the resources of the institution concerned.

Again once patients have been hospitalized, the assumptions on which treatment is based may differ in a further respect. On the hospital ward it is assumed that there is a clear-cut distinction between health and disease. If the patients are not sick, what are they doing there? They should be discharged. In out-patient clinics, however, patients are more likely to be considered in relation to other people, and the line between health and disease becomes blurred.

None of this is to endorse the views associated with some of the extreme followers of R. D. Laing, that what we call madness is simply an artefact of society and social relations themselves. But it is to underline that, below the surface of confident diagnoses and reliance on accepted treatments, neither the causes of mental disorders nor the reasons for the apparent effectiveness of the treatments are at all well understood—and that is before we broach the still more disputed fundamental questions of the relations between the mind and the brain, the mental and the physical.

The boundary between the criminal and the sick is also deeply contentious. Ian Hacking's work on what he calls human kinds is suggestive here. In a series of pioneering studies (1991, 1992, 1995) he showed how the very discourse of deviance may contribute to creating the phenomena it describes. He has examined the history of such notions as that of child abuse and multiple personality disorder and illustrated how in both cases there is a feedback effect, from the invention of the kind to the incidence of its occurrence. Once such a kind exists, that affects the perceptions of those who use it and of those liable to be so labelled.

Moreover as he also points out, the invention of the kind is often accompanied by determined efforts to divest it of moral content, specifically by biologizing or medicalizing the phenomena. The demand, in some quarters, is then to find the gene or the diet that may be held responsible. Child abusers are then not to be treated as wicked, just as sick and in need of help—or else the kind may be recategorized euphemistically, as when 'teenage pregnancy' was renamed 'early parenting'. Not only are there powerful preconceptions of what is normal at work in the construction of the kind, but the type of abnormality in question may be deeply controversial, as between criminality on the one hand, disease on the other. Different interest groups, social workers, the police, the judiciary, even journalists, express quite diverging views on what should be done, in particular cases and in general, arguing with great passion over 'diagnoses', understandably so, given that decisions about people's lives and issues of natural justice are at stake.

Finally how satisfactory are the explanations we can give of our deepest emotions, our aesthetic experience, or of human creativity? Here too we continue to be faced with considerable unknowns, even though there have been advances in the understanding of the physical correlates of psychic activities. We do not have recourse to the vocabulary of *katharsis*, but have little to offer by way of accounts of creative genius. One of the legacies of the Romantic movement is a stark contrast between intellect and the emotions, with creativity often being located on the side of the latter rather than of the former. Yet that must be said to be profoundly unsatisfactory both for empirical and for philosophical reasons. First, it does not allow for the intense variety that exists between different modes of creativity as exemplified in poetry, say, or music, or science. Should we even expect to be able to encompass that variety within a single rubric? Speculations about the factors contributing to the genius of Shakespeare or Beethoven or Einstein generally just reflect the preconceptions of those who would set themselves up as the guardians and interpreters of particular traditions. Once again it is notions of the normal and the abnormal that make the running (as they do with mental illness and criminality), though in the case of creative genius, there is this difference, that the abnormal is valorized, not condemned.

As for the philosophical problems, the Romantic dichotomy between the intellect and the emotions leaves quite unresolved a variety of problems to do with the interactions between thought and feeling, and in the process seems to have mislaid an important Aristotelian insight, namely that the manner in which people reason about the situations they are in often reflects their character or disposition. This is not just a matter of blatant rationalizations, but also, for example, of how wishes, hopes, and expectations influence the very perception of the options for action that are open. Practical reasoning, as he called it, is never a matter just of the analysis of certain well-formed formulae. The ability to sum up a situation involves a skill precisely like that of an artist, a gift for seeing connections that, in a way that Forster would have applauded, Aristotle considered to be one of the marks of the poet. But if we can appreciate certain negative points, about what creative genius is *not*, quite what we should offer by way of a positive account is as much a subject of myth-making as it ever was.

On these issues, then, it is worth while pondering how other cultures, at other times, with other presuppositions, got on. The Greeks found the discourse of health and disease a resource to tackle these issues, and the ingenuity with which they exploited its potentialities reflects not least their lack of unanimity on how to do so. It is in the spirit of learning from that variety that I have undertaken this investigation.

BIBLIOGRAPHY

AMUNDSEN, D. W. (1982) 'Medicine and Faith in Early Christianity', *Bulletin of the History of Medicine* 56: 326–50.
ARTELT, W. (1937) *Studien zur Geschichte der Begriffe "Heilmittel" und "Gift"*, Leipzig.
BAMBROUGH, R. (1967a) 'Plato's Modern Friends and Enemies', in R. Bambrough (ed.), *Plato, Popper and Politics*, Cambridge, 3–36.
——(1967b) 'Plato's Political Analogies', in R. Bambrough (ed.), *Plato, Popper and Politics*, Cambridge, 152–69.
BEHR, C. A. (1968) *Aelius Aristides and the Sacred Tales*, Amsterdam.
BETZ, H. D. (1986) *The Greek Magical Papyri in Translation*, Chicago.
BLACK, M. (1962) *Models and Metaphors*, Ithaca, NY.
BROCK, R. (2000) 'Sickness in the Body Politic: Medical Imagery in the Greek Polis', in V. M. Hope and E. Marshall (eds.), *Death and Disease in the Ancient City*, London, 24–34.
BURKERT, W. (1979) *Structure and History in Greek Mythology*, Berkeley.
COHN-HAFT, L. (1956) *The Public Physicians of Ancient Greece*, Smith College Studies in History 42, Northampton, Mass.
DEAN-JONES, L. A. (1994) *Women's Bodies in Classical Greek Science*, Oxford.
DEICHGRÄBER, K. (1970) *Medicus gratiosus: Untersuchungen zu einem griechischen Artzbild*, Mainz.
DEMAND, N. (1996) 'Medicine and Philosophy in the Attic Orators', in R. Wittern and P. Pellegrin (eds.) *Hippokratische Medizin und attische Philosophie*, Hildesheim, 91–9.
DERRIDA, J. (1981) *Dissemination*, trans. B. Johnson of *La Dissémination* (Paris, 1972), Oxford.
DETIENNE, M. (1996) *The Masters of Truth in Archaic Greece*, trans. J. Lloyd of *Les Maîtres de vérité dans la Grèce archaique* (Paris, 1967), New York.

DEUBNER, L. (1907) *Kosmas und Damian, Texte und Einleitung*, Leipzig.
DILLON, M. P. J. (1994) 'The Didactic Nature of the Epidaurian *iamata*', *Zeitschrift für Papyrologie und Epigraphik* 101: 239–60.
DINKLER, E. (1980) *Christus und Asklepios: zum Christustypus der polychromen Platten im Museo Nazionale Romano*, Sitzungsberichte der Heidelberger Akademie der Wissenschaften, Philosophisch-historische Klasse 1980 (2), Heidelberg.
DODDS, E. R. (1951) *The Greeks and the Irrational*, Berkeley.
DONINI, P. (1998) 'La tragedia senza la catarsi', *Phronesis* 43: 26–41.
DOUGLAS, M. (1966) *Purity and Danger*, London.
EDELSTEIN, E. J. and EDELSTEIN, L. (1945) *Asclepius*, 2 vols., Baltimore.
FERNANDEZ MARCOS, N. (1975) *Los Thaumata de Sofronio*, Madrid.
FERRARI, G. R. F. (1987) *Listening to the Cicadas*, Cambridge.
FOUCAULT, M. (1970) *The Order of Things*, trans. of *Les Mots et les choses* (Paris, 1966), London,
——(1972) *The Archaeology of Knowledge*, trans. A. M. Sheridan Smith of *L'Archéologie du savoir* (Paris, 1969), London.
FREDE, M. (1987) *Essays in Ancient Philosophy*, Minneapolis.
GIRARD, R. (1986) *The Scapegoat*, trans. Y. Freccero of *Le Bouc émissaire* (Paris, 1982), Baltimore.
GOODY, J. (1977) *The Domestication of the Savage Mind*, Cambridge.
GRAF, F. (1992) 'Heiligtum und Ritual: das Beispiel der griechisch-römischen Asklepieia', in O. Reverdin and B. Grange (eds.), *Le Sanctuaire grec*, Entretiens Fondation Hardt 37, Geneva, 159–99.
HACKING, I. (1991) 'The Making and Molding of Child Abuse', *Critical Inquiry* 17: 235–58.
——(1992) 'Multiple Personality Disorder and its Hosts', *History of the Human Sciences* 5(2): 3–31.
——(1995) 'The Looping Effects of Human Kinds', in D. Sperber, D. Premack, and A. Premack (eds.), *Causal Cognition*, Oxford, 351–83.
HANSON, A. E. (1990) 'The Medical Writers' Woman' in D. M. Halperin, J. J. Winkler, and F. I. Zeitlin (eds.), *Before Sexuality*, Princeton, 309–37.
HARTOG, F. (1988) *The Mirror of Herodotus*, trans. J. Lloyd of *Le Miroir d'Hérodote* (Paris, 1980), Berkeley.

Bibliography

HAVELOCK, E. A. (1982) *The Literate Revolution in Greece and its Cultural Consequences*, Princeton.
HERZOG, R. (1931) *Die Wunderheilungen von Epidauros*, Philologus Suppl. Bd. 22(3), Leipzig.
JAEGER, W. (1957) 'Aristotle's Use of Medicine as Model of Method in his Ethics', *Journal of Hellenic Studies* 77(1): 54–61.
KALLET, L. (1999) 'The Diseased Body Politic: Athenian Public Finance and the Massacre at Mykalessos (Thucydides 7.27–9)', *American Journal of Philology*, 120: 223–44.
KAPLAN, H. I. and SADOCK, B. J. (1996) *Pocket Handbook of Clinical Psychiatry*, 2nd edn. Baltimore.
KING, H. (1983) 'Bound to Bleed', in A. Cameron and A. Kuhrt, (eds.) *Images of Women in Antiquity*, London, 109–27.
——(1993) 'Once upon a Text: Hysteria from Hippocrates', in S. Gilman et al. (eds.), *Hysteria beyond Freud*, Berkeley, 3–90.
——(1998) *Hippocrates' Woman*, London.
KING, R. A. H. (2001) *Aristotle on Life and Death*, London.
KINGSLEY, P. (1995) *Ancient Philosophy, Mystery, and Magic*, Oxford.
KNOX, B. M. W. (1964) *The Heroic Temper*, Berkeley.
——(1998) *Oedipus at Thebes*, 2nd edn. (1st edn. 1957) New Haven.
KOLLESCH, J. (1965) 'Galen und seine ärztlichen Kollegen', *Das Altertum* 11: 47–53.
KOLLMANN, B. (1996) *Jesus und die Christen als Wundertäter*, Göttingen.
KUDLIEN, F. (1967) *Der Beginn des medizinischen Denkens bei den Griechen*, Zurich.
——(1979) *Der griechische Arzt im Zeitalter des Hellenismus*, Akademie der Wissenschaften und der Literatur, Mainz, Abhandlungen der geistes- und sozialwissenschaftlichen Kl., Jahrgang 1979(6), Wiesbaden.
KURIYAMA, S. (1999) *The Expressiveness of the Body*, Princeton.
KUTSCH, F. (1913) *Attische Heilgötter und Heilheroen*, Religionsgeschichtliche Versuche und Vorarbeiten 12.3 (1912–13), Giessen
LAÍN ENTRALGO, P. (1970) *The Therapy of the Word in Classical Antiquity*, trans L. J. Rather and J. M. Sharp of *La curación por la palabra en la Antigüedad clásica* (Madrid, 1958), New Haven.
LAKOFF, G., and JOHNSON, M. (1980) *The Metaphors We Live By*, Chicago.
LANZA, D. (1977) *Il tiranno e il suo pubblico*, Turin.

LÉVI-STRAUSS, C. (1968) *Structural Anthropology*, trans. C. Jacobson and B. C. Schoepf of *Anthropologie structurale* (Paris, 1958), London.
LEAR, J. (1988) 'Katharsis', *Phronesis* 33: 297–326.
LEWIS, G. (1975) *Knowledge of Illness in a Sepik Society*, London.
LLOYD, G. E. R. (1979) *Magic, Reason and Experience*, Cambridge.
——(1983) *Science, Folklore and Ideology*, Cambridge.
——(1987) *The Revolutions of Wisdom*, Berkeley.
——(1988) 'Scholarship, Authority and Argument in Galen's *Quod Animi Mores*', in P. Manuli and M. Vegetti (eds.), *Le Opere psicologiche di Galeno*, Naples, 11–42.
——(1990) *Demystifying Mentalities*, Cambridge.
——(1991) *Methods and Problems in Greek Science*, Cambridge.
LLOYD-JONES, H. (1983) *The Justice of Zeus*, 2nd edn., Berkeley.
LONG, A. A. and SEDLEY, D. N. (1987) *The Hellenistic Philosophers*, 2 vols., Cambridge.
LONIE, I. M. (1973) 'The Paradoxical Text "On the Heart"' *Medical History* 17: 1–15, 136–53.
LORAUX, N. (1980) 'Thucydide n'est pas un collègue', *Quaderni di Storia* 12: 55–81.
——(1993) *The Children of Athena*, trans. C. Levine of *Les Enfants d'Athéna* (Paris, 1981), Princeton.
LUHRMANN, T. M. (2000) *Of Two Minds: the Growing Disorder in American Psychiatry*, New York.
MANULI, P. (1980) 'Fisiologia e patologia del femminile negli scritti ippocratici dell'antica ginecologia greca', in M. Grmek (ed.), *Hippocratica*, Paris, 393–408.
MOULINIER, L. (1952) *Le Pur et l'impur dans la pensée des Grecs*, Etudes et commentaires 12, Paris.
NUSSBAUM, M. (1986) *The Fragility of Goodness*, Cambridge.
——(1994) *The Therapy of Desire*, Princeton.
NUTTON, V. (1988) *From Democedes to Harvey*, London.
PADEL, R. (1992) *In and Out of the Mind*, Princeton.
——(1995) *Whom Gods Destroy*, Princeton.
PARKER, R. (1996) *Miasma*, 2nd edn., Oxford.
PARRY, A. (1969) 'The Language of Thucydides' Description of the Plague', *Bulletin of the Institute of Classical Studies* 16: 106–18.
PRICE, S.R.F. (1990) 'The Future of Dreams: From Freud to Artemidoros', in D. M. Halperin, J. J. Winkler, and F. I. Zeitlin (eds.), *Before Sexuality*, Princeton, 365–87.

Bibliography 251

Pucci, P. (1977) *Hesiod and the Language of Poetry*, Baltimore.
Rawlings, H. R. (1975) *A Semantic Study of PROPHASIS to 400 B.C.*, Hermes Einzelschriften 33, Wiesbaden.
Rosaldo, M. Z. (1980) *Knowledge and Passion: Ilongot Notions of Self and Social Life*, Cambridge.
Rousselle, A. (1980) 'Images médicales du corps en Grèce: Observation féminine et idéologie masculine', *Annales ESC* 35: 1089–115.
Sabbatucci, D. (1978) *Il Mito, il rito e la storia*, Rome.
Segal, C. (1981) *Tragedy and Civilization: An Interpretation of Sophocles*, Cambridge, Mass.
——(1995) *Sophocles' Tragic World: Divinity, Nature, Society*, Cambridge, Mass.
Sherwin-White, S. M. (1978) *Ancient Cos*, Hypomnemata 51, Göttingen.
Simon, B. (1978) *Mind and Madness in Ancient Greece*, Ithaca, NY.
Sivin, N. (1987) *Traditional Medicine in Contemporary China*, Ann Arbor, Mich.
Smith, W. D. (1979) *The Hippocratic Tradition*, Ithaca, NY.
Sorabji, R. (2000) *Emotion and Peace of Mind*, Oxford.
Staden, H. von (1989) *Herophilus: the Art of Medicine in Early Alexandria*, Cambridge.
——(1992) 'Women and Dirt', *Helios* 19: 17-30.
——(1996) '"In a Pure and Holy Way": Personal and Professional Conduct in the Hippocratic Oath?', *Journal of the History of Medicine and Allied Sciences* 51: 404–37.
Taylor, A. E. (1928) *A Commentary on Plato's Timaeus*, Oxford.
Temkin, O. (1973) *Galenism: the Rise and Decline of a Medical Philosophy*, Ithaca, NY.
——(1991) *Hippocrates in a world of Pagans and Christians*, Baltimore.
Vegetti, M. (1966-9) 'Platone e la medicina, I, II, III, IV', *Rivista critica di storia della filosofia* 21: 3–39, 22: 251–70, 23: 251–67, 24: 3–22.
——(1981) 'Modelli di medicina in Galeno', in V. Nutton (ed.), *Galen: Problems and Prospects*, London, 47–63.
——(1983) *Tra Edipo e Euclide*, Milan.
Vernant, J. P. and Vidal-Naquet, P. (1988) *Myth and Tragedy in Ancient Greece*, trans. J. Lloyd of *Mythe et tragédie en Grèce*

ancienne (Paris, 1972) and *Mythe et tragédie en Grèce ancienne deux* (Paris, 1986), New York.
WILSON, E. (1952) *The Wound and the Bow*, 2nd edn., London.
WINKLER, J. J. (1990) *The Constraints of Desire*, London.

INDEX

abnormalities 186, 190, 244–5
abortion 43
Aeschylus 12, 90, 97, 151, 187
aetiology 23, 50, 115–16
Alcmaeon 155
Alexandria 41, 203
Amphiaraus 53
analogies 147, 181–7, 192, 208–9, 238
  between body and soul 142–4, 146, 209–12
  between body and state 143–4, 146, 148, 179–80, 192, 212
  between doctor and statesman 145, 149–50
  between medical and political purging 148, 185
animals 48, 177–80, 186–7, 192 n. 3, 202–3, 206
Anonymus Londinensis 25, 42, 152–3, 157, 178
Aphrodite 19, 22, 26, 95, 117
Apollo 14–17, 51, 53, 86–7, 216
appearance versus reality 84, 147, 184, 237
Aristides, Aelius 41, 54, 56, 212–16
Aristophanes 54
Aristotle 8–9, 11, 41–2, 47 n. 8, 48, 152, 176–93, 202–3, 206–7, 235–7, 245–6
  History of Animals 179
  Nicomachean Ethics 181–4
  On Respiration 177
  On the Movement of Animals 179–80

On the Parts of Animals 178, 203
On the Senses 177
On the Soul 206
Physics 178
Poetics 187–90, 193
Politics 180, 186, 188–93
Topics 178
Artemis 17, 50, 95
arteries 203
Asclepius 11, 17, 40–1, 51–7, 85, 90–1, 213–16, 232–3, 237, 239
Asia 92, 119
atheists 48 n. 5, 148
Athena 16, 19, 48, 214
Athens 23, 40–1, 59, 85, 89, 120, 122, 124, 218–19, 234
authority 2, 5–7, 16, 21, 50, 57, 84, 121, 142, 149, 157, 176, 181, 185, 192, 204, 234, 237–9, 241–2

Bacchants 92–4, 190, 241
Bambrough, Renford 148
bench, Hippocratic 215–16
bile 46–7, 124, 126, 146, 154–5, 204
biomedicine 1–2, 241–2
blindness 54, 85, 88, 116–17
body, variety of ideas about 3
  politicization of 154–7
body politic 7, 148, 179–80, 185–6, 192, 238, 240–1
brain 47, 203

Calchas 15–16, 18, 21, 57, 126
Cambyses 117–18, 241

case histories 42, 56–8, 120, 124–5
causation 5–6, 23–5, 40, 42–3,
  45–50, 84, 88, 120–1, 123–4,
  126, 147, 149, 153, 156,
  177–80, 187, 192, 204, 206,
  209, 218, 236, 238, 241–2
cauterization 55–6, 58, 143, 182,
  215
character 178, 183, 210–11, 215
  interdependence of, with
  reasoning 184, 206, 245
charlatans 43, 87
charms 10, 25–6, 41, 48, 58, 145
childbirth 17, 20, 51, 96, 215
China 4
Christianity 217, 232–4, 236
Chrysippus 207–10, 238, 241
Circe 48
city-state 180, 186, 190, 192–3
Cleanthes 208
Cleomenes 117–19, 241
Cnidos 25
competition 51, 120, 214, 216; see
  also rivalry
constitutions:
  of animals 178
  in *Epidemics* 123, 126
  physical 209–11
  political 12, 146, 176, 180,
  185–6, 190–2
Cos 40, 52–3
cosmology 8, 13, 142, 152–3, 156,
  209, 238
Craftsman, Platonic 156
creativity 245–6
criminality 244–5
critical days 124
Cyprian 233

Delphi 87, 116
democracy 122, 146, 186
Demosthenes 12
depletion/repletion 154, 204

Derrida, Jacques 10
despondency 59, 124–5, 218–19
determination, double 22–3, 116
Detienne, Marcel 27
diet 44, 47, 145, 211, 216, 244
Dionysus 92–4
disease versus illness 1–2
disorder 12, 142–3, 146, 150, 152,
  154–6, 212, 238, 241
dissection 47, 179, 202–3, 213 n. 8,
  234
divination 123, 213 n. 8, 217
diviners 15, 237
Douglas, Mary 9
dreams 13, 54–6, 58–9, 213–15,
  217, 237
drugs 10–11, 17–19, 24–5, 56, 58,
  94, 145–8, 182, 189, 214–17,
  240, 243

earthquakes 48–9, 116
education 14, 122, 147, 152,
  188–9, 191, 211, 234–5
Egypt 18–19, 115–16, 118
elements 24–6, 155, 204, 235
elites 4, 41, 85, 213, 234–5
emotions, *see* feelings
Empedocles 21, 24–7, 44, 90
Empiricist doctors 205
Epicureans 202, 206, 218–19
Epicurus 219
Epidaurus 40, 54, 214, 232–3, 237
epideixis 42, 153, 178
epidemics 120, 125
epilepsy 43, 46–7, 58
Epimenides 21, 23–4
equality 155
Erasistratus 47 n. 4, 203
ethics 181–2, 191–2, 205–6, 211,
  235, 238, 240
  medical 42, 52
etiquette, medical 42, 52
eugenics 145

Index

Euripides 91–7
evil 8, 11, 19–20, 84, 89, 91, 95–6, 142, 146, 150, 156, 208–10, 219, 236, 238
experts 4, 6, 18, 96, 142, 147–9, 157, 176, 181, 192, 236–8, 242

Fabricius 236
failure 50, 54, 58; *see also* helplessness
faith 233–4, 239
feelings 11, 22, 188–92, 207–9, 239, 245
Ferrari, John 151
fever 22, 124, 144, 209, 239
foreigners 18, 92, 94
foreknowledge 57, 90, 121, 126
Forms, Platonic 144, 150, 181–2, 184–5

Galen 11, 25, 202–4, 208–13, 234–6, 238–9, 241
gender differences 5, 8
geography 115
gods 11, 23–6, 48 n. 5, 49–50, 52, 59, 85, 88–91, 94–7, 116–17, 125, 148, 187, 218, 239–40
 and blessings of madness 150–2
 as causes of diseases 6, 16–18, 43–9, 52, 90, 116, 119, 126, 217, 233, 236
 as healers 16, 40, 43, 52–6, 58–9, 85, 91, 212–17, 232–3, 236, 239
 as sanctions of oaths 51
good 8, 84, 89, 157, 180–2, 184, 191–2, 236, 238, 240
Goody, Jack 4

Hacking, Ian 244
happiness 206, 219
harmony 7, 142, 156, 206
Hartog, François 115

Harvey, William 203, 236
heart 179–80
 valves of 203
Hecataeus 114–15, 119
helplessness 58–9, 85, 91, 97, 126, 149, 238–9
Hephaestus 19, 26, 54
Heracles 53, 90, 210, 232
herbs 24, 55
heroes 53, 89, 232; *see also* Asclepius; Heracles
Herodotus 13, 114–20, 123, 241
Herophilus 47 n. 4, 203
Hesiod 16–17, 19–22, 57, 90, 114
Hippocrates 41–2, 52, 152, 157, 204, 234–6
Hippocratic treatises 25, 40–52, 54–9, 85, 96, 115–16, 121, 124–5, 147, 149, 153–7, 178–9, 215–16, 238, 241–2
 Epidemics 42, 54, 57, 58 n. 7, 120, 123–4, 126
 Law 42, 52
 Oath 42–3, 51–2, 55
 On Airs Waters Places 43, 117, 210
 On Ancient Medicine 179
 On Diseases of Women I 51
 On Diseases of Young Girls 50, 52
 On Joints 58 n. 7
 On Regimen 42 n. 2, 52 n. 6, 56
 On Regimen in Acute Diseases 41
 On the Art 42
 On the Eighth Month Child 51
 On the Nature of Man 42, 204
 On the Sacred Disease 43–52, 56, 58–9, 87, 117, 177, 237
 Prognosis 57
historiē 115
Homer 14–21, 23, 48
humours 25, 124, 156, 204, 235

ignorance 43, 45, 85, 116, 122, 147, 156
incantations 26, 41, 43, 58
infallibility 55, 214, 241
India 4
intellect 184, 207–8, 211, 245
intelligence 178
Ister 87, 119

judgements, Stoic idea of 207–8, 210, 239
justice 6, 17, 20–1, 90, 142–4, 146, 152, 181, 245

knowledge 27, 43–4, 85, 88, 94, 126, 149–50, 184–5, 207, 218

Laing, R. D. 244
lectures 42, 153
Lévi-Strauss, Claude 5
Lewis, Gilbert 3
Libya 45–6
literacy 4–5
Loraux, Nicole 115
love 10, 12, 22, 95–6, 150–2, 239
 in Empedocles 24, 26
Lucretius 202, 218–19
Luhrmann, Tanya 243
Lysias 13

Machaon 17–18, 53
madness 12, 50, 92–5, 117–19, 150–1, 156, 239–40, 242–4
magoi 43, 87
Masters of Truth 27, 49, 57, 120, 123
mean, in Aristotle's definition of virtue 181–3
menstruation 9, 56
metaphor, problem of 8–10, 147
Methodist doctors 205, 216 n. 12
midwives 41
morale 120, 122

morality 119, 121–3, 125–7, 148–9, 156, 181–5, 187, 212, 242, 244
Muses 16, 21, 57, 114, 151
music 188–9, 191
mysteries 52
myth 19–20, 114–16, 145, 246

nature 21, 40, 43, 46, 48–51, 56, 59, 93, 117, 122, 177–80, 186–7, 191–3, 206, 212, 217, 233, 236–7, 239
 hierarchy of 206
 human 114, 121–2, 125, 145, 241
nerves 203–4
Nile 115, 117, 119–20
Nutton, Vivian 232–3

objectivity 2, 121, 147, 149–50, 176, 181–5, 192, 238, 241–2
Oedipus 85–90, 151, 241
oligarchy 146, 186
oracles 26, 88
order 142–5, 152, 155–7, 180, 238
Oribasius 234

Padel, Ruth 3
pain 18, 25, 143, 219, 240
Pandora 19–21
pathos 11–12, 147, 188, 207, 209, 211–12, 239
penalties 52, 125, 148
Pentheus 92–4, 241
Pergamum 40, 214, 233
Pericles 122–3
Persians 115–16
persuasion 156, 216
pharmakon 10, 17, 24–5, 93–4, 145–8, 189
pharmakos 11, 88
Pheretime 116
Philistion 25, 153, 157

Philoctetes 89–90, 151
Philolaus 25, 153, 157, 178
philosopher-kings 145, 149, 157, 181, 184, 238
philosophy as therapy 210, 218–19, 238, 240
phlegm 46–7, 49, 126, 146, 154–5, 204
phronesis 181–2, 185–6, 207 n. 4, 238
piety 11, 45–6, 125, 217, 237
Pindar 53
plague 1, 20, 91, 96, 123, 126, 202, 233, 236
  at Athens 23, 59, 84–5, 120–6, 202, 218–19, 238
  in the *Iliad* 14–17, 85, 120, 236
  at Rome 202
  at Thebes 85–6, 88
Plato 7, 23, 41, 44, 142–57, 178–9, 181–2, 184–5, 187, 190, 192, 204, 206–8, 210–12, 235, 237–8, 240–2
  Gorgias 142–4
  Laws 44, 48 n. 5, 148, 154, 156, 185
  Phaedrus 150–2, 190, 204
  Republic 44, 144–7, 150, 152, 154, 156, 179, 185, 187
  Sophist 146–7, 212
  Symposium 184
  Timaeus 142, 152–7, 178, 211, 238
pleasure 181, 183–4, 189, 191–2, 206
poetry 150–1, 187–91, 218
poets 19, 21, 246
poisons 10, 146–7, 215, 240
politics 7, 88, 93, 122, 125, 142–6, 148–9, 156, 185–7, 191–2, 238, 240, 242
pollution 6–7, 9, 23–5, 85–9, 96, 148, 151, 241

Polybus (son-in-law of Hippocrates) 42, 204
Poseidon 48–9, 116
Posidonius 208–9
prayer 6, 14, 16, 52 n. 6, 59, 85, 151, 217, 237, 240
pregnancy 50–1
priestesses and priests 7, 14–17, 21, 23, 50–2, 55, 126, 217, 237, 240
prognosis 56–8, 122, 237
Prometheus 19, 90–1
prophecy 15, 25, 85–7, 90, 150
prophets 15, 21, 57, 88, 93, 95, 126, 237
proportion 155–6, 178
psychotherapeutics 210–11
public physicians 53
pulse 213
punishments 16–17, 20, 53, 59, 116–19, 143–4, 147–8, 181, 217, 233
purging 6–7, 56, 58, 146–8, 155, 157, 187–90, 237
purification 6, 9, 23–5, 43–5, 56, 58, 87, 126, 147, 150–1, 157, 187, 189, 191–3, 237
purifiers 24, 43–9, 52, 56, 87, 191, 237
Pythagoreans 25, 44
Pythia 23, 118

reason 7, 142, 144, 146, 150–2, 156, 190, 206–11, 239, 241
regularities 48–9, 122, 187, 191
religion 25, 40, 45, 85, 148, 187, 189–91, 232–4
responsibility 5–6, 16, 22–3, 45, 48–9, 84, 95, 209
retribution 21, 116, 119–20, 236
riddles 85–7
ritual 6, 25, 116–17, 126, 187, 189, 193, 217, 237

rivalry 4, 51, 56, 58, 61, 120, 123–4, 153, 177, 232, 237
Rome 202, 232
rule 144, 150, 152, 180–1, 206–7
rulers 145, 148, 186

sacrifices 6, 15–16, 23–5
sanctuaries 54, 123, 218, 232; *see also* shrines; temples
Sappho 21–3, 26, 150
saviours 87, 215
scepticism 4–5
Scythia 115–17, 119
seers 15–16, 94
semantic stretch 9–10, 147
Semonides 19–20, 22
shrines 40, 51, 53–5, 232–3, 237
sin 6, 20, 59, 151
society, diseases of 7, 146–8, 240–1; *see also* body politic
Socrates 181, 207, 210
Sophocles 41, 84–91
soul 3, 142–4, 146–8, 151, 156, 179–81, 188, 190, 206–12, 219
Sparta 118–19
spells 10, 25, 94, 145, 189, 240
stasis 7, 122, 146, 154–5, 212
state, ideal 144, 157, 241
Stoics 11, 206–12, 219, 239
surgery 42, 55, 58–9, 143, 182, 204, 215–16
Sydenham 236

Teiresias 87–8, 92–4, 126
teleology 234, 236
temples 23, 46, 117–18, 214, 218
medicine practised in 11, 40–1, 51–6, 58–9, 216–17, 232
Tertullian 233–4
Thebes 85–9, 91–2
theodicy 6, 117
Thucydides 13, 59, 85, 114–15, 120–7, 153, 218, 238, 241
tragedy, Aristotle's account of 187–93
trainers 143, 145
tyranny 12, 146, 186

values 145, 181, 240, 242
veins 46–7, 49, 117
venesection 47, 214
verifiability 179
Vesalius 236
Vidal-Naquet, Pierre 84, 90 n. 2
virtue 144, 157, 181–2, 184, 207, 211
vivisection 203

war 121–3
in the body 155
women 18–23, 50–1, 92–3, 96
diseases of 8, 17, 42, 51, 96
as healers 19, 41
word, healing by 2, 25–6, 44

Xenophon 13
Xerxes 116

Zeno of Citium 208
Zeus 15, 19–21, 23, 48, 53, 90, 95

Ingram Content Group UK Ltd.
Milton Keynes UK
UKHW041841040423
419514UK00001B/12